Essentials of Mental Health and Psychiatric Nursing

Volume 2

Essentials of Mental Health and Psychiatric Nursing

Volume 2

KP Neeraja

MSc (N), MA, PhD
Vice Principal
Navodaya College of Nursing
Raichur, Karnataka
India

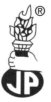

JAYPEE BROTHERS MEDICAL PUBLISHERS (P) LTD

New Delhi • Ahmedabad • Bengaluru • Chennai • Hyderabad • Kochi • Kolkata • Lucknow
• Mumbai • Nagpur

Published by

Jitendar P Vij

Jaypee Brothers Medical Publishers (P) Ltd

B-3 EMCA House, 23/23B Ansari Road, Daryaganj, New Delhi 110 002 INDIA
Phones: +91-11-23272143, +91-11-23272703, +91-11-23282021, +91-11-23245672
Rel: +91-11-32558559   Fax: +91-11-23276490, +91-11-23245683
e-mail: jaypee@jaypeebrothers.com   Visit our website: www.jaypeebrothers.com

Branches

❑ 2/B, Akruti Society, Jodhpur Gam Road Satellite,
Ahmedabad 380 015, Phones: +91-79-26926233, Rel: +91-79-32988717
Fax: +91-79-26927094 e-mail: ahmedabad@jaypeebrothers.com

❑ 202 Batavia Chambers, 8 Kumara Krupa Road, Kumara Park East
Bengaluru 560 001   Phones: +91-80-22285971, +91-80-22382956
+91-80-22372664, Rel: +91-80-32714073   Fax: +91-80-22281761
e-mail: bangalore@jaypeebrothers.com

❑ 282 IIIrd Floor, Khaleel Shirazi Estate, Fountain Plaza, Pantheon Road
Chennai 600 008, Phones: +91-44-28193265, +91-44-28194897
Rel: +91-44-32972089   Fax: +91-44-28193231
e-mail:chennai@jaypeebrothers.com

❑ 4-2-1067/1-3, 1st Floor, Balaji Building, Ramkote, Cross Road
Hyderabad 500 095   Phones: +91-40-66610020, +91-40-24758498
Rel: +91-40-32940929   Fax:+91-40-24758499
e-mail: hyderabad@jaypeebrothers.com

❑ Kuruvi Building, 1st Floor, Plot/Door No. 41/3098, B & B1, St. Vincent Road
Kochi 682 018 Kerala   Phones: +91-484-4036109, +91-484-2395739
Fax: +91-484-2395740   e-mail: kochi@jaypeebrothers.com

❑ 1-A Indian Mirror Street, Wellington Square
Kolkata 700 013, Phones: +91-33-22651926, +91-33-22276404
+91-33-22276415, Rel: +91-33-32901926   Fax: +91-33-22656075
e-mail: kolkata@jaypeebrothers.com

❑ Lekhraj Market III, B-2, Sector-4, Faizabad Road, Indira Nagar
Lucknow 226 016   Phones: +91-522-3040553, +91-522-3040554
e-mail: lucknow@jaypeebrothers.com

❑ 106 Amit Industrial Estate, 61 Dr SS Rao Road, Near MGM Hospital, Parel
Mumbai 400 012   Phones: +91-22-24124863, +91-22-24104532
Rel: +91-22-32926896,   Fax: +91-22-24160828
e-mail: mumbai@jaypeebrothers.com

❑ "KAMALPUSHPA" 38, Reshimbag, Opp. Mohota Science College, Umred Road
Nagpur 440 009 Phone: Rel: +91-712-3245220   Fax: +91-712-2704275
e-mail: nagpur@jaypeebrothers.com

Essentials of Mental Health and Psychiatric Nursing (Volume 2)

© 2008, Jaypee Brothers Medical Publishers

This book has been published in good faith that the material provided by author is original. Every effort is made to ensure accuracy of material, but the publisher, printer and author will not be held responsible for any inadvertent error(s). In case of any dispute, all legal matters are to be settled under Delhi jurisdiction only.

First Edition: **2008**

ISBN 978-81-8448-329-1

Typeset at   JPBMP typesetting unit
Printed at   Replika Press Pvt Ltd

Dedicated to
"Sree Shiridi Sai Baba"
and
"Bhagwan Sree Sathya Sai Baba"

Foreword

The Author deserves to be congratulated for preparing two volumes of *"Essentials of Mental Health and Psychiatric Nursing"*. We have immense pleasure in presenting the Foreword for the two volumes, brought by Dr KP Neeraja, who was our student.

Ever since, Nursing profession has recognized the 'Wholistic Approach', the importance of 'Mental Health and Psychiatric Nursing' is growing and the core concept is well recognized. The knowledge related to Mental Health Nursing is essential to guide the people to move towards the wellness of health.

Dr Neeraja has taken genuine interest to bring forth this important information, which will be useful 'Informative Material' to the students as well as to the teachers. We are sure, every Nursing Professional will be benefited by these volumes to enhance their knowledge, attitude and practices in their professional career. It can be widely read by the Health Care Professionals and the people, who have a desire to learn the importance of Mental Health. We are certain that these two volumes will help in dealing with the individual clients in specific and their families in all settings in general.

The contents of the Volumes 1 and 2, covered the syllabi of Undergraduate, Diploma in General Nursing and Midwifery Training Programmes, are definitely helpful for the Nursing Students at different levels, throughout the Globe. We are confident, these volumes will benefit the Nursing Professionals in a broader outlook. We are delighted that these two volumes are published in right moment, when the students need most in applicable manner.

Ms B Lucy Sarojini
Principal, SVS College
of Nursing
Mahabubnagar, AP

Ms G Mary Kamala
Professor in Nursing (Retd)

Preface

Essentials of Mental Health and Psychiatric Nursing Volume 2 is a continuation of volume 1. The content in this volume, is mainly focussed on 'Clinical Psychiatry', which is helpful for the nurses and the other professionals to enhance and utilize their knowledge in the Clinical Field. The psychiatric disorders are described in wide ranging manner, like the Definitions, Incidence, Prevalence, Risk Factors, Aetiological Factors, Clinical Manifestations, Diagnostic Features, Management (Medical, Nursing), etc. in respective chapters. I have made sincere and hard effort to bring out these two volumes in an understandable and applicable manner for Health Care Professionals to practice Psychiatric Nursing. Constructive criticisms and valuable suggestions are solicited on my e-mail ID: kpn21@indiatimes.com

KP Neeraja

Acknowledgements

I would like to express a deep sense of gratitude to the *"Almighty"* who is continuously giving the moral support and guidance required in all my deeds.

I owe a great deal of thanks to my beloved teachers Ms B Lucy Sarojini and Ms G Mary Kamala who had at the very first request whole heartedly accepted to write the Foreword and also is the spirit of Inspiration in taking up this project. I would like to express my gratitude to my friends, Mr Bejoice Thomas, Ms Aaina Amrish, Dr R Vasundhara and Ms Anitha P who lend their support in accomplishing the task. I like to acknowledge and thank all my family members especially my brother, KP Rajesh and my son Chi V Balasubramanyam who gave continuous cooperation and valued assistance in bringing out this book. Their expertise in drawing and creating graphics and diagrams is of great help.

I would also like to thank all the staff of Jaypee Brothers Medical Publishers, New Delhi, in particular Mr V Venugopal, Manager and Mr Ravi Kumar, Assistant Sales Manager, Bengaluru Branch for their moral support in bringing out this book.

Contents

Volume 1

Interview Technique

Definitions, Purposes, Characteristics, Attitude of Interviewer; Interview Skills, Qualities of an Interviewer; Essential Conditions for Interviewing; Guidelines for Conducting Interview; Techniques used for Conducting Interview

Observation, Recording and Reporting

Aims, Classification of Therapies

Physical Therapies – Electro Convulsive Therapy, Chemical Convulsive Therapy; Abreaction Therapy; Insulin Therapy

Psychotherapy – Individual Psychotherapy, Group Psychotherapy; Supportive Psychotherapy, Reeducative Psychotherapy; Interpersonal Psychotherapy, Behaviour Therapy, Hypnosis, Psychoanalysis, Psychosurgery; Psychodrama, Counselling, Family Therapy – Self Help Groups; Halfway Homes

Social Therapy/Case Work

Restitutive Therapy

Activity Therapy – Occupational Therapy, Play Therapy, Recreational Therapy, Art Therapy

Music Therapy, Dance Therapy

Narco Analysis and Narco Synthesis

Milieu Therapy – Therapeutic Community

Drug Therapy

Psychiatric Rehabilitation

Crisis

Definitions, Crisis Proneness; Characteristics; Developmental Phases; Types; Crisis Continuum, Signs and Symptoms, Therapy, Indications, Settings, Techniques of Crisis Intervention

Grief

Definition, Types; Theories of Grieving Process; Risk Factors; Manifestations; Resolution of Grief Responses; Management; Application of Nursing Process

Psychiatric Emergencies

Definition, Concept and Meaning, Common Psychiatric Emergencies; Objectives of Psychiatric Emergency Intervention; Characteristics; Management

Suicide

Risk Factors, Prevalence and Incidence; Definitions, Causes, Classification, Assessing the Degree of Suicidal Risk; Recognition of Suicidal Ideas or Facts, Methods of Committing Suicide; Nursing Management; Prevention

Anger, Hostility, Aggressive Behaviour

Terminology, Onset and Clinical Course, Aggression Cycle; Aetiology; Treatment, Nursing Management

Violent Behaviour

Risk Profile, Aetiology, Manifestations, Management

Hysteria
Definition, Aetiology, Incidence, Psychopathology, Symptoms, Prognosis, Treatment, Nursing Management
Withdrawn Behaviour
Definition, Associated Conditions, Psychodynamics, Nursing Management

Volume 2

Depression – Mild, Moderate, Severe; Nursing Management of A Client with Depression, Differences Between Exogenous and Endogenous Depression; Mania – Definition, Incidence, Aetiology, Clinical Manifestations, Types – Hypomania, Dysphoric Mania, Acute Mania, Delirious Mania, Treatment, Outcome, Nursing Management; Involutional Melancholia, Dysthymia, Cyclothymia

Definition, Classification, Causes, Clinical Manifestations, Treatment, Prognosis, Differences Between Psychosis and Neurosis, Types of Neurosis – Anxiety Disorder and its Types; Hypochondriasis, Depersonalization, Neurasthenia, Obsessive Compulsive Neurosis, Phobia and its Types, Post Traumatic Stress Disorder

Definition, Classification, Incidence, Risk Factors, Aetiology, Diagnosis, Treatment, Complications, Types of personality Disorders and its Management – Psychopathy, Sociopathy, Antisocial Personality Disorder, Paranoid Personality Disorder, Borderline Personality Disorder, Histrionic Personality Disorder, Obsessive-Compulsive Personality Disorder, Dependent Personality Disorder, Narcissistic Personality Disorder, Avoidant/ Anxious Personality Disorder, Schizoid Personality Disorder, Impulsive Aggressive Personality Disorder

Definition, Classification
Mental Retardation : Definition, Incidence and Prevalence, Classification, Predisposing Factors, Causes, Clinical Manifestations, Diagnosis, Management, Rehabilitation, Complications, Prevention, Nursing Management, Prognosis
Autism, Selective Mutism, Speech Disorders – Cluttering, Fluency Disorders – Unclear Speech, Stuttering; Movement Disorders – Mannerisms, Tic Disorder, Attention Deficit Hyperactivity Disorder, Eating Disorders – Classification, causes, Treatment, Nursing Management; Types of Eating Disorders – Obesity, Anorexia Nervosa, Bulimia Nervosa, Differences Between Anorexia Nervosa and Bulimia Nervosa, Pica
Behavioural Problems and Its Management (in General), Specific Behavioural Problems – Sleeping Problems, Conduct Disorders, Anxiety Disorders, Problems in Toilet Training – Enuresis, Encopresis, Bipolar Disorder, Violent Behaviour, Childhood Schizophrenia, Child Guidance Clinic
Therapeutic Modalities used in Child Psychiary, Nursing Management of Child with Psychiatric Disorders

Definition, Causes, Classification, Clinical Manifestations, Treatment, Nursing Management Types of Organic Brain Disorders – Dementia, Alzheimer's Disease, Senile Dementia, Senile Psychosis, Delirium

11

Nursing Process

DEFINITION

'It is an organized, systematic provision of rendering individualized nursing care to meet the wholistic needs of the client by utilizing problem-solving approach in the field of nursing'.

Steps in Nursing Process

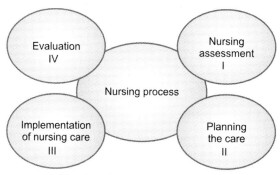

Fig. 11.1: Steps in nursing process

STEPS

I. Nursing Assessment

To identify the clients' problems and felt needs, the following methods will be used (collection of data)

The collection of data can be obtained through different sources:

1. Primary source–collecting the data directly from the patient and his relatives or friends (significant personalities)
2. Secondary source–collecting information through records and reports. For example, Process recording, nurses report etc.
   a. *To obtain 'subjective data'/'demographic data':* of the client and related general information through 'history collection' either from client, family members or significant personalities by systematic, structured interview method.
   b. *To obtain 'objective data':* The following methods will be adopted:
      • Physical examination (to exclude physical illness–the physician will conduct 'head to foot' examination by 4 techniques viz., observation/inspection, auscultation, percussion, palpation for assessing general health status of an individual.
      • Mental status examination and mini-mental status examination (psychological assessment to observe mental functioning capacities).

- Clinical investigations (routine and specific) as per doctor's advice and based on clients' manifestations.
- Social assessment.
- Family assessment (interaction pattern, relationship, bonding behaviour, family's perception of the problem).
- Nurse establishes and maintain therapeutic nurse patient relationship, after gaining confidence of client; explores the information of the client by vigilant observation and with keen interest, nurse will gather the data in a systematic manner by interview method. The data includes–demographic information/identification such as: age, gender, educational status, occupation, family monthly income, family size, religion, caste, type of family, marital status, marital duration.
- Clients' perception about problem, family's perception related to clients' problem.
- Through history, the actual or existing problems and potential problems of the client will be identified.

c. *Classification and Analysis of data:*
By incorporating and utilizing scientific principles and knowledge the clients' data will be critically classified and analyzed to identify the needs (felt and demand) of the client and formulate nursing diagnosis. Need assessment can be made by using varied approaches like Henderson and Maslow's hierarchy of needs. After collecting data, the nursing needs of the client can be grouped into different categories viz.,

- Identification data, e.g. Demographic data, date of hospital admission.
- Physical needs like feeding, bathing, care of bladder and bowel, rest and sleep, protection of the client from physical injuries etc.
- Psychosocial needs like love and belonging, sense of security, bondage, interaction and

communication, socialization, need of self-esteem, interpersonal needs.
- Intellectual needs, e.g. Cognition–thought, memory, intelligence, imagination, perception, attention and concentration.
- Spiritual needs, e.g. Arranging for spiritual meetings and prayers.
- Recreational needs, e.g. Exercises, relaxation.
- Discharging needs, e.g. health education, follow up and continuity of care.

d. *Nursing Diagnosis:* Identification of problem/need stating nursing problems related to client needs (actual and potential problems) based on which nursing interventions will be planned, e.g. Nursing Diagnosis/needs/medical diagnosis concern/nursing problems.
For example, Defective cognitive abilities-dementia.

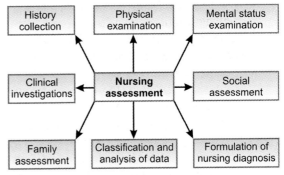

Fig. 11.2: Nursing assessment

II. Planning the Care

In planning nursing care of the client, nurses will involve the client, his family and members of health team (refer flow chart p. 365).

a. *Priority setting*–after identifying and listing out the clients' wholistic needs, nurses will keenly analyze the information related to needs and prioritize the clients' needs (highest to lowest) to provide immediate attention.

b. *Goal setting*–stating short term, intermediate and long term goals, which has to be achieved through systematized nursing care.

- Short term goals, can be achieved immediately, e.g. protect the client from self injury in suicidal tendency cases
- Intermediate goals can be achieved within few hours to few days, e.g. takes initiation in performing the activities in moderate depression cases
- Long term goals take long time to achieve, e.g. attaining self-esteem.

Factors to be considered when setting goals for nursing care:

- Patient centred, e.g. takes adequate rest
- Concise, brief
- Use action/verbs, e.g. promotes, enhances, obtains, follows etc.
- Type of behaviour expected from the patient must be qualified, e.g. performs the activities independently.

c. *Deciding or selecting the nursing activity*– Nursing activities or tasks will enable the nurse to attain specified nursing goal, e.g. Goal-maintains physical hygiene.

Nursing activities:

- Assisting the client to maintain personal hygiene (activities of daily living, cultivation of good relaxation techniques)
- Nursing interventions may not be necessary for certain illness, where clients can be able to manage, e.g. mild depression cases, the clients can be able to manage the routine activities.

d. *Developing or writing nursing care plan*– Plan must be used upto date SOAPIE format is an acronym suggested to guide the management of problem.

S – Subjective data
O – Objective data
A – Assessment
P – Plan the intervention
I – Implementing nursing activities or interventions

E – Evaluation/outcome of implemented nursing interventions

Basic components of written nursing care plan

- Assessment of clients' needs
  - Objective data
  - Subjective data
- Stating nursing diagnosis
- Goal/objectives
- Nursing activities/nursing actions
- The outcome criteria/expected behavioural outcome of the client.

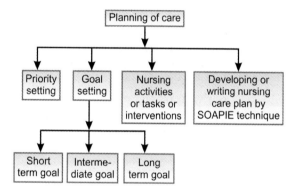

III. Implementation of Nursing Care

When planning is put into action, i.e. providing comprehensive nursing care to the client to meet wholistic needs of client. Nursing actions are client-oriented and goal directed, based on scientific and interdisciplinary principles nurse has to possess professional skills in implementing nursing activities.

Nursing actions are of 2 types:

- *Dependent nursing actions:* Actions derived from the doctor's prescriptions, e.g. administration of medications
- *Independent nursing actions:* Based on nursing diagnosis and plan of care, e.g. motivating the client to catharsizes or ventilate the internal conflicts.

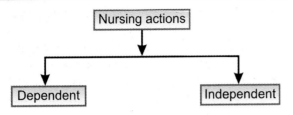

IV. Evaluation

It is the final step in nursing process. It is ongoing and continuous. It helps us, the outcome of nursing activity, whether the client relieved from problem or still existing. Nurse will be able to assess (visualize) how far the nursing activities are helpful to relieve clients' problems. Is it appropriate and able to plan or modify the strategy to achieve the targets or desired goals. Evaluation is the feedback mechanism for judging the quality of nursing care.

Advantages of Nursing Process

* Assesses relevant/needed data in a scientific and systematic manner
* Classifies and analyzes the data
* Delegates the nursing care aspects to various health team members
* Enhances decision making process
* Ensures standards of nursing care
* Attains specified objectives through nursing action
* Provides continuity of care and follow up care.

PROCESS-RECORDING/ INTERPERSONAL RELATIONS RECORDING/PATIENT-NURSE INTERACTION INTERVIEWS

Introduction

Process-recording is a tool used by professionals in the field of Psychiatry, Clinical Psychology, Nursing, Social Work and in Teaching. It helps and guides in the acquisition of the skills, 'self-reflection'. It focusses on one's thoughts, beliefs, actions and reactions in relation to practice. A good process recording will capture the various facets of a 'practice moment' and allow for identification of what one performed and where improvement is needed. The process recording addresses and examines the content and the process of the interaction with the client/client system.

The art of effective communication is a dynamic process. Nurses are continuously attempting to cope up with the wide range of human experiences. Nurses effectively uses the interpersonal techniques based on their intellectual level, maturity of judgement and capacity for adaptability.

Definitions

'A verbatim account of a visit for purposes of bringing out the interplay between the nurse and the patient in relation to the objectives of the visit'.
—*Walker*

'An exact written report of the conversation between the nurse and the patient during the time, they were together in psychiatric set-up'.
—*Hudson*

'It is a record of the nurse's feeling about what was going at the time and as far as possible, how the patient said, what he did'.

'Written description of the dynamic interaction of an interview or other encounters with a client system. It is expected to reveal facts, feelings, observations, responses and interactions of the client and the student nurse. It expands into an analysis of the student's observations of and reaction to the interview or encounter and graduates into analytical thinking and intervene planning'.

Objectives/Purposes/Goals

Process recording will be used as a
* Teaching tool
* Communicative tool
* Self evaluation tool
* Diagnostic tool
* Therapeutic tool
* A prerequisite for nursing process.

a. For Client

- Plays a vital role in establishing and maintaining therapeutic nurse-patient relationship
- Gains competence in maintaining good interpersonal relationship
- Clients can be helped more efficaciously by the nurse, who have the knowledge and dynamics of human behaviour and skills in using their own behaviour as a therapeutic tool
- Helps in identification and understanding of clients' total needs and the methods of assisting clients to workout solutions to their health and related problems are being recognized
- Workout solutions for clients' health problems and related other problems.

b. For Student Nurse

- Serves as a basic instrument in guiding the student nurses' learning by addressing learning areas
- Structures thinking related to professional practice
- Helps the student nurses to clarify thinking about the purpose of an interview and their role in it
- Conceptualizes thinking and develops abilities in organizing ongoing activities and transactions with client systems
- Applies nursing theories into practice
- It is a basic tool which stimulates communication and self awareness
- Assists in planning, structuring and evaluating the interaction at a conscious level rather than in an intrutive level
- Heightens awareness of oneself in action and as a part of transaction
- Distinguishes 'facts' from judgements and impressions
- Aids in identification of strengths and weaknesses, areas where the student-nurse needs improvement, without feeling of threatened or exposed

- Gains competence in communication, interaction and related skills
- Becomes as a base of assimilation of new knowledge and skills associated with it
- Provides an opportunity to gain ease and freedom in written expression that are important for professional development
- Gains deeper insight and feedback in his/her practice
- Offers a base for developing summarized and other styles of recording required by the agency and other educational institutions
- Helps in rethink each interview with the consciousness that the experiences and interactions with client must come through clearly to the field instructor who reads the recordings
- To gain competency in interpreting and synthesizing raw data under supervision
- Aids to learn and identify the thoughts and feelings in relation to others
- Increases the ability to identify problems and gain skills in solving them.

c. For Field Instructors

- Provides an opportunity to individualize both student-nurse and client with whom the students are working
- Assesses quickly the students' ability to respond to the feeling content of interviews or activities with the client
- Reflects the extent to which student nurses are able to integrate theory gained from previous experiences, classroom courses and outside readings
- Provides direction and a structural framework for the supervisory conferences and evaluation conferences.

Prerequisites

- Psychiatric clinical setting
- Consent of the client
- Winning the confidence of the client to obtain cooperation for process recording.

Elements of communication studies through process recording are:

- Observational skills
- Interpersonal skills
- Interviewing skills
- Verbal skills and non-verbal clues to the clients' needs
- Awareness of behaviour in relation to the client and to the self
- Control of behaviour as a result of awareness
- Identification of recurrent themes in the nurse client interaction
- Generic experiences out of which the inter-action patterns arises.

Outline of Process Recording

Clients' identification data/introductory material/ Client background information

- Name
- Age
- Gender
- Race
- Educational status
- Occupation
- Religion .... Caste ....
- Monthly family income
- Ward No
- Bed No
- ORD No
- H/o any health problems
- Date of admission
- Length of stay in hospital
- Date, time and place of interaction
- Number of visits made by nurse in what capacity and context
- I. Personal history
  - Past medical history
  - Past psychiatric history
  - Present medical history
- II. Family history
- III. Socio-economic history
- IV. Provisional diagnosis (if any)
- V. Presentation of complaints

- According to the patient
- According to the relatives
- VI. Aims and objectives of interview
  - Patient point of view
  - Student-nurse point of view
  - Short term goal (in the beginning)
  - Long term goal (working phase)
    - Corrective psychodynamics
    - Preparing the family for future plans
    - Follow-up
    - Rehabilitation

Recording the interaction between student-nurse and the client

- What the nurse said and did
- What the client said and did
- Non-verbal behaviour clues, e.g. eye-to-eye contact, changing the position frequently, biting the nails, pacing, nurses' non-verbal behaviour, nurses' thoughts and feelings, self evaluation

First interview: Date ..... Time ..... Duration .....

- Specific objectives
- Participants
- Conversation
- Inference
- Interview techniques used
- Introspective observation.

Analysis of the Interaction

- Interpretation of verbal and non-verbal behaviour of the client
- How the student-nurse understands the client system's situation and behaviour
- Clients' thoughts and feelings
- Communication techniques used, briefly characterize role(s) in the transaction
- Evaluation based on objectives, effect of techniques used
- What intervention skills were useful and were not useful
- Plans made for further interaction
- Did you achieve your purpose/goals? If not why?

- Recording time: 20–30 mts (while interacting with the client, nurse makes short note of it and after interaction, immediately written, conclusion are made.
- Tuning in: What do you think the client is expecting from this interaction? What are you expecting or anticipating (describe your thoughts and feelings prior to interaction).
- Even though video or cassette recording gives accurate information, the impact of these instruments will make an unnatural influence.

Verbatim

Ward:

Bed no:

Date and time of interview:

Situation:

Specific objectives:

- Overall assessment: how effective the student-nurses' interaction pattern and performance
- Points/comment where improvement is needed – signature with date and time.

FINAL POINTERS FOR STUDENT-NURSES WHO ARE MAINTAINING PROCESS RECORDING

- Remember the focus is on you, i.e. the student-nurse, not the client. It is important to remember what is communicated (verbal and non-verbal)
- Ability to recall will improve overtime
- Remember that you are writing honestly about the interaction for professional development
- Be sure to leave room throughout (e.g. wide margins) for comment from field instructor as they have to review and provide feedback before

Person	Verbatim (Conversation)	Non-verbal communication	Inference
			– Signature

Conclusion – Overall Impression of the Interview, follow-up Visit

Summary

- Phases of one-to-one relationship
- Clients' behaviour – physiological, psychological, emotional and social
- Evaluation – whether objectives achieved or not
- Interview tactics used with illustrations and outcome
- Areas needs improvement
- Evaluation of clients' condition at the time of termination of relationship
- Clients' response to various therapies intervened
- Plan/contract for future interventions–'how you and your client have decided to work on'; indicate next steps–signature of student-nurse
- Comments of instructor on students' performance

you submit the process recording to the field liaison

- Editing to be done before submitting to the instructor.

APPROACHES

- *Purpose of client contact.* The student-nurse should be directed toward formulating a statement of purpose in concise, clear and specific in relation to the proposed interview or encounter. It shows the relatedness between this meeting and the previous contact and should reflect the student-nurses' awareness of the particular function of the agency and of the clients' capacity and motivation.
- *Observation.* This section of the recording will vary in length and content in accordance with the stage of the student-client relationship. More detail is likely to be needed in relation to the

initial contacts. The student record general impressions of the physical and emotional climate at the outset of meeting, and its impact on the client. Significant changes in the client's appearance and/or surroundings are also important.

- *Content.* The actual description of the interactions during the planned contact. Although each student develops their own style of writing, this section should include the following:
  - A description of how the interview/activity began
  - Pertinent factual information and responses of both the client and the student in relation to it
  - A description of the interaction between the client and student in dealing with the purpose and concerns identified in the client contact. This includes fact and feelings revealed by both client and student-nurse
  - Description of the client's preparation for the next interview/activity, and a statement of how the contact ended.
- *Impressions.* As early as the student's first contact with the client. They have to make a statement of impressions based on the facts. This process gradually develops into analytical thinking as the student begins to integrate course content and gains understanding of the interaction between self and the client
- Worker's role. Highlight the student's activity with the client and reflect use of the professional skills and techniques. The student should include and evaluate of their effectiveness as a helping person in each interview or encounter with the client
- *Plan.* The student should make a brief statement of plans for the next contact and record some of their thoughts about the long-range goals for the client.

PROFESSIONAL SKILLS SETS

Generic professional work skills (apply throughout all phases and processes)

Self-understanding

- Self-esteem
- Acceptance of others
- Responsible assertiveness
- Self control

Talking and Listening

- Voice, speech and language
- Body language
- Active listening

Ethical Decision Making

- Understanding the legal duties of professional helpers
- Understanding the fundamental values and ethics of social work
- Identifying ethical and legal implications
- Ethical decision making.

PHASES OF SPECIFIC SKILLS

Preparing for

- Reviewing
- Exploring
- Consulting
- Arranging
- Empathy
- Self exploration
- Centering
- Preliminary planning and recording.

Beginning

- Introducing
- Describing initial purpose
- Discussing policy and ethical factors
- Seeking feedback.

Exploring

- Probing
- Seeking clarification
- Reflecting content

- Reflecting feelings
- Reflecting meaning
- Partializing.

Assessing

- Organizing descriptive information
- Formulating a tentative agreement.

Contracting

- Reflecting
- Sharing your view
- Specifying what to work on
- Establishing goals
- Developing and approach
- Identifying action steps
- Planning for evaluation
- Summarizing the contract.

Working and Evaluating

- Rehearsing action steps
- Reviewing actions steps
- Evaluating
- Educating
- Advising
- Reframing
- Confronting

- Pointing out
- Transitions/endings
- Progress recording.

Ending

- Reviewing the process
- Final evaluating
- Sharing ending feelings and saying goodbye
- Recording the closing summary.

—Cournoyer's (1999)

REVIEW QUESTIONS

1. Process Recording. (5M, 10M, RGUHS, 99, 2000, 2001, 02, 03, 04, 05, 06).
2. Four purposes of Process Recording. (2M, RGUHS, 1999, 2006).
3. What is the importance of Process Recording in Nursing Profession. (5M, MGRU, 2002).
4. Explain the role of Nurse in implementing Process Recording as self understanding therapeutic tool. (10M, MGRU, 2002).
5. Describe the Nursing Process in Psychiatric Nursing. (5M, RGUHS, 04).
6. Describe various methods of assessment in psychiatry. (5M, RGUHS, 02).
7. Prepare a Proforma to collect basic data on Psychiatric in patients in a mental hospital. (5M, 10M, RGUHS, MSc(N), 2006).
8. Purpose of Nursing Process in the Psychiatric setting. (5M, RGUHS, 2007).

12

Psychosis

INTRODUCTION

The term, 'Psychosis' is derived from 2 Greek words 'Psyche' (mind) and 'osis' (diseased or abnormal condition). The word 'Psychosis' was first used by Ernest Von Reuchtersleben in 1845, as an alternative term for 'insanity' and 'mania'. Today, the difference in uses for the terms, 'psychosis' and 'insanity' is vast, the term 'insanity' is employed primarily in a legal setting to denote that a person cannot be criminally held responsible for his/her actions in a court of law, due to psychological distress.

Psychotic episodes might affect a person with or without a mental disease. It is believed to be more of a symptom than a diagnosis; but it is not a mental illness in its own right. According to DSM, psychosis is a symptom common to several other mental illness categories. Psychosis is a generic psychiatric term, used for a mental state often described as involving a 'loss of contact with reality'.

DEFINITION

'A severe mental disorder, with or without organic damage, characterized by derangement of personality and loss of contact with reality and causing deterioration of normal social functioning'.
—*Stedman's Medical Dictionary*

Risk Factors and Incidence

- Psychosis can affect by psychiatric condition, e.g. schizophrenia or bipolar disorder usually starts during the teen years or in early adulthood, having a family history of schizophrenia is at risk
- In young people, psychosis can be mistaken for normal teenage rebellion or can be associated with drug and alcohol use
- Depression related psychosis typically begins after adolescence and may appear during second or third decade.

Causes

Psychosis can result from a variety of psychiatric or medical problems
1. Psychoactive drug intoxication or withdrawal. For example, Alcohol, prescribed drugs like barbiturates, benzodiazepines, anticholenergic drugs (atropine, scopolamine) certain antihistamines at high doses, antidepressants, antiepileptics, etc. street drugs like cocaine, amphetamines, hallucinogens (LSD, mescaline cannabis, etc.) symptoms will fade after the intoxicating effect of the substance has worn off, adverse drug reaction will also cause psychosis.

2. Physical illness 'organic' cause: that interfere with brain function can cause psychosis known as, 'secondary psychosis'. For example, Brain infections, brain tumours, metabolic abnormalities, nutritional deficiencies, dementia and lewy bodies, multiple sclerosis, sarcoidosis, lyme disease, neuro-syphilis, Parkinson's disease, hypoglycaemia, AIDS, lupus, leprosy, malaria, leucoencephalopathy, electrolyte disorders, hypocalcaemia, hypernatraemia, hyponatraemia, hypokalaemia, hypermagnesaemia, hypercalcaemia, hypophosphatemia, etc.

3. Functional causes/Psychiatric illnesses: due to psychological causes. For example,
   - Anxiety
   - Severe clinical depression
   - Delusional disorder
   - Schizophrenia
   - Bipolar disorder–mania and depression
   - Severe psychosocial stress.

4. Reaction to extreme stress is known to contribute to trigger psychotic states. For example, history of psychological traumatic events affects a person's psychosocial well being may trigger episodes and the recent experience of a stressful event, can both contribute to the development of psychosis. For example, witnessing a violent act or being sexually abused. Major life stress (death in a family); postpartum psychosis, subjected to a violence, sleep deprivation.

Types of Psychosis

I. Based on Duration

- Brief reactive psychosis–short lived psychosis triggered by stress, clients may spontaneously recover normal functioning within two weeks
- Full blown psychosis–in rare cases, individual may remain in a state of 'full blown psychosis' for many years or have attenuated psychotic symptoms, e.g. low intensity hallucinations, present at most times.

II. Based on Causes

- Functional psychosis–For example, schizophrenia
- Affective psychosis–For example, either bipolar disorder or unipolar, i.e. extreme mania, severe clinical depression
- Organic psychosis–organic brain disorders: Acute and Chronic
  - Acute organic psychosis–For example, drug intoxication, nutritional deficiencies, mild head injury
  - Chronic organic psychosis–For example, permanent brain tissue destruction as a result of brain injury, degenerative disease of CNS. For example, senile dementia, Parkinson's disease, drug intoxication, intracranial space occupying lesions.

Manifestations

- Psychotic individual may be able to perform actions that require a high level of intellectual effort in clear consciousness.
- A psychotic episode can be significantly affected by mood. For example, people experiencing a psychotic episode in the context of depression may experience persecutory or self blaming delusions or delusion of worthlessness or hallucinations.
- People experiencing a psychotic episode in the context of mania may form grandiose delusions.
- In paranoid state or disordered thinking–people may have false beliefs that are paranoid in nature. For example, they experience somebody is watching them.
- Psychosis may involve delusions or paranoid beliefs. Karl Jaspers classified psychotic delusions into primary and secondary types:
  - Primary delusions–arising out of the blue and not being comprehensible in terms of normal mental processes
  - Secondary delusions–being influenced by the person's background or current situation,

e.g. ethnic or sexual discrimination, religious or superstitious beliefs.

- In schizophrenic disorders–(psychotic behaviour lasts for atleast 6 months) and schizophrenic form disorder (psychotic behaviour that lasts for less than 6 months) typically cause visual and auditory hallucinations. E.g. the experience of hearing voices, hallucinated voices may talk about or to the person and may involve several speakers with distinct persons. Visual hallucinations. For example, more meaningful experiences like seeing and interacting with fully formed animals and people; kinesthetic hallucination (tactile sensations, olfactory, hallucinations, gestatory hallucinations also seen) delusions, the ability to socialize and function typically becomes impaired (personal, social and occupational functioning is impaired) inappropriate and incongruent affect, mute pressure of speech, talking or laughing to self, withdrawn or restlessness or hyperactive, sleep disturbance, waxy flexibility, phases of excitement (hostility, abusive, assaultive behaviour)
- Formal thought disorder: An underlying disturbances to conscious thought in the form of confused or muddled thoughts (impairment of a person's ability to think clearly), it may have effect over speech and writing, e.g. affected persons may show pressure of speech (speaking incessantly and quickly, mute) derailment or flight of ideas (switching topic mid sentence or inappropriately) thought blocking and rhyming or punning
- Altered emotions (overly emotional; not showing any emotion at all; depression, mania, radical shifts in emotions and behaviour, e.g. the patient might become incredibly happy and over active or severely depressed and lethargic; or unusual behaviour like client may laugh at odd times or become angered and upset for no apparent reason
- Experiences change in personality

- Neglects personal hygiene
- Inability to function
- Lack of interest in daily activities
- Inability to understand clearly, i.e. reality and behave appropriately
- Lack of insight into the unusual, strange or bizarre nature of the person's experience or behaviour
- In acute psychotic cases, people may be completely unaware that their vivid hallucinations and impossible delusions are in any way unrealistic.

Diagnosis

- A careful history to explore the cause viz. functional, organic, affective; as the patient may not be able to communicate reliably; relatives and friends have to accompany the patient to the physician to provide accurate information
- Physical examination, neurological assessment includes sensory and motor functioning, psychological assessment to identify underlying illness, e.g. reflexes, gait
- Radiological studies/brain imaging studies, e.g. X-ray, CT scan, MRI (to reveal structural problems in brain)
- Blood tests and urinalysis (to identify hormonal and metabolic problems, infection or drug use, vitamin deficiency).

Treatment

- When psychosis stems from mental illness, it is best handled by a psychiatrist
- Family Physician or Neurologist can manage cases of psychosis that are triggered by an underlying medical problem
- Drug therapy–antipsychotic medications, e.g. Neuroleptics
- Cognitive behaviour therapy
- Family therapy–to support the client in times of stress to understand the illness and cope-up with their own frustrations

- Psychotherapy–directs to cope up with stressful event to regain behaviour pattern and to function normally
- When other treatments for psychosis are ineffective, electroconvulsive therapy may be helpful to relive the underlying symptoms of psychosis, e.g. in schizophrenia and depression cases
- Animal assisted therapy can contribute to the improvement in general well being of people with schizophrenia
- In extreme cases, periods of hospitalization may be required or psychotic clients who behave in ways that put themselves or others in danger have to be hospitalized
- Follow-up is essential to discuss the problems and they arise and to cope-up with the situations and guides them to handle gently
- With proper treatment, people suffering from psychosis frequently improves, some even recover
- If underlying problem is treated, the client will typically recovers, once the problem is addressed
- When the origin of psychosis is psychiatric in nature, the prognosis is not always promising, e.g. when schizophrenia starts later in life, prognosis tends to be better, if family history of schizophrenia, early onset and poor functioning prior to the symptoms generally do worse.

SCHIZOPHRENIA

Introduction

In 1896, Krapeline gave clinical description of "Demention praecox" and classified into Hebephrenic, Catatonic, and Paranoid types. In 1911, Eugene Bleuler, a Swiss Psychiatrist. Coined the term, 'schizophrenia', which is a combination of two Greek words, 'Schizo' means 'split' and 'phren' means 'mind'. Bleuler described simple schizophrenia.

Bleuler explained split occurred between the cognitive and emotional aspects of the personality. The age of onset is from late childhood to late middle age, frequent onset is adolescent and early adulthood. It is one of the serious or major psychotic disorders having primary and secondary symptoms. It is a type of functional psychotic disorder.

Definitions

"A group of disorders manifested by fundamental disturbances or distortions in thinking, mood and behaviour, last for at least a month of active phase symptoms like delusions, hallucinations, disorganized speech, grossly disorganized or catatonic behaviour, negative symptoms such as shallow or flat affect, alogia or avolition and incongruous mood".   —*ICD–10; DSM–W*

"Disturbance in thinking is marked by alteration of concept formation, which may lead to misinterpretation of reality, hallucinations and delusions. Mood changes include ambivalent, constricted, inappropriate emotional responsiveness, or blunted effect. Lack of empathy with others, disturbance in behaviour may be withdrawn, regressive and bizarre".   —*American Psychiatric Association*

"The schizophrenic disorders are characterized in general by fundamental and characteristic distortions of thinking and perception, and by inappropriate or blunted effect. The most intimate thoughts, feelings and acts are often felt to be known or shared by others; explanatory delusions may develop, to the effect that natural or supernatural forces are at work to influence the affected individual's thoughts and actions in ways that are often bizarre".   —*K.Lalitha, 2007*

"A group of mental illness characterized by specific psychological symptoms leading to disorganization of personality of an individual. The symptoms chiefly interfere with the patient's thinking, emotions and behaviour in a characteristic way".   —*LP Shah and Hema Shah, 1997*

"A group of mental disorders chiefly characterized by distortion or disturbances in mood, thinking and behaviour leading to disorganization in the personality of an individual".

Classification (ICD–10; F_{20}–F_{29})

F_{20}– Schizophrenia
$F_{20.0}$– Paranoid Schizophrenia
$F_{20.1}$– Hebephrenic Schizophrenia
$F_{20.2}$– Catatonic Schizophrenia
$F_{20.3}$– Undifferentiated Schizophrenia
$F_{20.4}$– Postschizophrenic depression
$F_{20.5}$– Residual Schizophrenia
$F_{20.6}$– Simple Schizophrenia
$F_{20.8}$– Other Schizophrenia
$F_{20.9}$– Unspecified Schizophrenia.

To classify the clinical course:
X_0– Continuous
X_1– Episode with progressive deficit
X_2– Episode with stable deficit
X_3– Episode remittent
X_4– Incomplete remission
X_5– Complete remission
X_8– Other
X_9– Course uncertain, period of observation too short.

Incidence

- Eldest child is more vulnerable
- 15–30 years the peak incidence
- Common in both sexes
- Overcrowding, slum areas, low
- Low socioeconomic groups
- Child born from consanguineous parents and schizophrenic parents.

Aetiological Factors

- Influence of Neurotransmitters
  For example, Dopamine, serotonin have influence in the pathophysiology of schizophrenia
  Pathophysiology of schizophrenia

- Glutamate, nor epinephrine and gamma amino butyric acid will also have effect over the causation of schizophrenia
- Vitamin B1, B6, B12 and C deficiency
- Genetic:
  – Uniovular twins, monozygotic twins. Schizophrenia is very common
  – Relatives of client are commonly suffer with disease
  – Transmission is probably through one or more autosomal recessive genes
  – Parents to offsprings though genes
  – Genes apparently provides a predisposition or vulnerability to develop the disease
  – Most of the chromosomes (5, 11, 18–long arm; 19 short arm) have been affected in schizophrenic cases
- Neuro developmental factors:
  – Viral infections affecting antenatal mothers (in 2nd and 3rd trimesters of pregnancy)
  – Any conditions that injure or impair the developing brain causes schizophrenia
- Neuro psychological factors:
  – Organic brain dysfunction or damage, e.g. frontal lobe atrophy
  – Brain infections
  – Poison
  – Trauma
  – Metabolic disorders
- Family factors:
  – High level of expressed emotions in the family, e.g. hostility, over indulgence, critical attitude weak and submissive father, dominant and aggressive mother, improper communication leading to double blind and contradictory messages
  – Parent blaming
  – Broken homes, disorganized families or rejection by the parents
  – Over protection
  – Deprived parent child relationship
  – Pathogenic family interaction

- Environmental factors
  - Stressful environmental influence
  - Traumatic experiences
- Psychological factors
  - Impaired ego functioning
  - Intra-psychic conflicts
  - Unstable persons
  - Low IQ levels
  - Exposed to crisis situations
- Social factors
  - Community disorganization
  - Industrialization
  - Strained interpersonal relationship
  - Urbanization
  - Defective interaction
  - Social isolation; deprived social network
  - Pathological communication, e.g. Double bound communication
  - Acculturation; minority status
- Personality
  - Schizoid personality or aesthenic perso-nality type a social, shy, reserved, eccentric, oversensitive, fond of books, having very few friends
- Endocrinal, metabolic, biochemical distur-bances
- Transitional periods in life, e.g. pregnancy, childbirth.

Psychopathology

- Not clearly known
- Phenomenon of regression, i.e. going back to infantile and childhood patterns of psycho-logical living
- A state of organization, where reality does not exist, e.g. to resolve psychological conflicts by denying the harsh, painful reality world and living in a fantasy world with full of pleasures
  - Primary type–arouse directly from the patho-physiology of schizophrenia
  - Secondary symptoms–results from some other cause, e.g. drug side effects; depres-sion, etc.

- Intra-psychic influence–Negative effects, e.g. hostility, guilty, worthlessness of parent, emotional detachment, etc.
- Triggering life events, e.g. death of a loved person exacerbate a crisis and emotional collapse for the person
- Interpersonal influence
  Lack of adequate supportive systems, lack of adequate feedback mechanisms, uncorrected values, attitudes and understanding
- Pathologic communication within the family, two opposite messages from the parents and both views have to be followed
- Expressed attitudes about the client.

Clinical Manifestations

Bleuler has explained
- Primary/Fundamental symptoms
- Secondary/Accessory symptoms.

Fundamental Symptoms

- Associative disturbances or looseness
- The person does not think logically; ideas have little or no connections, shift from one point to another very quickly, thinking will become bizarre, illogic and chaotic
- Disturbances of thinking and perceiving
  I. Stream of Thought–incoherence or absence of link between ideas; audible thoughts; thought broadcasting; thought insertion; impaired abstraction, concreteness, etc.
    - The person does not think logically; ideas have little or no connections, shift from one point to another very quickly, thinking will become bizarre, illogic and chaotic
    - Poverty of ideas, thought block, thought withdrawal, flight of ideas, etc.
  II. Content–irrelevant and meaningless thoughts; circumstantiality; pseudo-philosophical, pseudo-religious and pseudo-scientific ideas, neologism, word salad; lacks concrete thinking

III. Delusions–Somatic, grandiose, paranoid, persecutory, reference, control

IV. Difficulty in concentration, emptiness, blankness of mind
- Depersonalization, change of personality
- De-realization
- Autism

Patient is preoccupied with ideas deriving from fantasy; emotionally detached from the world. Muttering, spells, of laughter and crying without reason; regression; client passes urine and stools in clothes, plays with his own excreta; absent mindedness, mistakes in inattentiveness resulting forgetfulness, deterioration in studies and in work.

Affective in congruity or disturbances in Mood pattern or Inappropriate Moods:
- Flat or blunt mood, inappropriate, no emotions; (apathy) shallowness of affect (diminished intensity of emotional experience; hypersensitiveness or insensitiveness of feelings (Depressive or euphoric mood changes); feelings of emotional impoverishment; temperament; callousness, anhaldonia
- Ambivalence: Experiencing two contradictory or opposing feelings, attitudes or wishes towards same person.

Secondary or Accessory Symptoms

- Disorders of perception:
  - Hallucinations–Auditory, Visual, Gestatory, Kinaesthetic olfactory
  - Voices commenting
  - Illusion
- Disorders of Activity:

Echopraxia (Imitation of the interviewer's movement automatically, even when asked not to do so); catatonia; increased psychomotor activity or excitement; stupor, negativism, automatic obedience, stereotype, perseveration, mannerism, mutism, change in work habits absenteeism, neglect of work, reduction in efficiency and productivity.

Waxy flexibility, impulsiveness, somatic passivity experiences; extreme motor agitation;

Deteriorated appearance and Manner: Disinterested towards grooming and self care.

Disturbance in attention:
Client is unable to hold attention for long time
Lives in his own autistic world

Disturbances in behaviour:
Irrelevant and inappropriate behaviour

Awkward and eccentric actions:
- Rowdy, violent, abusive, assaultive and destructive behaviour
- Agitation, bizarre
- Neglect of personal toilet, social obligations and responsibilities
- Suicidal and homicidal tendencies
- Criminal behaviour
- Sexual over activity
- Perversions
- Addiction, e.g. alcohol abuse, substance abuse.

Disturbances of volition or will:
- Blunting of will power (anergia)
- Reduction of drive and desire to carry out routines
- Aloofness (avoiding mixing with family and friends)
- Inability to take decisions
- Sudden, vague, undefined interest in religion, philosophy, metaphysics, etc.

Disturbances in Speech Pattern

- Neologism
- Looseness of association
- Echolalia (repeating the words of examiner)
- Clang association
- Word salad
- Poverty of speech (decreased speech production)
- Poverty of ideation (speech amount is adequate, but content will have little information)
- Preservation (preexistent repetition of words or themes beyond the point of relevance)
- Verbigeration (senseless repetition of words again and again).

Other Symptoms

- Disequilibrium of ANS
- Cold hands and feet
- Blotchy skin
- Widely dilated pupils
- Loss of weight (acute phase of illness)
- Gain in weight (chronic illness)
- Loss of ego boundaries
- Loss of insight
- Poor judgement
- Commits suicide due to depression, impulsive behaviour, hallucinations
- No disturbance of consciousness, orientation, attention, memory and intelligence.

TREATMENT OF SCHIZOPHRENIA

The mode of treatment is based on the type of schizophrenia and the predominant symptoms of the client.

1. Drug Therapy

- Antipsychotics, e.g. major tranquilizers or Neuroleptics.

Action

- Acts on specific areas of brain reduces psychotic symptoms like perceptual thought disturbances, passivity phenomenon, ideas of reference, inappropriate moods
- Produces calming effect within 4–6 hours of administration of drug.

Types of Antipsychotic Drugs

- Phenothiazines, e.g. Chlorpromazine 300–1500 mg/day or 50–100 mg/day I.M
- Butyrophenones, e.g. Haloperidol 5–100 mg/day or 5–20 mg/day I.M
- Diphenylbutyl piperidines, e.g. Pimozide
- Thioxanthines, e.g. Flupenthixol
- Benzamides, e.g. Sulpiride

- Atypical new antipsychotics, e.g. Clozapine 25–450 mg/day
- Anti-parkinsonian agents can be added to prevent extrapyramidal symptoms side effects
- Clients are treated prophylactic with antipsychotics for 1–2 years after the 1st episode, 3–5 years after multiple episodes
- Long acting preparations–Depot neuroleptics, e.g. Fluphenazine decanonate 25–50 mg I.M every 3 weeks once to have improved compliance.

Side Effects

- Dysphoria–c/o uneasiness, body pains
- Acute dyskinesia–contraction of one or more muscle groups, e.g. neck, trunk, tongue
- Tardive dyskinesia–involuntary movements which may affect the mouth, lips, tongue, arms, legs or trunk
- Parkinsonism–lack of motivation, restlessness, tremors, rigidity of extremities
- Akathisia–inability to remain still, legs swinging, foot tapping, hand wringing, walking up and down, restless legs syndrome, motor restlessness, repetitive purposeless movements
- Hypotension–giddiness, fatigue, falls
- Endocrinal dysfunctioning.

2. Physical Therapy

Electroconvulsive therapy–to control excitement, aggressive behaviour, violent reactions in acute cases ECT will be given. Combination of therapies are helpful to have better effects. For example, ECT, drug therapy, rehabilitation, family therapy, psychotherapy, etc.

3. Psychotherapy

To enhance self-esteem and to provide comfort to the client, therapist has to utilize different psychological processes and varied psychological approaches.

a. Individual Psychotherapy

Therapist has to follow certain principles:
- Provision of warmth and reassurance
- Avoid anxiety stimulants
- Maintain a state of 'delicate balance' therapeutic approach are employed
- Encourage honesty, self confidence, self worth, commitment, persistence, hope
- Enhance tolerance for error, uncertainty, madness without becoming frightened or rejecting.

b. Group Therapy

It is a form of psycho-social treatment benefits the patient by enhancing social interaction and social cohesiveness.

c. Behaviour Therapy

To improve psycho-social adaptation, vocational functioning and subjective well being behaviour modification techniques (based on learning principles) are used.

d. Family Therapy

Relapse rates for schizophrenia are higher in families with high expressed emotions, hence family education is essential. Therapist teaches the techniques to significant personalities for reducing family expectations, tensions, comment and to enhance adaptation of client to family environment.

4. Milieu Therapy

It provides non-threatening democratic environment to the clients, they will feel free to express their feelings through talking and relearn certain social skills, decision making skills, managing skills and a sense of responsibility are enhanced, slowly the client learns to adopt to the living situations.

5. Psycho-social Rehabilitation

a. Social Skills Training

The skills related to personal care, communication skills, problem solving skills, interpersonal skills, etc. will be taught to the client to promote independent living. Variety of teaching methods will be used to enhance the client's social skills. For example, psychodrama, role play, modeling, instruction, etc.

b. Cognitive Therapy

To improve cognitive skills like attention and concentration, training programmes are organized.

c. Prevocational Skills Training

It helps the client to fit for normative occupational functioning. The skills like punctuality, grooming pattern, communication skills, interactional pattern, need for assistance, ways of approaching, proper utilization of time are trained up.

d. Vocational Training

- Advise the client to enroll or occupy themselves in less stressful jobs
- Vocational training to improve the health status, socioeconomic status of the client, existing skills, competence
- Enhances social contacts, coping and competence strategies
- Utilize the family support and plans for supportive therapy
- Client will learn new living and social skills, structures the activities of an individual
- Insist the client to follow continuation of treatment
- After improvement of client's condition and possession of working skills, client may be recommended either open employment or sheltered employment based on client's abilities and needed situation
- Guidance and counselling services as to be organized based on client's need and demand.

NURSING MANAGEMENT OF THE CLIENT

Nursing Assessment

Obtain the history from primary sources. For example, both the client and from significant personalities. For example, family members, relatives or close friends who are in a position to report the progression of client's behaviour and also from the secondary sources like old records, registers

- Find out the client is having first psychotic episode or an exacerbation of chronic disorders
- Assess the functioning capacity of an individual
- Assess whether the client is able to perform his self care activities on his own or required assistance
- Physical examination is done to exclude any physical illness
- Observe for any perceptual disturbances, its frequency, nature and type; psychiatric emergency behaviour like suicidal tendency, purposefully ignoring basic needs due to negligence or suspiciousness, the necessity of hospitalization or treating as OPD case
- Mental status examination includes appearance, hygiene, eye contact, behaviour, perceptual behaviour, thought disturbances, sensory and motor aspects of behaviour, time of the day when the disturbances are more, client's response to the problems, withdrawal tendency
- Process recording–mention the therapeutic goals, symptoms of illness, explore the verbal and non-verbal behaviour of the client
- Assist for the investigations like neuro-imaging studies like CT and MRI scan; microscopic histopathology, collect the report and inform the psychiatric team member.

1. Nursing Diagnosis

Altered thought process evidenced by perceptual disturbance like hallucinations, delusions, loss of reality, autism and associative problems.

Goals

- The client will be able to improve his thought process, lives in reality and enjoys productive life.

Interventions

- Accept the client as he is

- Encourage the client to perform assertiveness techniques and reality based activities by orienting him with short term plans
- Approach the client calmly, gently, focus on current behaviour; establish therapeutic relationship with the client
- Provide structured guidelines and routines
- Motivate the client to talk about real events and present situation
- Make short and brief statement, avoid physical contact or threatening environment; sit and interact with the client
- Explore the feelings of the client related to anxiety or frustration
- Don't show concentration or attention to the event which provokes hallucination or delusion
- Discourage long discussions related to irrational thinking
- Avoid laughing, arguing, whispering near to the client
- Be honest and try to keep all promises, use the same staff to provide care to the client
- Never criticize the client
- Listen to the client and find out the relationship with hallucinations and delusions and his present behaviour
- Try to distract the client from perceptual disturbances and involve him in interpersonal activities and actual situations.

2. Nursing Diagnosis

- Impaired verbal communication related to disordered thinking process, poor judgement
- Social isolation related to withdrawal tendency.

Goals

- Gain confidence and communicates effectively with others
- Improves social interaction and exhibit appropriate behaviour.

Interventions

- Never ignore the client, have patience and understanding

- Develop trust, establish rapport, utilize friendly approach, initiate conversation
- Provide a comfortable, trustworthy, conducive environment when the client is exploring his feelings
- Encourage the client to verbalize openly at his own pace, ventilate his feelings through catharasis
- Utilize the communication techniques. For example, pin-pointing, clarifying, reflecting, summarizing, etc.
- Ask the client to clarify, restate the communication
- Start a calm, reassuring, brief, simple, direct statement by which the client will initiate to interact slowly with others by starting with one or few and to the group
- Appreciate and reinforce the client when he is communicating effectively; permit him to spend more time with others
- Arrange for brief and frequent contacts
- Encourage the client to participate in social activity
- Maintain a honest and consistent approach; use supportive statements in a non-threatening manner
- Identify the client's interest and encourage it to maximize and develop competence if appropriate
- Encourage the client to develop efficient coping strategies
- Give the client gentle feedback for their appropriate and inappropriate behaviour
- Ensure the client that he can leave the social situation any time, if it is threatening
- Utilize role model approach in communicating
- Anticipate and fulfill the needs of the client and maintain frequent contact, so that the client will feel free to communicate
- Exhibit positive unconditional friendly regard.

3. Nursing Diagnosis

Disturbed personal identify related to disorganized thinking process.

Goal

Mobilize the client to participate in therapeutic milieu.

Interventions

- Explain the routines, procedures to the client
- Protect the client from harming either to himself or to others
- Remove the client from the group, when he is having bizarre behaviour
- Accept the client as he is, nurse in-charge will allocate the client to different nursing personnel working in the ward based on the needs and requirements of the client
- If the client's behaviour is aggressive and disturbing to other clients in the ward, nurse has to explain to the other clients that it is due to illness and request their cooperation
- Set limits to the client's behaviour, when he is able to follow; if he is unable to follow the limits don't punish him, it may be because of his illness
- Avoid increased stimuli in the environment, the psychotic client may not be able to respond to it
- Spend some time with the client, let him know your interest and concern in caring, reorient the client
- Don't give any false hopes, promises and reassurances; make him to understand and realistic things to do
- Provide safe, non-stimulating environment to the client
- Develop one-to-one interaction
- Never do challenging or confrontational statements or arguments with the clients
- It is better to maintain a safe distance with the client to avoid injury as sometimes the client may go into aggressive behaviour
- Avoid to keep sharp instruments nearer to the client, to prevent self harm by the client, provide safety measures
- Administer PRN medications, if anything prescribed

- Never give support for misperceptions
- Assist the client in desirable activities
- Set goals based on client's needs and requirements, plan daily routine and intervene specific activities.

4. Nursing Diagnosis

Self care deficit related to withdrawal and cognitive impairment and perceptual disturbances.

Goal

- Client will develop independent living skills, daily care living activities (ADL)
- Meet the total needs of the client, if the client is severely withdrawn and not taking care of his activities
- Structured schedule and creative approaches can be adopted in meeting his daily needs like elimination, rest, sleep and nutritional needs. For example, regular sleeping, bowel and bladder habits
- Avoiding frequent naps in the noon time
- Switch of main lights at 10 pm, keeping dim-light, soft music, serving a glass of warm milk before going to bed
- Provide a clean environment and serve the food in neat, attractive and appealing manner
- Pursue the client to eat the food by himself
- Explain the family members and involve them in provision of care and meet daily living activities of the client.

5. Nursing Diagnosis

Non-adherence to treatment due to psychotic condition.

Goal

Assist the client to recover by explaining the importance of compliance to treatment aids in recovery and maintains health.

Interventions

- Administer the drugs as per doctors prescription and maintain drug chart
- Observe for side effects and take necessary or appropriate action
- Allow the client to interact with team members to disclose his problems
- Assist the team members in implementation of therapeutic activities
- Explain the client and his relatives the importance of following therapeutic interventions which will aid for early recovery.

6. Nursing Diagnosis

Inability to develop self concept related to poor judgement and attention deficit.

Goal

To develop a sense of worthiness.

Interventions

- Insist the client to do the activities on his own for achieving a sense of accomplishment and worthiness
- Allot the client specific assignments and perform specified responsibilities
- Help the client to take and implement proper decisions on his own in appropriate manner.

7. Nursing Diagnosis

Activity deficit related to psychotic conditions.

Goal

Divert the mind from sickness to well being.

Interventions

- Assist the client to cultivate the hobbies which will recreate his mind and to recover early from his sickness

- Encourage the client to develop normal pattern of living by developing a sense of achievement and satisfaction
- Motivate the client to participate in activities of his interest and choice.

If the client is spiritually deprived, arrange for daily prayers, counsel him, encourage him to participate in festival celebrations and religious functions.

8. Nursing Diagnosis

Insecurity related to altered affect, impulsiveness.

Goal

Implements right decisions based on reality.

Interventions

- Try to avoid unnecessary or excessive stimuli from the environment
- Make the client to understand the difference between perceptional problems and reality situations
- Directly communicate with the client, avoid gestures
- Provide comfort, conducive environment to the client where he can feel secured
- Insist positive reinforcement, show appreciation for the desirable behaviour
- Motivate the client to communicate his ideas, feelings openly so that, the care providers will interact with the client and adopts appropriate measures to overcome difficulty
- Exhibit acceptance, concern, love, therapeutic touch compassion to overcome the client's perceptional disturbances, allow him to adopt adequate coping strategies
- Show honest in responding to the client's questions.

9. Nursing Diagnosis

Client will be able to protect himself and does not harm others.

Interventions

- Remove sharp instruments or dangerous objects from the client's surroundings
- Maintain adequate or low level of stimuli in the client's environment
- Adequate monitoring of client's behaviour and reaction to different stimuli in essential
- Redirect the client's behaviour into productive activities
- Staff has to maintain consistent approach and calm, positive attitude in rendering client's care
- Encourage him to verbalize the feelings of aggression, frustration and conflict
- Provide structured environment with specified scheduled activities of daily living
- One-to-one association may be necessary
- Formulate realistic goals and help him to divert his energy in productive activities
- Behaviour modification techniques can be implemented.

10. Nursing Diagnosis

Maladaptive family coping strategies related to disturbances in family relationships.

Goals

Family adopts adequate coping strategies to provide care and support to the client.

Interventions

- Assess the level of functioning or roles exhibited by family members, communication and interaction pattern, supportive systems, interpersonal relationship among family members, problems solving techniques adopted by family
- Organize family education programmes in which the client's condition and prognosis, role of supportive system in client's prognosis, therapeutic modalities, involvement of family members in rendering client care services, etc. will be discussed

- Encourage the family members to accompany the client during hospitalization and support the client in the hour of need
- Advise the family members not to overprotect, criticize or show rejection towards the client
- Arrange client interaction sessions with other clients and their family members
- Exhibit certain teaching methods, e.g. role play, sociodrama, psychodrama, behaviour modification techniques, team approach to uplift the knowledge of clients and their relatives
- Client centered education programmes can be carried out, when acute manifestations will subside
- Consistent approach is always needed in provision of care
- Teach self help techniques and cognitive techniques to the client to modify their behaviour
- Clarify the doubts of family members related to client care; introduce them with local rehabilitation centres and community agencies, local support groups to utilize them in needed times
- Recognize families beliefs and if it is desirable provide adequate support, incorporate them in the client's care.

SUB-TYPES OF SCHIZOPHRENIA

1. Simple Schizophrenia

The onset is early in life, gradual, progressive, manifestations includes negative symptoms, disturbances in affect, motor activity and human relations; associative looseness is present, does not show interest in schooling or any occupation, never care for any criticisms, going on changing jobs frequently (migratory workers) likes to enjoy idleness, wandering tendency, aimless activity tendency, poor prognosis.

2. Hebephrenic Type (Disorganized schizophrenia)

Early, insidious onset between 15–25 years, associated with poor morbid personality, the manifestations are: severe disintegration of personality,

emotionally person will act indifferently, senseless giggling, silly smile, inappropriate, shallow laughter after little or no provocation, bizarre child like behaviour, fantasy and fragmentary delusions, tendency to regress, enuresis, encopresis, self care deficit, masturbates openly, marked thought disturbances, incoherent, severe loosening of associations, social impairment, mirror gazing, grimacing, odd mannerisms, disorganized speech, poor prognosis.

3. Catatonic Schizophrenia

Acute or sudden onset, early in age, common between 15–25 years, characterized by marked disturbance in motor behaviour. It has two forms:

A. Catatonic Stupor/Retarded Catatonic

Depression, apathy, non-reactive, not communicating, lacks interest, preoccupied with his own thoughts, poverty of ideas, thoughts, feelings, mute, extreme resistant to all instructions, stupor does not react to surroundings, mimics as if he is unaware of the situation. Masking the ideas, staring or closing of eyes, immobile, whole day sits, lie down in same position for long days, negativism, somatic disturbances, catalepsy or waxy flexibility (keeping in the same position all body parts, Echopraxia (repeating the actions), ambivalent, automatic obedient (follows every command) refuses to eat or greedily eats (if no one is observing, enuresis, encopresis, dribbling of urine, will give account of all activities slowly, suddenly, without inhibitions, assumes different postures for long time, rigidity, severe physical immobility, stereotyped environment, echolalia (mimics the same words).

B. Catatonic Excitement

Wild behaviour in a unpredictable manner (raging from restlessness, agitation, excitement, violent) aggressive motor activity without any emotional expression, cold approach, impulsive, suddenly attacks nearby people, destroys the articles, tears the clothes, remains nude, loosening of association ranging from Mutism to flight of ideas, negativistic, auditory and visual hallucinations, sleeplessness, dehydration, assaultive, homosexual prone, not consistently joyful, increased in speech production, frank incoherent, sometimes it will go in severe form with rigidity, hyperthermia, dehydration, collapse due to exhaustion called as, 'lethal catatonia or pernicious catatonia'.

4. Residual Schizophrenia

Chronic form of schizophrenia, client can be able to do his routine work normally, as they attained a 'social recovery' but symptoms may persist after acute phase like blunting of emotions, eccentric behaviour, illogical thinking, social withdrawal, loosening of associations, disorganized speech, catatonic behaviour, negativistic symptoms, unusual perceptions, absence of social contacts, poor personal relationships, apathy, not talkative.

5. Undifferentiated Schizophrenia

Features of more than one sub-type are exhibited, delusions, hallucinations, disorganized speech, catatonic behaviour, negative symptoms.
Chronic undifferentiated type.
Thought, affect and behaviour will be affected.

6. Post-schizophrenic Depression

Depressive symptoms will develop in active schizophrenia and are associated with suicidal tendency.

7. Acute Schizophrenic Type

Sudden onset, it may be acute or sub-acute form, clouding of consciousness; fantasy, ideas of reference, emotional turmoil, depression, fear, massive breakdown, fragmented, suffering with nightmares.

8. Latent Schizophrenia

Schizophrenic symptoms present, lacks any full blown type.

9. Schizoaffective Type

Combination of MDP and schizophrenic symptoms, hypo-manic, ideation is like schizophrenia.

10. Childhood Type

Appears before adolescent life, preoccupied mind, fantasy, withdrawn, atypical behaviour.

11. Paranoid Schizophrenia

It is the commonest form, (ICD-10, $F_{20.0}$). The word 'paranoid' means 'delusional', the terms are interchangeably used. Majority of time, acute onset observed after 30 years of age. The term, 'paranoid' is commonly used for 'suspiciousness'.

The personality deterioration is minimal, the individual can lead normal productive life. Good prognosis, if treated early. The clinical manifestations are: client lacks trust, extremely suspicious, delusions of jealousy, hypochondrical, persecution, depressive, grandiosity, ideas of reference, erotomanic, somatic delusions are marked. Auditory hallucinations, disturbances of volition, speech and motor behaviour, poor interpersonal relationship, distrustful, withdrawn, argumentative, sarcastic, resentful, disturbances in associations also noticed, mood disturbances. For example, anger, fear, etc. are observed. These clients markedly use projection and regression defense mechanisms in place of rejection, inadequate reality testing, preservation of ego functioning, hostile, high expectations can cause frustration to the child, sets unrealistic goals, failure rate is common.

NURSING MANAGEMENT

1. Nursing Diagnosis

Hyper-anxiety related to unrealistic goals, repeated failures, high expectations from the caretakers.

Goal

To decrease anxiety level and frustration.

Interventions

- Allow the client to establish trusting inter-personal relationships with fellow beings, thereby social isolation will be avoided
- Staff has to use client's language to make them to understand
- Advise them to avoid or lessen anxiety produ-cing stimuli
- Permit the patient to move around and talk to others
- Briefly respond to the questions and clarify their doubts consistently
- Never pressurize the client to establish new contacts
- Motivate the client to participate in therapeutic activities.

2. Nursing Diagnosis

Altered perception related to delusions.

Goal

To reduce the delusions and to promote perceptions.

Interventions

- Maintain and establish therapeutic nurse-patient relationship
- Develop positive attitude
- Assist the client to interact with others
- Show mild concern, provide support, security
- Involve the client in social activities
- Allow the client to move freely and talk effec-tively
- Assist the client in therapeutic activities
- Make him to understand between reality and the present behaviour
- Explain the client, the differences between hal-lucinations, illusions and its effects, if he is able to understand.

3. Nursing Diagnosis

Impaired communication due to perceptual deficit.

Goal

To reduce frustration and conflict, enhances socia-lisation process.

Interventions

- Motivate the client to initiate conversation
- Develop positive attitude
- Encourage the client to participate in social activities
- Utilize communication techniques
- Do not provoke personalized questions, agita-ting questions in the beginning
- Never argue or criticize with the client, related to delusions
- Orient the client about ward routines, policies, therapeutic procedures to be carried out
- Talk with the client clearly, specifically
- Explain to the client, the reason of his behaviour and the attitude.

4. Nursing Diagnosis

Altered thought process which predisposes for insecurity.

Goal

Provision of secured and safe environment.

Interventions

- Develop a sense of security, adequacy and trust feeling
- Provide safe and comfortable environment, therapeutic touch
- If it is desirable try to implement his desires into action, e.g. changing of room or close the doors, making relative to stay along with the client
- Avoid over-crowding in the ward by placing unnecessary furnitures.

5. Nursing Diagnosis

Self care deficit related to inability to meet his daily care living activities and needs.

Goal

To maintain physical health.

Interventions

- Serve the food in small and frequent feeds
- Provide adequate nutritious diet
- Encourage the client to have food along with group members to avoid suspiciousness
- Record the weight daily
- Encourage the client to cultivate regular habit related to hygiene (bladder, bowel, eating, dressing, appearance, etc.)
- Always keep one person to safeguard the client by protecting from persecutory delusions
- Promote regular sleeping habits, be near with the client when he is sleeping, switch on the lights, if it is not disturbing
- Assess the mental status, behaviour of the client, e.g. Hostility
- Explain to the family members, the condition of the patient and obtain needed support
- Try to divert the mind of client by spending the time in useful solitary recreational activities, e.g. Drawing, painting, etc. later it can be progressed to group activities
- Constant monitoring of the client is needed
- Meet the spiritual needs by arranging prayers and spiritual meetings to get satisfaction and relief to the client.

6. Nursing Diagnosis

Need for discharge advice, ready to go home and adjust to family environment.

Goal

Gain family support and able to adjust with family and its environment.

Interventions

- Help the client to adjust to the family surroundings

Encourage the client to develop positive attitude and achieving self confidence
- Family and situational support will help them to become normal and it reduces stress, adopts to the family situation
- Plan for involving the client gradually in family activities so that he feel secured
- Arrange for discussions with client, their family members and health care team members
- Allow the client to go along with family during parole time and ask the family members to observe and report the client's behaviour
- Educate the need of continuity and follow-up services, identify the community agencies which will help them for employment and follow-up services.

7. Nursing Diagnosis

Non-adherence to treatment.

Goal

Accepts and follows the therapeutic advices and treatment.

Interventions

- Advise the client to follow the importance of treatment and enjoys its beneficial effects
- If the client expresses any doubts, clarify and give correct information
- Administer the drugs, observe for side effects of drugs and prepare drug chart
- Encourage the client to follow the therapeutic advices and its combinations
- Explain the client, the need of taking treatment regularly and continuously until complete cure.

MOOD DISORDERS (AFFECTIVE DISORDERS/PSYCHOSIS)

Terminology

Affect

Is related to the feelings, mood or emotional tone of an individual. It is an eternal expression of an internal emotional content.

Mood

Internal emotional state of an individual.

Classification of Mood Disorder

1. Unipolar disorder–Recurrent episodes of depression or mania
   Bipolar disorder–Recurrent episode of depression and mania
   Type I Bipolar–Episodes of mania and major depression
   Type II Bipolar–Episodes of mania, hypomania and major depression
   Type III Bipolar–Episodes of major depression
   Type IV Bipolar–Consists of all other forms of bipolar disorders
2. Affective disorders
   Manic depressive psychosis
   Mania
   Depression
   Circular reactions
   Involutional psychotic reactions
3. ICD -10 classification of affective (mood) disorders
   F_{20}–F_{29}
   Unipolar depression
      Major depression
      Recurrent depression
      Psychotic depression
      Dysthymia
      Postpartum depression
   F_{30}–F_{39}
   Mood (Affective) Disorders
   F_{30} –Manic episode
   $F_{30.0}$ –Hypomania
   $F_{30.1}$ –Mania without psychotic symptoms
   $F_{30.2}$ –Mania with psychotic symptoms
   $F_{30.8}$ –Other manic episodes
   $F_{30.9}$ –Manic episodes, unspecified
   F_{31} –Bipolar affective disorder
   $F_{31.0}$ –Bipolar affective disorder, current episode hypomania

$F_{31.1}$ –Bipolar affective disorder, current episode manic with psychotic symptoms
$F_{31.2}$ –Bipolar affective disorder, current episode manic with mixed in remission.

Psychotic symptoms
$F_{31.3}$ –Bipolar affective disorder, current episode mild or moderate depression
   .30 Without somatic syndrome
   .31 With somatic syndrome
$F_{31.4}$ –Bipolar affective disorder, current episode severe depression without psychotic symptoms
$F_{31.5}$ –Bipolar affective disorder, current episode severe depression with psychotic symptoms
$F_{31.6}$ –Bipolar affective disorder, current episode mixed
$F_{31.7}$ –Bipolar affective disorder, current episode currently in remission
$F_{31.8}$ –Other bipolar affective disorder
$F_{31.9}$ –Bipolar affective disorder, unspecified
F_{32} –Depressive episode
$F_{32.0}$ –Mild depressive episode
   .00 Without somatic syndrome
   .01 With somatic syndrome
$F_{32.1}$ –Moderate depressive episode
   .10 Without somatic syndrome
   .11 With somatic syndrome
$F_{32.2}$ –Severe depressive episode without psychotic symptoms
$F_{32.3}$ –Severe depressive episode with psychotic symptoms
$F_{32.8}$ –Other depressive episodes
$F_{32.9}$ –Depressive episode, unspecified
F_{33} –Recurrent depressive disorder
$F_{33.0}$ –Recurrent depressive disorder, current episode mild
   .00 Without somatic syndrome
   .01 With somatic syndrome
$F_{33.1}$ –Recurrent depressive disorder, current episode moderate

.10 Without somatic syndrome

.11 With somatic syndrome

$F_{33.2}$ –Recurrent depressive disorder, current severe episode without psychotic symptoms

$F_{33.3}$ –Recurrent depressive disorder, current severe episode with psychotic symptoms

$F_{33.4}$ –Recurrent depressive disorder, currently in remission

$F_{33.8}$ –Other recurrent depressive disorders

$F_{33.9}$ –Recurrent depressive disorder, unspecified

F_{34} –Persistent Mood (Affective) disorders

$F_{34.0}$ –Cyclothymia

$F_{34.1}$ –Dysthymia

$F_{34.8}$ –Other persistent mood (affective) disorders

$F_{34.9}$ –Persistent mood (affective) disorders, unspecified

F_{38} –Other mood (affective) disorders

$F_{38.0}$ –Other single mood (affective) disorders

.00–Mixed affective episodes

$F_{38.1}$ –Other recurrent mood (affective) disorders

.01–Recurrent brief depressive disorders

$F_{38.8}$ –Other specified mood (affective) disorders

F_{39} –Unspecified mood (affective) disorder I.V. According to DSM III

Major affective disorders. For example, Manic episode, major depressive episode, bipolar disorders.

Specific affective disorders. For example, Cyclothymic disorders, dysthymic disorders, atypical affective disorders.

Definitions

'Mood disorder is a condition whereby the prevailing emotional mood is distorted or inappropriate to the specified circumstances'.

'Affective disorders are group of disorders in which fundamental disturbances or changes in mood occur accompanied by overall change in level of activity'. For example, Elation or depression–IGNOU Manual.

'Clinical conditions in which mood change is predominant and persistent, associated with cognitive, psychomotor, psycho-physiological and behavioural difficulties or its related changes like excitement/elation or depression and occurrence of such manifestations based on client's *mood*'.

BIPOLAR DISORDER

'It is a brain disorder that cause unusual shifts in a person's mood energy and ability to function. It is a long term illness which has to be carefully managed throughout a person's life'.

Incidence

- Per 1000 population 3–4 cases will occur
- 3:2 male:female
- MDP cases are observed more in
  - High social classes
  - Unmarried
  - Widowhood
  - Professionals
- Age: 20–35 years (mania)
  - 35–50 years (depression)
  - more common in identical twins; genetic predisposition observed
- Depression is more common in women than in men
- 5.7 million American adults or about 2.6 per cent of total population aged 18 years and above in any given year are having bipolar disorder. It develops typically in late adolescence or early adulthood and runs throughout life. (Source: Health, 2007)
- Brain image studies shown, the brains of bipolar disorders will be varying from normative individual.

Spectrum of Illness or Magnitude of Illness

Bipolar disorder is a mood disorder described by alternating periods of depression and mania. It distorts moods, thoughts and destroys the basis of rational thought and too often erodes the desire and will to live. It is almost unendurable suffering. It

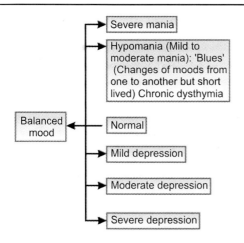

causes dramatic mood swings from overly 'high' irritable mood to sad and hopeless and then back again. Severe changes in mood, behaviour, energy. The periods of 'high' and 'low' are called episodes of mania and depression (refer the above flow chart).

These disorders tend to be recurrent. Some may experience recurrent depressive reactions, few exhibit elation in mood, some manifest behavioural reactions in alteration between the two affects.

AETIOLOGICAL FACTORS

I. Biological Factors

Heredity

Genetic predisposition is common, life time risk is noticed in first degree relatives of the client. If one parent suffers, 25 per cent chance for children to have the disorders, if both parents are suffering, 50-75 perc cent chances to occur in children. Twins are more predisposed, higher percentage (40-70%) is observed in identical/monozygotic/uniovular twins than dizygotic twins (20%).

Neuro-physiological Factors

Imbalance in excitatory and inhibitory processes may predispose MDP. Obliteration of excitatory functions leads to mania, inhibitory functions may lead to depression.

Physical Factors

Viral infections. For example, Hepatitis, mononucleosis.

Biochemical Factors

Imbalances in catecholamine (Norepinephrine, dopamine) levels or its functions obliterate results into MDP. If catecholamine amounts are increased mania, will occur; decreased levels predisposes for depression.

Deficiency in serotonin levels results in MDP.

Deficiency in GABA, acetylcholine contributes for mania occurrence.

These deficits interfaces with transmission of nerve impulses from one cell to another resulting in an affect.

Neuro-hormonal Factors

Decreased cortisol secretions; alteration in hippocampus functions predisposes for MDP.

Due to non-adrenergic receptors dysfunction in nocturnal period, alteration in pineal gland hormonal secretion (melatonin hormone) results into MDP (Excess secretion leads to mania; decreased secretions leads to depression).

II. Social Factors

- Stressful life events, traumatic or unpleasant or disturbing life experiences
- Social pressures
- Rejection of children by parents
- Difficult or strained interpersonal relationships; interpersonal loss, interpersonal role dispute or transition or deficits
- Sociocultural factors
- Loss of loved one (real or symbolic)
- Financial difficulties
- Unemployment, poor job opportunities
- Criticism and rejection
- Failures in life, defeat, hardship in scholastic environment

- Faulty interactions within the social environment
- Environmental stress
- Uncontrollable events or factors
- Maladaptive behaviour
- Unhealthy comparison
- Parental influence
- Trying to escape from reality.

III. Physiological Factors

- Felling of helplessness, hopelessness, inadequate, worthlessness
- Premorbid personality pattern–ambitious, energetic, social, will not express hostile feelings, endomorphic in their built, uncontrollable impulsive behaviour, lack of energy, breakdown under stress, introversion, insecurity, tendency to worry always, dependency, obsessionality
- Psychoanalytical factors–hostility, loss, conflicts within the self, borderline personality traits predisposes for depression
- Cognitive factors–faulty cognition, Beck has described 'cognitive traid' which predisposes for depression as
  - Perceiving oneself as defective as demanding and punishing
  - Expecting failure, defeat and hardship
  - Negative cognitions, i.e. negative expectations of environment, self, future.

CLINICAL MANIFESTATION OR PSYCHODYNAMICS OF MOOD DISORDER

Depression

A form of affective manifestation in which the client will exhibit mood disturbances related to self and his environment.

Depressive episodes–The classical symptoms in depression are:

Depressed Mood–Ranges from mild, acute or severe depression.

a. Mild Depression

Rigid, sensitive to criticism, fatigue, flattened of mood, blunt affect, dullness, sad, anxious, empty mood, physical complaints with no organic cause, blue spells, lacks confidence in himself, lack of interest in activities once enjoyed, including sex; reduced energy, lowered activity performance, inadequacy, exhibits aversion to activities, spends alone, finds difficulty in performing ordinary activities, sleeping disturbances, anorexia, feeling of hopelessness/helplessness, pessimism, worthlessness, unreasonable guilt, self blaming, low self-esteem.

b. Psychomotor Retardation; Slow in Activities and Moods

Poverty of ideas, retarded in thinking, preoccupied with gloomy thoughts, always sees the dark side of things, no enthusiasm for daily activities, no zest for living and no pleasure in everyday things, loss of libido, incongruent moods, lack of reactivity and confidence, difficulty in concentration, remembering, decision making.

c. Acute or Severe Depression

Client feels tensed, unable to relax, anxious, low or poor concentration, lack of attention, poor memory, guilty, inadequacy feelings, loss of energy, tired, exhausted, vague feeling of bodyaches, severe headache, GIT manifestations, restlessness, irritability, cannot concentrate for longer period, diurnal variations (depression is more in early morning and in late evenings).

Stooped posture, downward facing of looks, no interest, retarded thoughts, monosyllable, express with low tone.

GIT manifestations. For example, Dryness of mouth, constipation, anorexia or eats more, (unintended weight loss or gain) menstrual or sexual disturbances; responds with great difficulty, as if he has used more energy to respond it; sleeping too much or can't sleep, chronic pain, persistent bodily symptoms that are not caused by physical illness or injury, suicidal tendency and attempts; thoughts of death, if not treated, they may go into stupor.

d. Depressive Stupor

Intensive form in which the client will have acute dementia, mute, clouded sensorium, preoccupied mind, hallucinations, depersonalization, derealization, delusion, progresses into death.

Diagnosis: A depressive episode is diagnosed if five or more of these symptoms persist most of the day, nearly every day, for a period of 2 weeks or longer.

Treatment: Combination of approaches are effective rather than single approach. Severely depressed patient with an idea of suicide required constant medical supervision and need to be hospitalized.

TREATMENT

i. Pharmacotherapy–Antidepressants

Tricyclic antidepressants (TCAs)–Imipramine 75–300 mg/day

or

Monoamino reuptake inhibitors–Amitriptyline 75–300 mg/day
Clomipramine 75–80 mg/day
Selective serotonin reuptake inhibitors (SSRIs)–
Fluoxetine 10–80 mg/day
Sertraline 50–200 mg/day
Fluvoxamine 50–300 mg/day
Dopaminergic antidepressants. Fluvoxamine 50–300 mg/day
Atypical antidepressants. Amineptine 100–400 mg/day
Mono aminooxidase inhibitors (MAO). Isocarboxazid 10–30 mg/day
Miscellaneous newer antidepressants. Venlafaxine 150–375 mg/day
Bupropion 150–450 mg/day

Based on the symptoms of the client, type of depression, choice of psychiatrist the drugs will be prescribed.

Mechanism of Action

- Increases catecholamine level in the brain
- TCAs block the reuptake of norepinephrine or serotonin at the nerve terminals and increase its level at the receptor site. 2–3 weeks will be taken to decrease the depressive symptoms; weight gain
- MAOs degrade the catecholamine after reuptake and increases brain amine level 5–10 days it will take to bring down depressive symptoms
- SSRIs act by inhibiting the reuptake of serotonin and increases its level at receptor site.

Side Effects

- Anticholenergic reaction: Dry mouth, constipation, distress, mydriasis, urinary retention, blurred vision, delirium
- Sexual dysfunction: Impaired ejaculation, priapism, impotence
- CNS effects: Fine tremors, sedation, extra pyramidal symptoms, withdrawal syndrome, seizures, precipitation of mania reflecting bipolar illness
- Cardiovascular effects: Postural or orthostatic hypotension, palpitation, arrhythmias, ECG changes (QT lengthening), myocardial depression
- In IHD cases AV block, sudden death may occur
- Hypertensive crisis with MAOs.

Nursing Intervention

- Administer and record the drugs as per order
- Monitor action and if any side effect of the drugs observed, report to the authority immediately
- Advise the client not to take any medication of his own or position is required
- Monitoring and recording of vital signs is essential, specially blood pressure
- Ask the client to take sips of water, apply glycerine or vaseline on lips to prevent dryness of lips
- Advise to high fibre diet and more fluids to prevent constipation.

ii. Electroconvulsive Therapy

- ECT is indicated to have rapid action and remission of symptoms. In major depression cases it will be given as initial treatment and fosters antidepressant action.

iii. Psychotherapeutic Approach

Supportive Psychotherapy

Client will be guided for regularity of schedules and fixation of appointments. Various psycho-therapeutic processes like ventilation, reassurance and relaxation technique guidance, counselling, education sessions will be planned to improve the morale and support to the client. Discourage the client, not to expose to major changes, if they are prone for depression. Involve the client in diversional, purposeful activities, where he can relax his mind and concentrate for productive and independent activities.

Psychoanalysis

Free association or word association, motivation, guidance and counselling techniques are used to have stabilized environment, to maintain self esteem to resolve emotional conflicts, to improve self-esteem and insight, to reduce depressive symptoms, to prevent acute episodes.

Group Therapy

In mild depression cases group therapy is helpful to overcome negative feelings and to develop good interpersonal skills, by enhancing emotional growth and support.

Interpersonal Therapy

It improves social functioning, resolves psycho-social conflicts, explores precipitants predisposing MDP. For example, Losses, conflicts, transitions, etc. maintenance phase will be maintained.

Family Therapy

Provides support, reduces the depressive symptoms, relapses occurrence, resolves interpersonal and familial disputes or conflicts or problems. Psycho-education, guidance and counselling are the essential approaches used in family therapy.

Marital Therapy

To resolve marital conflicts, interpersonal, emotional conflicts among the couple and within the family and to attain family cohesiveness, counselors will give intensive advices to both partners.

Behaviour Therapy

Learning principles, varied techniques like social skill training, problem solving techniques, self control methods activity scheduling, decision making, assertiveness training, etc. will be used. Maintenance phase, this technique is helpful.

iv. Cognitive Therapy

To replace negative emotions with positive means by developing adequate coping skills and strategies; cognitive therapy is helpful. Specific learning experiences will be provided, where the client will be given training to learn specific tasks, assignments and accomplishes the work in scheduled time. The methods like role playing, positive reinforcement, modelling, practicing, rehearsal, etc. will be used to attain life time achievements. Maladaptive techniques will be replaced with adaptive procedures like activity schedules, graded task assignment, mastery and pleasure ratings, cognitive appraisal, rehearsal, negative reinforcement techniques will be used.

NURSING MANAGEMENT OF A CLIENT WITH DEPRESSION

I. Nursing Assessment

Obtain the general history of the client both from the client (Primary source) and from other reliable source (significant people like family members, close friends: secondary sources like previous records).

a. General or demographic information: Age, sex, health status, nativity/residence, date of admission.

b. Socio-economic history:
   i. Education: Educational status, pattern of education, scholastic environment and any difficulties experienced, any history of repeated failures, scholastic upheavals.
   ii. Occupation: Age at which he started responsibilities and earning, type of job, work, cultural pattern, schedule and work environment, stress associated with it.
   iii. Economy: Financial status, type of class, financial stability, commitments, experiencing difficulty in meeting economic needs
   iv. Marital history: Married, single, widowed, married but staying alone, marital relationship, duration of marital life.
   v. Family history: Type of family, size of family, relationship with family members, interaction within the family, involvement of family members, provision or level of moral support, pattern of family living conditions.

c. Past medical history: Number of episodes, type of depression experienced, place and type of treatment obtained, history of hospitalization, pattern of manifestation, duration, course of prognosis and recovery.

d. Present medical history: manifestation, duration, associated conditions. Type of illness, effect of disorder on other people, performance of social activities, clues of deterioration, seeking assistance, type of activities and behaviour during sickness. Explore the causes, situational support available to the client. Assess the severity of the disorder. For example, Type, associated illness or factors, emotion pattern. Assess the effects of disorder over the client, his family and their social environment.

Physical examination of client to exclude any physical illness, environmental surroundings, safety.

II. Nursing Interventions

1. Nursing Diagnosis

High risk for violence related to suicidal tendency.

Goal

Protect the client from suicidal tendency and self harm.

Interventions

- Vigilant observation of the client for any clues (active or passive) and disturbed behavioural pattern or related activities, etc is required
- Provide safe environment, pace the patient near to the nurses station to have constant monitoring and immediate care
- Remove all potentially harmful objects in the client's unit or near to the client's surroundings
- Administer the medications as prescribed, observe for side effects specifically extra pyramidal symptoms and if any observed, report immediately
- Counsel the client, show concern, love, care at the time of need, discuss in detail with the client, provide moral support
- Never allow the client to be alone, if provision is there, permit the relative to stay near to the client or one-to-one observation may be needed
- Encourage the client to ventilate the feelings or emotions openly
- Emphasize positive attitude; needed observational skills, pros and cons pattern, related to suicidal plans.
- Establish and maintain positive contracts, counsel the client frequently, provide guidance and support
- Assist the client in finding meaning to the real life situation and teach coping strategies

- Encourage the family to provide support and to inform pleasant events to the client; need of his presence or his company
- Educate the client to gain deeper insight in his own behaviour, new ways of problem solving techniques.

2. Nursing Diagnosis

Alteration in mood pattern related to reduced self esteem, self concept, guilty feelings.

Goal

Client will be able to express positive aspects of life and tries to adopt new coping strategies to uplift him which will enhance the self esteem and self concept.

Interventions

- Accept the client as he is
- Spend some time leisurely with the client, express concern, support, well wishes, etc.
- Encourage the client to verbalize/ventilate his feelings openly, never pass any comments or disturb the process of ventilation
- Motivate the client to perform the activities in which he is confident, appreciate or give reward for his self accomplishment, provide assistance whenever needed
- Emphasize the client to participate in group activities
- Inform the client about the progress made in accomplishing the activities, which enhances self confidence
- Involve the family members to provide support, concern and not to make the client to undergo or experience difficulty in situations
- Assist the client to enjoy satisfaction and meaning to life
- Motivate the client to appreciate areas of change and provide needed guidance and assistance.

3. Nursing Diagnosis

Ego deficit related to lack of confidence, repeated failure in achieving goals.

Goal

Raise the self-esteem, self confidence to strengthen client's ego processes.

Interventions

- Permit the client to take decisions and perform the activities without any assistance effectively
- Provide related resources to gain confidence through interaction
- Discourage the client to have the thoughts which hampers his growth and efficiency
- Provide conducive environment, repeated opportunities to expose themselves to stressors.

4. Nursing Diagnosis

Variation in life style pattern due to defective coping strategies or lack of control over any type of life tragedies or situations.

Goal

Develop adequate coping strategies to enjoy the life situations.

Interventions

- Explain the reason for the changed situation
- Educate the client to utilize adoptive coping strategies, assertive techniques to enhance the ego strengthening
- According to the situation, use either positive or negative reinforcement techniques and other behaviour modification techniques to face the reality
- Encourage the client to take decisions and set realistic goals and work for its achievement
- Motivate the client to express his inabilities

- Teach new coping strategies skills, allow them to participate in group activities, where they can interact and share their feelings and listen to others.

5. Nursing Diagnosis

Inappropriate expression of emotional feelings due to emotional upset.

6. Nursing Diagnosis

Altered attention and concentration due to thought disturbances.

Goal

Client will be able to verbalize his feelings and diverts his mind in constructive activities, which improve attention and concentration.

Interventions

- Assist the client to facilitate catharsis process and ventilate his feelings
- Assess the extent of depressive feelings, secondary gains and its effects over the life
- Motivate the client to participate in group therapy and its process; to develop the ability to observe, how the other clients are ventilating their experiences and adapting coping strategies by utilizing the resources
- Allow the client to participate in social activities whereby he can divert his mind and learn to utilize varied techniques to attack the problem
- Identify the areas of interest and if it is desirable, encourage him to perform it effectively, e.g. allow the client in playing games and sports and achieving skills and mastery over it
- Help the client to frankly discuss his feelings; ask the client not to hesitate to ask for assistance to achieve skills in it
- Clarify the doubts of the client
- Reorient the client to adopt to the new life style.

7. Nursing Diagnosis

Impaired cognition due to increased sensitivity to the environmental stressful stimuli.

Goal

Enhance the cognitive abilities and improve thought process, utilizes appropriate adaptive skills to overcome stress.

Interventions

- Encourage the client to utilize the available resources to enhance the abilities, strengths and weakens the failure process
- Assist him to learn new assertive techniques and to adopt coping strategies adequately
- Permit the client to engage in purposeful activities in a constructive manner
- Expose the client to environmental stimuli in non-graded manner and simultaneously allow him to utilize problem solving techniques effectively and tries to adopt to the situation efficiently.

8. Nursing Diagnosis

Impaired communication and socialization pattern related to withdrawal tendency, fears and other stressors.

Goal

Improve communication process and socialization pattern, diverts his mind in constructive activities.

Interventions

- Nurse will utilize the different psychological processes and approaches, varied modes of communication techniques and strategies, while talking to the client
- Approach the client in an active friendly manner
- Be brief in conversation

- Motivate the client to respond adequately
- Nurse will act as an active listener, good supporter, guide, motivator and an effective communicator
- Educate the client appropriate communication techniques to converse or interact efficiently with others
- Explain the client, how failures will help the individual to develop 'will power' and 'efficiency in making efforts' and strategies to overcome the deficiencies
- Accept the client's inner feelings and narrate the related events, how others have gone though the same pattern in their life situations and methods adopted to achieve their goals
- Observe the non-verbal communication pattern and the method of interaction of the client
- Motivate the client to observe the social situations thoroughly, where he has to participate shortly
- Teach the client, the importance of adequate socialization
- Gradually make the client to actively participate in social activities which enhances socialization process and self confidence
- Help the client to identify and approach significant members either from family or friends to have situational support and for establishing good interpersonal relationship.

9. Nursing Diagnosis

Alteration in activities of daily living or self care deficit related to mood disturbances.

Goals

Able to perform the self care, daily living activities independently.
- Utilize the maxims of teaching in guiding the client
- Teach the behaviour modification techniques and motivate to sue it appropriately
- Assist whenever the need arises, emphasize the importance of taking care of all body parts

- Plan the daily care activities, provide conducive environment and encourage the client to take care of himself and ensure his activities
- Appreciate the client when he appears neat and tidy and able to perform self care activities effectively
- Encourage the client to participate in ward activities.

10. Nursing Diagnosis

Altered nutrition, weight loss due to irregular eating pattern and disturbed behavioural pattern.

Goal

Gains adequate improvement in nutritional status and appears healthy way.

Interventions

- Try to explore the likes, dislikes or preferences of client's food items
- Educate the client the importance of nutrition (in maintaining physical health) and hazards of malnutrition
- Serve small and frequent feeds; meet the dietary requirements of clients to prevent the deficiencies
- Be with the patient and serve the food, talk to him while he is eating, pursue him to take total/required food
- Try to incorporate his best preferred foods and see that it will meet the daily requirements
- Encourage him to develop regular eating habits with adequate nutrient supplementation and balanced diet
- Check and record the weight, bowel pattern daily
- If the client is in 'stupor', Nasogastric tube feeding may be necessary and maintain intake and output chart
- Teach the client to take adequate amount of nutrients and fluids

- Plan the next day menu by discussing with the client
- Give one glass of warm milk to the client before going to bed.

11. Nursing Diagnosis

Alteration in sleep pattern due to emotional upset, inadequate adaptation process.

Goal

Improves sleeping pattern thereby rest and comfort will be enhanced.

Interventions

- Help the client to plan the schedule (day time activities) in order of priority
- Don't allow the client to sit 'idle' or 'sleep' in day time
- Encourage the client to do the activities simple to complex, appreciate after accomplishment of a given task
- Provide a calm/conducive environment, dim light, soft music to facilitate sleep
- If the client is spiritually deprived, assist him in spiritual activity by arranging prayer, consoling, warm support, provide materials/books related to spirituality/yoga and meditation
- Administer PRN medications if prescribed
- If the client desires, allow the relative to stay along with him to feel security and comfort
- Explain the client to make himself busy in day time, thereby getting fatigue, which enhances sleep at night
- Encourage the client to let out his emotions freely to the 'confident people' and take their assistance in implementing comfortable activities
- Provide the discharge advices to the client, including follow-up visits and continuation of treatments.

12. Nursing Diagnosis

Dysfunctional grieving related to real or perceived loss or threat of loss.

Goal

Expresses his feelings outwardly; exhibits associated behaviours related to grieving process.

Interventions

- Asses the pattern of loss and stages of grieving associated with it
- Accept the client feelings and make him to understand the situation, encourage him to express his feelings openly to ventilate and catharsis
- Explain crisis interventions and assist him to adopt appropriate activities to accommodate and adjust to the inevitable situation appropriately
- Allow sometime to relax and cope-up, teach the client to utilize appropriate behavioural techniques for coping up the situation
- Never allow him to stay alone, motivate him to divert the mind by utilizing his time in productive activities, permit him to enjoy its fragrance and ask the client to share all types of feelings to the person whomever he gained the confidence.

Differences Between Endogenous and Exogenous Depression

(Refer table p. 400).

Involutional Melancholia

Occurs in women in late middle life or during the menopausal period.

Causes: Psychological stress, environmental stressors

Clinical manifestation

Severe depression, agitation, apprehension, despair feelings-worthlessness, insomnia, fatigue, anorexia.

Differences between endogenous depression and exogenous depression	
Endogenous/Major/Biological/Psychotic depression/Autogenous	*Exogenous/Reactive/Neurotic depression*
Caused due to factors within the individual, i.e. biological and personality deficit factors	External stimuli play a significant role in manifestation of disease. For example, Environmental stressful stimuli
Mild or absence of precipitating factors	Presence of precipitating factors
Incidence: Common in lower socioeconomic group and working groups	Commonly observed in middle and upper socioeconomic class, men, sometimes both sex are exposed for it
Personality type: Pyknic and mesomorphic body built	No specified physique
Premorbid personality: Cyclothymic or dysthymic	Anxious, obsessive or inadequate when exposed to stressful environment
Manifestations: Psychomotor retardation, unable to fulfill their roles. For example, Familial, social or occupational	Less intensity, able to manage all the functions effectively
Late insomnia, early awakening, suicidal tendency is common in late and early hours	More sleep disturbance, experience difficulty in getting sleep. Feels more sad in late evening
Feels depressed in early hours, as the day passes improves, again in night disturbances	Less depressed in early morning, as the day progresses depression also progresses
Severe thought disturbances, experiences delusions, hallucinations	Restlessness, more attention seeking, psychomotor agitation
Not having desire or interest in sexual activities due to decreased libidinal energy	Feels comfort or relief when indulging in sexual activities, interested in it
Alteration in self care activity functioning, lack of insight in his own activities	Can take care of themselves with good insight
Feels comfort when alone and ventilates by crying	Feels better in group
Slowing down of physiological process. For example, Anorexia, constipation, sad appearance, slow walking, poor posture	Physiological process and mood changes according to the environmental stimuli
Alteration in psychological processes, poor intellectual functioning, suicidal is common	Suicidal threats are common
Diagnosis Needs good insight and skillful in psychoanalysis technique to identify the cause Psychoanalysis Interview Keen observation Process recording	Explorational skills are required to identify the cause Interview and Observation
Therapy Electro-convulsive therapy Drug therapy For example, Mood stabilizers; antidepressants; and psychotics, benzodiazepines	Psychotherapy Social therapy Drug therapy. For example, Antimanics Milieu therapy
Prognosis Relapses are common	Relapses are uncommon

Delusions-persecutory, hypochondriacal, nihilistic.
Treatment
Electroconvulsive therapy
Pharmacotherapy. For example, antidepressants.

MANIA

True mania people can be described by 'frantic'
'hyperactive' 'over-excited' 'tangents of thoughts
and ideas'.

Definition

It is a psychiatric medical condition in which client
manifests a clinical syndrome characterized by
extremely elevated mood, energy, hyperactivity,
unusual thought process with flight of ideas and
acceleration in speaking process.

Incidence and Epidemiology

- 0.6–1 per cent adults will have mania during
  their life time
- Onset is most common in late adolescence or
  early adulthood
- Incidence is more in
  - Unmarried, separated or divorced cases
  - Urban, upper socioeconomic groups
  - Positive family history, monozygotic twins
  - Drug induced manic disturbances
  - Male:Female ratio 1:1 (Bipolar disorder;
    males tend to have manic episode first,
    cycling with depressive episode; females
    tend to have depressive episode first circle
    with mania later).

Aetiology

- Heredity, genetic predisposition
- Interference in neurotransmitter functioning and
  regulation
- Stressful life events. For example, bereavement.

Secondary mania can occur due to a variety of
- Neurological conditions, e.g. Multiple sclerosis,
  brain tumors, epilepsy, brain trauma

- Metabolic disorders
- Endocrinal disorders, e.g. Hyper-adreno-
  corticalism, hyperthyroidism
- Conditions which affects brain functioning
- Drug induced: Corticosterids, androgenic
  steroids, L-dopa, anti-depressants, stimulants
- Co-morbid illnesses adversely affect the outlook
  for mania, e.g. alcoholism and substance abuse.

Types

I.
  - Acute mania
  - Hypomania or mild to moderate mania
  - Delirium mania or severe mania

II.
  - Primary mania
  - Secondary mania due to organic cause

III.
  - Description of recent manic episode
  - Mania without psychotic symptoms
  - Mania with psychotic symptoms
  - Unspecified manic episode
  - Mania with catatonic features
  - Mania with postpartum episode

IV.
  - Mania
  - Hypomania
  - Mixed state or dysphoric mania.

Clinical Manifestations

An excess in behavioural activity, mood states, self-
esteem and confidence. Manic behaviour seems to
begin abruptly or over the space of few hours or
few days.
- Changes in mood for a distinct period of time
  Based on severity of manic episode changes in
  mood elevation is observed.

1. Mild Mania or Hypomania

Episode will be atleast for five days, euphoria or
expansive mood (stage-I) abnormal mood elevation,
cheerful, extremely happy, elevated sense of

psychological well being; happiness is not correlated with ongoing events, may tend to have more enthusiasm, emphasis on certain events (expensiveness). A sudden pleasant mood, lightening, positive energy, heightened feelings of well being with increased alertness and drive, sudden oscillation of moods, expansive sociability the individual is able to function well; inflated self esteem. Persistence and pervasive elated or irritable mood, thoughts and consistent behaviours, absence of psychotic symptoms.

- Confident on skills, abilities or strengths, thoughts
- Creative talents, most productive
- Total awareness; easily gets ideas, over flowing with new ideas; energetic, flight of ideas, charismatic
- Coherent thoughts, feeling pressure from within the thought process which keeps him to talk or racing thoughts
- Immune to fear and doubts.
  Talks to the strangers easily, offer solutions to problems, finds pleasure in small activities
- Sometimes hypomanic episodes can be dysphoric, irritable, ragful, may make poor choices and display little or no sympathy for others' emotions
- Inflated self-esteem or grandiosity
- Decreased need for sleep or disturbed sleep pattern, rapid eye movement is increased, but the client looks fresh
- Being more talkative than usual
- Easily distractable, attention deficit
- Increase in psychomotor agitation
- Involvement in pleasurable activities that may have a high potential for negative psychosocial or physical consequences
- Mild or severe form of obsessional behaviour
- Poor judgement relative to a particular situation's judgment
- Partially controllable
- Mild or severe recklessness
- Excessive spending money
- Involves in risky sexual activity

- Simply 'feels great'
- Increased assertiveness, denies if anything goes wrong
- Delusion of grandiosity
- Uninhibited in approach
- Oracious eater
- Intellectual
- Inability to tolerate criticisms, anger, aggressive, argumentative, more ambitious, poor interpersonal relationship among partners
- Bored with routines, lacks interest in specific topics
- Possesses humour and makes environment happy
- Oscillation in moods
- Extrovert, mischievous in behaviour.

2. Mixed Mood State/Dysphoric Mania

- Pronounced symptoms of both depression and mania coexist or alternate during different periods of the day. Increased probability of suicide in mixed state, as they have the energy needed to commit suicide.

3. Acute Mania

- Euphoria, elation (stage-II) and exaltation of moods (stage-III)
- Elation of mood–moderate elevation of mood, increased psychomotor activity, joyous excitement
- Exaltation of moods (stage-III); Intense elevation of mood, grandeur delusions (affective tonality), frequent variations in moods
- Unselective enthusiasm for interacting with people and surrounding environment
- Extreme irritability may easily be evoked especially when the person is stopped from doing what he is intended to do, however, they may be unrealistic
- Inflated self-esteem
- Over activity/increased activity, restlessness

- Obvious over talkativeness or pressured or rapid speech, used rhythmic, rhyming language, loudly speaks, difficult to interrupt
- Socially embarrassing behaviour, distress to family
- Inflated self-esteem or delusion of grandiosity, persecution, paranoid, delusion of control, reference, etc. may be seen
- Distractibility-easily attention will be drawn to irrelevant stimuli
- Indiscretion
- Flight of ideas, rapidly shifting from one to another, making it hard for others to understand
- Racing thoughts and perceptions lead to frustration-rapid thoughts that the patient finds it hard to keep-up with them or express them
- Decreased need for sleep, sleep deprived psychosis-only few hours of sleep is needed daily for the client to feel rested, do not look fatigued
- Humorous and teasing
- Frequently denies if anything is wrong with them
- Encourage high energy, increased perception of need or ability to sleep
- Impulsively taking part in activities
- Potentially harmful to self and others
- Anger or rage, provocative, aggressive, intrusive demanding, revengeful, arrogant
- Hypersensitivity
- Hypersexual drive
- Hyper religious
- Increased stress in personal relationship, problems at work
- Increased goal directed activity, pursues with specific goals at work
- Fragmented and psychotic
- Excessive involvement in pleasurable activities with high potential for negative consequence
- Common problem areas: spending sprees, sexual indiscretion, increased substance abuse (cocaine tranquilizers), investing more money in unreasonable manner

- Distributes money or articles to unknown persons
- Excessively 'high', overly good
- Unrealistic beliefs in one's abilities and powers
- Lacks judgement skills, impaired attention, concentration, poor insight
- Denial tendency
- Children with mania are more prone for destructive tantrums
- Neglects hygiene, disorganized dressing
- Impulsive, sociable
- Decreased food intake eventhough increased appetite, as he may not time to eat, hence client will loss weight
- Crispy speaking, noisy sounds, hilarious, changes in pitch while speaking
- He will be giving free suggestions, e.g. how to run a social organization
- Hallucination may occur, but not common
- Sad, crying
- Psychotic symptoms: occasionally severe episodes of mania or depression include psychotic manifestations. For example, Perceptual disturbances-hallucinations, delusions, grandiosity in mania, delusion of guilt will appear in depression.

4. Delirious Mania

- Rarely it will occurs
- Client will be out of contact with external world
- Word salad, incoherent speech
- Client will be active without any aim or goal
  - Perceptual problems, i.e. hallucination, delusion, may be extreme
  - Self care deficit, unable to concentrate
  - Client may die as a result of physical exhaustion.

Treatment

- Involuntary admission may be required until client stabilizes, to prevent harm to themselves or others. Tactful persuasion is necessary, involve the family members in making the client to agree for the admission.

- Acute mania is bipolar disorder is typically treated with mood stabilizers and antipsychotic medication. Careful monitoring and administration of prescribed drugs are needed to prevent harmful side effects. For example, malignant syndrome with antipsychotic medications.
- When the symptoms of severe mania subside, long term treatment focusses on prophylactic treatment, a combination of approaches may be required to stabilize the client's emotion.

a. Pharmacotherapy

- For example, Valproic acid, Carbamazepine 600–1800 mg/day, and benzodiazepines (600–2600 mg/day) may be added for sedation and to restore sleep
- Calcium channel blockers. For example, verapamil; if lithium must be discontinued, gradual reduction over a few weeks is associated with a lower risk of relapse than abrupt discontinuation.

b. Electroconvulsive Therapy

- If the client is not responding to antipsychotic medications (when client is having acute mania symptoms) or in early pregnancy to avoid the risk of birth defects due to drugs; ECT may be given.

c. Psychotherapy

- Marital therapy, behaviour therapy, family therapy and cognitive therapy certainly useful as adjunctive therapies. To enhance interpersonal relations, family cohesion, ensures continuation of treatment and adequate drug compliance, reduces stressors to modify the behaviour, restores self esteem, adapts a new range of emotions and workout to overcome/to prevent relapses.

d. Maintenance Therapy

- Call to medical attention, before things moves 'out of control' as severe mania cannot be managed by self, assistance from professional mental health care team is necessary. Attend the client as soon as possible.
- Insist the client to take regular prescribed medications.
- Instruct the client to handover his credit card, cheque, excess money to someone he can trust, as the client may have the chance to spend it more.
- Encourage the client to use defense mechanism, such as nomadism, sublimation, identification, etc. to overcome stressful environment.
- Advise the family members to be supportive to the client and to place the client in non-stimulating surroundings.
- Provide guidance and counselling, show love and concern to the client.
- Instruct the client to prepare a schedule of activities to be performed, and inform him to maintain it.
- Teach the relaxation techniques, rest and comfort measures and ask him to follow, keep the thought in a focussed manner rather than obsessive way.
- Insist on taking nutritious, well balanced diet.
- Extend support to family members and to monitor their coping abilities.

Course or Outcome

- Most manic episodes remit with treatment within few months.
- Majority cases may have recurrences. Considerable variability in outcome is noticed.
- Many individual show enduring difficulties in some areas of social adjustment.
- Childhood or adolescent onset may follow a more severe course in early years.
- Manic episodes are more likely receive clinical attention.

- Positive family history of mania is predictive of more manic recurrences overtime.
- In women, rapid cycling is associated with antidepressant use, possibly with hypothyroidism.
- Mild hypomania was observed during the first week of postnatal period, associated with a higher risk of depression in subsequent months.
- With holistic treatment approach, hypomania can be curable, if no treatment it may go into severe mania or depression (bipolar disorder).

NURSING MANAGEMENT OF THE CLIENT WITH MANIA

Nursing Assessment

Obtain the general history of the client, both from the client (primary source) and from other reliable source (significant people like family members, close friends: secondary sources like previous records).

a. General or demographic information: Age, sex, health status, nativity/residence, date of admission.

b. Socioeconomic history:

 i. Education: Educational status, pattern of education, scholastic environment and any difficulties experienced, any history of repeated failures, scholastic upheavals.

 ii. Occupation: Age at which he started responsibilities and earning, type of job, work, culture, pattern, schedule and its environment, stress associated with it.

 iii. Economy: Financial status, type of class, financial stability, commitments, experiencing difficulty in meeting economic needs.

 iv. Marital history: Married, single, widowed, married but staying alone, marital relationship, duration of marital life.

 v. Family history: Type of family, size of family, relationship with family members, interaction within the family, involvement of family members, provision or level of moral support, pattern of family living conditions.

c. Past medical history: Number of episodes, type of depression experienced, place and type of treatment obtained, history of hospitalization, pattern of manifestation, duration, course of prognosis and recovery.

d. Present medical history: Manifestation, duration, associated conditions. Type of illness, effect of disorder on other people, performance of social activities, clues of deterioration, seeking assistance, type of activities and behaviour during sickness. Explore the causes, situational support available to the client. Assess the severity of the disorder. For example, Type, associated illness or factors, emotion pattern. Assess the effects of disorder over the client, his family and their social environment. Physical examination of client to exclude any physical illness, environmental surroundings, safety.

1. Nursing Diagnosis

Non-compliance to treatment carries an increased risk for relapses.

Goal

Takes regular medications.

Interventions

- Explain to the client and his family members the importance of medicine and continuation of medication as per prescription and treatment plans, effects or complications, if not consuming drugs, etc. in an understanding, simple manner; it is good to convey the message in their own language

- Administer the drugs according to doctors order and monitor for side effects, record and report the drugs administered, and if any side effects observed

- While the client is on lithium prescription, monitor the level of serum lithium levels periodically, advice salt restricted diet

- Encourage the client to perform productive activities
- Provide calm and quiet environment
- Denial, reluctance are common in mania cases, report the changes to the doctor, make changes in medication prescription.

2. Nursing Diagnosis

Potential for self injury or causing harm to others.

Goal

Defend/guard the client from injury or causing harm to others.

Nursing Interventions

- Establish calm and quiet, non-provocative or non-stimulating environment.
- Keep sharp instruments away from the client.
- Provide supportive environment.
- Keep the client aside from stressful environment.
- Do not provoke or argue with the client or others in the client's unit.
- Protect the client by engaging in useful activities.
- Divert the client's mind by asking him to participate in calm activities like watching TV, playing with children, reading spiritual materials or interest of his own.
- Never allow violent patients stay together or nearby place in the same environment.
- Establish reliable, framed environment, set priorities and goals for everyday activity.
- Administer if any PRN prescribed medication, teach its importance.
- Educate the client the coping strategies and deep relaxation techniques to overcome aggressive feelings.
- Never leave the client all alone, one person has to accompany to observe and guide or assist the patient to perform useful activities. Observe

the client's interactions and restrict him to involve in group destructive activities.

- Keep the music volume low, and dim light in client's room.
- Avoid slippery floor to prevent accidents.

3. Nursing Diagnosis

Prone for violence resulting causing harm to himself or to others related to manic excitement and perceptual disturbance.

Nursing Interventions

- Provide peaceful, safe, environment, establish and maintain low stimuli in client's unit.
- Monitor the client's behaviour every 15 minutes once and maintain process recording of it, report it to appropriate health care professional.
- Remove all hazardous material in client's unit.
- Motivate the client to verbalize his feelings openly, thereby internal conflicts and hesitation will be reduced.
- Encourage the client to perform deep breathing exercises, meditation and interested activities in a desirable manner.
- Promote physical outlet for violent behaviour.
- Accept the client's feelings, be with him, show positive attitude, concern, and make him to understand that nurses are their well wishers and caretakers. Be brief, clear, direct speech in conversation, make the client to ventilate the emotions.
- Administer the drugs as per order and explain to the client and his relatives its importance.
- Always some nursing staff should be ready to handle the client in the time of need (violent behaviour or exciting if needed placement of restraints may be necessary.
- If restraints are placed, gradually remove one by one by observing his behaviour.
- Maintain adequate distance with the violent client and be ready to exit during violent behaviour.

- Exhibit consistency behaviour at all times.
- Never hurt inner feelings of the client, do not do any unhealthy comparisons.
- Review the incident with client after he gained control over his behaviour.
- Restrict or limit the client's negative feelings or activities.
- Define specified tasks, schedule it, orient and reinforce the client to perform his scheduled activities without postponing, insist for implementation of activities in a desirable manner.
- Encourage the client to participate in group activities and in small discussions.
- Provide minimum furniture.

4. Nursing Diagnosis

Alteration in thought process related to flight of ideas and delusions.

Goal

Recovers from perceptual and thought disturbances.

Interventions

- Be with the client, reorient him to the present situation
- Reduce the environmental stimuli in client's environment
- Engage the client's mind in pleasurable thoughts, encourage to participate in useful activities, appreciate for desirable behaviour
- Teach the problem solving techniques, suggest alternative methods
- Increase the frequency of activities in an expected manner based on performance and a sense of tolerance
- Warm approach is required in handling the client
- Provide support and motivate him to ventilate his inner feelings, use low voice, positive concern, feedback for client's behaviour
- Do not dig personnel issues in the beginning, talk general issues, gain confidence then the client will automatically verbalize his inner feelings
- Make the client to live in reality.

5. Nursing Diagnosis

Impaired communication, social isolation related to low coping skill, unsatisfactory environment.

Goal

Maintain good interpersonal relationship through adequate interaction.

Interventions

- Maintain good therapeutic interpersonal relationship
- Teach social skill and communication skills training
- Spend some time with the client; initiate brief conversation, directly speak to the client
- Encourage the client to interact with others, facilitate interaction process grading from individual to group interaction, motivate to talk clearly and slowly
- Provide feedback to the client, pursue him to involve in group activities (small to large)
- Motivate the client to inculcate good hobbies, plan the activities according to his interest
- If needed, obtain consultation from speech therapist
- Try to explore the supportive people, agencies to receive situational support
- Provide scheduled activities
- Keep limits for client behaviour and monitor it, as client may have flight of ideas ranging from anger to aggressive or rage, excited behaviour. Record the observations made
- Explain and orient the client for ward routines, procedures, policies
- Never argue or discourage with the client, when he is in a disturbed mood
- Provide stress free environment to calm the client's mind, protect the client from over flowing of thoughts

- Give positive reinforcements for non-manipulative behaviour
- Insist the client to verbalize his feelings whether positive or negative
- Explain the client, what is expected from him
- Teach problem solvation techniques, the ways of communicating its results; the skills required through regular selected activities
- Demonstrate specific behaviour modification techniques to ensure security feelings
- Provide positive reinforcement for the desired behaviour.

6. Nursing Diagnosis

Low self-esteem related to isolation, negative feelings, inferiority in thinking process.

Goal

Learn to live realistic environment.

Interventions

- Accept the client as he is, approach him in courteous way and friendly manner
- Assist the client to identify positive aspects, strengths in behaviour and reinforce it
- Initiate recreational activities and motivate the client to participate in activities related to his area of interest
- Provide opportunities, acknowledge the efforts and support in enhancing his skills
- Structure the schedule of activities to be implemented
- Gradually enhance the activities in acceptable, accomplished manner.

7. Nursing Diagnosis

Self care deficit related to hygienic needs.

Goal

Enable to perform activities independently and maintain personal hygiene.

Interventions

- Minimum assistance has to be provided to the client to perform his activities in prioritized manner
- Explain the importance of maintaining good attire, poise
- If the client is able to perform the activities independently, appreciate and encourage to meet his needs as soon as possible
- Assist for hygienic care and to choose the cloths as per seasons
- Insist to cultivate the regular bowel habits.

8. Nursing Diagnosis

Activity deficit, sleep disturbance perceptual problem due to fight of ideas.

Goal

Able to perform the activities without any difficulties related to perceptions.

Interventions

- Involve the client to do the activities in simple, short term projects to complex of activities
- Plan and implement the activities within the scope of client's achievement
- Never force the client to participate in challenging games
- Ask the client to perform 'gross motor activities', non-competitive, exercises to channelize the energy related to hyperactivity
- Provide calm and quiet environment; comfort measures can be followed. For example, minimize volume, dim light, warm milk, warm water bath
- Advise the client to have minimum 6–8 hours of sleep, which is necessary for maintaining good health.

9. Nursing Diagnosis

Alteration in nutrition related to improper food intake.

Goal

Able to consume adequate and balanced diet.

Interventions

- Provide 'finger foods', snacks, salads, fruits, juices intermittently
- For the client with lithium therapy, salt restricted diet has to be administered
- Provide high protein diet, as the client will be hyperactive, enthusiastic, more ambitious to accomplish tasks
- Minimize distraction, while the client is having food
- Record the weight and input and output chart
- Monitor bowel habits.

10. Nursing Diagnosis

Impaired intellectual processes related to alteration in cognitive functioning.

Goal

Improvement in cognitive functioning.

Interventions

- Accept client's feelings
- Help the client to focus on one idea at a time and encourage him to pay attention and concentration over a specific item or topic
- Never argue or challenge with the client
- Ignore client negative feelings, e.g. hostile, provocative, teasing, etc. instruct and guide him to develop positive feelings and attitudes
- If the client's conversation is not understandable, ask him to speak clearly and slowly
- Set limits for client's manipulative behaviour, make him to understand the consequences of the crossing the limits
- Do not reinforce delusions
- Create conducive and joyful atmosphere
- Never laugh at the client
- Give a pen and paper to the client to put their thoughts and feelings voluntarily

- Motivate to perform the intellectual activities creatively and modulate the activities to prevent exhaustion
- Try to enhance the attention span by emphasizing him to perform the activities in graded manner.

11. Nursing Diagnosis

Disturbed family process related to their defective coping ability for client's hyperactivity behaviour.

Goal

Family accepts and takes responsibility and develops their abilities in rendering supportive services to the client.

Interventions

- Assess the family living conditions; communication and behaviour pattern of family members, situational support, etc.
- Educate the family about cooing strategies, the problem-solving techniques and its clues, impact of situational support and effect of good interpersonal relationship to the client, handling of crisis situations, aspects of bipolar illness
- Stimulate and involve them in taking responsibilities related to care and rehabilitation of the client, provision of structured and consistent environment to the client.

12. Nursing Diagnosis

Knowledge deficit related to follow-up care and continuity of care and treatment.

Goal

Leads qualitative life.

Interventions

- Assess the self care abilities, interaction pattern, communication abilities, family support, situational guidance, etc.

- If permitted, send the client for trail visits to family environment, observe his adaptation to the situation
- Arrange for family gathering and spiritual meetings (whichever the client is interested), group work and observe how the client is able to participate and involve in it
- Make the client to utilize the time productively (like working hours, leisure time) schedule and prioritize the activities
- Educate the client and his family members regarding follow-up visits; continuation of medications; care at home; activities to be carried out to prevent and warning signs of new mood episode.

Diagnosis of Bipolar disorder

- Based on symptoms, course of illness, history of the client, physical examination, mental status examination has to be made.

Treatment of Bipolar disorder

Aims

- To assess and treat acute manifestations of episodes (exacerbation)
- To prevent relapses or recurrences
- To promote functioning capacity of an individual
- To provide assistance or support for both client and his family
- To establish and maintain therapeutic relationship
- To educate the client and his family members about the condition and its prognosis, follow-up care
- To promote treatment compliance
- To reduce morbidity and sequelae of bipolar disorder.

Type of Treatment

- Drug therapy
- Electroconvulsive therapy
- Psychotherapy.

Prognosis

- Usually manic episode lasts for 3–4 months, depressive episode lasts for 4–9 months
- Good prognosis will be observed in acute onset, with typical clinical manifestations, well adjusted personality and good response to treatment (95% of cases), 4 per cent of cases may progress to chronic illness; 1 per cent of cases will commit suicide
- Poor prognosis results in dysthymia, abuse, defective personality, stress and clients with psychotic features.

Follow-up Care

- Teach the client and his family about continuation of medication and regularity and its effect, action, side effects, check-up, warning signs and new episode, chronic episode, bipolar disorder, its course and prognosis, effect of untreated bipolar disorders on individual and family functioning, consequences of abuse
- Help the family to identify the community agencies and provide guidance to utilize those services in rehabilitation of the client
- Demonstrate the emergency care to be taken in need of hour, step to be followed in enhancing cognitive abilities; problem solvation techniques and coping strategies to be adopted
- Teach the family members to maintain drug chart.

DYSTHYMIA/DEPRESSIVE NEUROSIS

Dysthymia is a sub-clinical psychotic condition, it is derived from two Greek words, 'dys' means abnormal or disordered, 'thymia' means 'interpretation or feelings'. Dysthymia was not considered a specific disorder, but the name was given to any type of depression in general.

In ICD-10 (F.34.1), ICD-9 (300.4) dysthymia has been described. Dysthymia is a form of mood disorder in which chronic mild neurotic/reactive depression exists atleast for 2 years. It is also a paradoxical disorder, which fairly exhibits mild symptoms on a day-to-day basis. However, over a lifetime it can have severe effects, if major depression superimposes results into 'double depression'. It may occur alone or in conjunction with more severe depression. It usually lasts significantly longer than an episode of major depression.

Incidence

- Common in women
- Age of onset is last third decade
- 5 per cent of general population will be affected with disease.

Causes

Aetiology is based on a psychoanalytic theory, but probably applied to persisting mood depression of moderate to severe depression without psychotic symptoms.

- Psychological factors–Personality defects, ego disintegration
- Difficulty process in psychological adaptation especially in adolescence and young adulthood
- Internal conflicts
- Interpersonal disturbances
- Disappointments in life
- Threatened loss in adult life
- Disparity between real and fantasized situations.

Clinical Features

- Duration of the symptoms is much longer ranging from 2 months–2 years
- Depressed mood or appears to be depressed for most of the day
- Decreased or increased appetite
- Insomnia or hypersomnia
- Low energy, fatigue
- Poor self image
- Decreased concentration
- Indecisiveness
- Feels hopelessness, helplessness, worthlessness

- Ineffective personal or social or occupational functioning
- Client may feel consistently low
- Lack of enjoyment and pleasure in life continues for atleast 6 months
- A person suffering from dysthymia could go into major depression from a stressful event in their life like a death in family or divorce
- Low self-esteem
- Anhedonia, introversion, a different sense of reality may believe that they have a higher understanding of the world
- Sufferers usually antisocial
- Excessive guilt
- Poor concentration
- Difficulty in making decisions
- Emotional distress
- Diurnal variation–sadness, blues, lack of interest in daily activities
- Nihilistic delusion
- Brooding, demanding, complaining
- Psychomotor retardation
- Decreased sexual urges.

Diagnosis

Neuro-endocrine Studies

Majority of the clients with dysthymia disorder show abnormalities on thyroid axis.

Sleep Studies

- REM latency
- Increased REM density in the first part of sleep
- Moody person; exhibits 2 or more symptoms constantly for a longer time or long-lasting disabling.

Treatment

Pharmacotherapy

Antidepressants
Mono aminooxidase inhibitors
Serotonin specific reuptake inhibitors.

Psychotherapy

Cognitive therapy–To change the mindset of an effected individual. A brief, structured treatment is used to alter the dysfunctional belief and negative automatic thoughts of typical of depression. The techniques like identification, evaluation, modification of negative automatic thoughts, etc. will be used.

Behaviour therapy–Social skill training, graded task management, activities scheduling, etc. techniques are used to divert the mind and occupy with present tasks.

Interpersonal psychotherapy–To enhance the social contacts, interpersonal communication and interpersonal relationship.

Alternate Therapies

Meditation, yoga, relaxation exercises, acupuncture, herbal medicine.

Complications

- Work impairment, suicide, social problems like divorce, social isolation, unemployment.

CYCLOTHYMIA

It is a milder form of bipolar II disorder consists of recurrent mood disturbances between episodes of hypomania and dysthymic mood (mild depression).

Causes

Heredity

A significant genetic contribution is observed, common in twins (monozygotic and dizygotic), shows positive family history
Psychosocial factors
Stressful life events
Faulty living conditions
Interpersonal difficulties, losses
Marital difficulties
Unprovoked disagreement with family and coworkers.

Prevalence

- Early onset (late teenage or twenties) or late
- Life time prevalence 0.4–1 per cent
- Equal in both sexes, women often seeks treatment.

Clinical Manifestations

- Persistent instability of mood (mild depression and mild elation) develops early in life and pursues a chronic course; although at times the mood may be normal and stable for months
- Mood swings unrelated to life events
- Irritable
- Lack of control on moods causes distress
- Rapid, abrupt changes in mood
- Significant distress, work impairment, social and personal dysfunctioning.

Diagnosis

History collection
Observation of clinical manifestation.

Treatment

Pharmacotherapy
Low dose of mood stabilizers, e.g. Lithium.
Low dose of anticonvulsants, e.g. Carbamazepine, valporate.
Antidepressants are administered with caution to prevent manic attack.
Psychotherapy
Social therapy, family therapy, group psychotherapy, educational therapies are helpful to enhance the client's awareness and to prevent mood swings, to utilize coping techniques and strategies.

CIRCULAR TYPE–BIPOLAR DISORDERS

'Alteration of manic and depressed phases' rarely manic phases progresses into delirious mania or depression phase progress into depressive stupor.

Treatment: Bipolar disorders–Lithium; Unipolar patients–Imipramine.

REVIEW QUESTIONS

1. Describe the Aetiology, Clinical Manifestations, Treatment and Nursing Management of Schizophrenia. (15M, GULBU, 1994; 15M, NTRU, 1996; 10M, NIMS, 2001; 5M, NIMS, 1991).

2. a) Define Schizophrenia. (2M, GULBU; 2M, RGUHS).
   b) Discuss briefly the classification of Schizophrenia. (5M, MGRU, 1999).
   c) Develop a Nursing Care Plan for a patient with Catatonic Stupor. (2M+6M+7M, MGRU).

3. Describe the role of Nurse in the Management of Schizophrenia. (10M, RGUHS, 2004).

4. Schizophrenic disorder. (5M, RGUHS, 2002; 5M, BOARD, 1993, 98;10M, BOARD, 1999; 10M, PCBSc, 2002).

5. Dynamics of Schizophrenia. (2M, RGUHS, 2001; 2M, PCBSc, 2001).

6. Four types of Schizophrenia. (2M, 5M, RGUHS, 1999; 3M, MGRU, 1996; 5M, MGRU, 2000).

7. Catatonic Stupor and Catatonic Excitement. (2M, RGUHS, 2000; 2M, IGNOU, 2001).

8. Explain Schizophrenia under the following headings
   a) Causes
   b) Types
   c) Nursing management of paranoid schizophrenia. (15M, GULBU, 1995, 97; 15M, RGUHS, 1998, 99; 10M, RGUHS, 2000; 15M, MGRU).

9. Catatonic Schizophrenia. (10M, MGRU, 2002).

10. Describe the Aetiology. Clinical features and Nursing Management of a patient with Catatonic Schizophrenia. (11M, MGRU, 1996).

11. Care of the paranoid patient. (15M, MGRU, 1990).

12. Describe the role of a Nurse in the Management of Schizophrenia. (10M, RGHUS, 2004).

13. How will you develop rapport with a patient of suspicious behavior? (10M, 2001, 1999 RGHUS, MGRU).

14. Mental status examination findings of a patient with Paranoid Schizophrenia; discuss the caring management of such patient. (10M, RGUHS, 2001).

15. List the difference between Endogenous and Reactive Depression and Nursing Management of Endogenous Depression with Nursing Process. (10M, NTRUHS, 93; MGRU, 02).

16. Define Schizophrenia. (2M, RGUHS, 2004).

17. Discuss briefly the classification of Schizophrenia. (6M, 2003, RGUHS).

18. Manic disorders. (10M, RGUHS, 03, 05).

19. Dynamics of schizophrenia. (2M, RGUHS, 01).

20. Enumerate the specific clinical manifestations of Acute Manic state ; explain he Nursing Interventions in any one of them. (10M, RGUHS, 00).

21. Four types of Schizophrenia. (5M, MGRU, 00).

22. Causes, signs, and symptoms and treatment of Manic Depressive Psychosis; explain the nurse's role in taking care of such patient. (15M, Gulb. U. 95, 97; 10M, MGRU, 1998).

23. What are the symptoms of Hypomania, how will you manage a patient with Hypomanic reaction? (5+10M, Gulb, 95, 99).

24. Describe aetiology, clinical features and nursing management of a patient with Catatonic Schizophrenia. (10M, MGRU, 96).

25. How will you establish Therapeutic Relationship with a Depressed client? (5M, MGRU, 97).

26. How will take care of a patient, who is admitted to your ward with Mania. (15M, MGRU, 02).

27. Define affective disorder. Explain the clinical features of affective disorders, explain the manage-ment of a 30-year-old lady admitted for Affective disorder. (15M, MGRU, 99).

28. Define Dynamics of suspicious behaviour. (5M, MGRU, 90).

29. Write the nursing process for the first 24 hours for a patient who is admitted with an Acute Hypomania. (5M, MGRU, 90).

30. What is the Role of Psychiatric Nurse in the Management of a person with Acute Depression? (15M, MGRU, 85; 10M, RGUHS).

31. Discus the role of Psychiatric Nurse in the various Treatment available for Depression. (15M, MGRU).

32. State the types of Depression. List the common Nursing Diagnosis. Write the Nursing Intervention for any two Nursing Diagnosis. (15M, MGRU, 00).

33. Describe the various aspects of Bipolar Affective Disorder. (15M, MGRU, 03).

34. Describe Behavioural Manifestation, Treatment and Nursing Management of a patient with Acute Mania. (15M, MGRU, 99).

35. How will you develop a nursing care plan for a patient with endogenous depression? (10M, MGRU).

36. Discuss in detail the Nursing Management of patient with Severe Depression. Prepare a Nursing Care Plan. (10M, RGUHS, 06).

37. Discuss the Nursing Care of a patient with Paranoid Schizophrenia. (15M, MGRU, 2000).

38. Define Paranoid Schizophrenia. Explain Nurse's role in managing a patient with strong paranoid of his food being poisoned. (10M, RGUHS, 05).

39. List the different types of Depressive Disorders and plan the nursing care for Depressive patient. (7M, IGNOU, 99).

40. Define Hypomania. List the symptoms of Acute Mania. Write nursing intervention. (15M, IGNOU, 01).

41. Define Depression. List signs and symptoms of Depression. (7M, NIMS, 05).

42. Mr. 'Y' had been admitted with paranoid features. What are the expected signs and symptoms? Explain the role of nurse in the care of Mr. 'Y' with special emphasis on group therapy. (10M, NIMS, 00).

43. Define psychosis. Discuss aetiology and dynamics of Schizophrenia disorders. Explain nurse's role in managing the patient with paranoid schizophrenia. (10M, RGUHS, 99).

44. Chronic Schizophrenia. (5M, RGUHS, 00).

45. Paranoid. (2M, RGUHS, 06).

46. Endogenous Depression. (5M, RGUHS, 05).

13 *Neurosis*

INTRODUCTION

'A certain degree of neurosis is of inestimable values as a drive'.   —*Sigmund Freud*

Neurosis is a normal human experience, part of the human condition. The term, 'Neurosis' is derived from two Greek words, 'Neuron' means 'nerve' with the suffix 'osis' means 'diseased' or 'abnormal condition'.

The term was coined by Scottish Doctor 'William Culen' in 1769 to refer to 'disorders of sense and motion' caused by a 'general affection of the nervous system'. Neurosis has fallen out of favour along with the psychological school of thought, i.e. 'the field of psychoanalysis' founded by Sigmund Freud. Neurosis is psychiatry, a broad category of psychological disturbance encompassing various mild forms of mental disorder. Neurosis is a normal human experience, part of human condition, majority of people are affected by neurosis in some mild form or other. A psychological problem develops when neurosis begin to interfere with, but not significantly impair, normal functioning, does not prevent rational thought or an individual's ability to function in daily life.

Neurosis is an illness that represents a variety of psychiatric conditions in which emotional distress or unconscious conflict is expressed through various physical, physiological and mental disturbances which may include physical symptoms. For example, anxiety, hysteria, phobia, depression, obsessive compulsive tendencies.

DEFINITIONS

'Specific differentiation of the ego'.
                        —*Topographical Stand Point of view*

'Ego's embrace (under the influence of the super ego) of the reality principle, to the detriment of the pleasure principle and the id's instinctual demands and this leads to the emergence of castration anxiety'.
                        —*Dynamic Stand Point of view*

'Partly ineffective mobilization of the mechanism of repression against the id's instinctual demands'.   —*Economic Stand Point of view*

'Achievement of a symbolization of intrapsychic conflicts in accord with the oedipal model'.
    —*Developmental or genetic Stand Point of view*

'Any mental imbalance that causes distress, does not prevent rational thought or an individual's ability to function in daily life'.

'Poor ability to adapt to one's environment, an ability to change one's life patterns, and the inability to develop a richer, more complex, more satisfying personality'.

'A symbolic behaviour in defense against excessive psychologic pain is self perpetuating because symbolic satisfactions cannot fulfill real needs'.

'Thought and behaviour patterns that produce difficulties in living is neurosis'.

—Psychoanalytic theory

'A functional mental disorder characterized by a high level of anxiety and other distressing emotional symptoms such as morbid fears, obsessive thoughts, compulsive acts, somatic reactions, dissociative states and depressive reactions; the symptoms do not involve gross personality disorganization, total lack of insight or loss of contact with reality'. —*DSM-III*

'An exaggerated, unconscious method of coping with the internal conflict and anxiety they produce'.   —*DSM-III*

CLASSIFICATION OF NEUROSIS (ICD-10)

F_{40} – Phobic anxiety disorders
$F_{40.0}$ – Agoraphobia
       $_{00}$ – Without panic disorder
       $_{01}$ – With panic disorder
$F_{40.1}$ – Social phobias
$F_{40.2}$ – Specific (isolated) phobias
$F_{40.8}$ – Other phobic anxiety disorders
$F_{40.9}$ – Phobic anxiety disorder, unspecified
F_{41} – Other anxiety disorders
$F_{41.0}$ – Panic disorder (episodic) paroxysmal anxiety
$F_{41.1}$ – Generalized anxiety disorder
$F_{41.2}$ – Mixed anxiety and depressive disorder
$F_{41.3}$ – Other mixed anxiety disorders
$F_{41.8}$ – Other specified anxiety disorders
$F_{41.9}$ – Unspecified anxiety disorders
F_{42} – Obsessive-compulsive disorders
$F_{42.0}$ – Predominantly obsessional thoughts or ruminations

$F_{42.1}$ – Predominantly compulsive acts (obsessional rituals)
$F_{42.2}$ – Mixed obsessional thoughts and acts
$F_{42.8}$ – Other obsessive-compulsive disorders
$F_{42.9}$ – Obsessive-compulsive disorders, unspecified
F_{43} – Reaction to serve stress and adjustment disorders
$F_{43.0}$ –   Acute stress reaction
$F_{43.1}$ – Post traumatic stress disorder
$F_{43.2}$ – Adjustment disorders
$F_{43.20}$ – Brief depressive reactions
$F_{43.21}$ – Prolonged depressive reactions
$F_{43.22}$ – Mixed anxiety and depressive reaction
$F_{43.23}$ – With predominant disturbance of other emotions
$F_{43.24}$ – With predominant disturbance of conduct
$F_{43.25}$ – With mixed disturbance of emotions and conduct
$F_{43.28}$ – With other specified predominant symptoms
$F_{43.8}$ – Other reactions to severe stress
$F_{43.9}$ – Reaction to severe stress, unspecified
F_{44} – Dissociative (conversion) disorders
$F_{44.0}$ – Dissociative amnesia
$F_{44.1}$ – Dissociative fugue
$F_{44.2}$ – Dissociative stupor
$F_{44.3}$ – Trance and Possession disorders
$F_{44.4}$ – Dissociative motor disorders
$F_{44.5}$ – Dissociative convulsions
$F_{44.6}$ – Dissociative anaesthesia and sensory loss
$F_{44.7}$ – Mixed dissociative (conversion) disorders
$F_{44.8}$ – Other dissociative (conversion) disorders
$F_{44.80}$ – Ganser's syndrome
$F_{44.81}$ – Multiple personality disorder
$F_{44.82}$ – Transient dissociative (conversion) disorders
$F_{44.88}$ – Other specified dissociative (conversion) disorders
$F_{44.9}$ – Dissociative (conversion) disorder, unspecified

F_{45} – Somatoform disorder
$F_{45.0}$ – Somatization disorder
$F_{45.1}$ – Undifferentiated somatoform disorder
$F_{45.2}$ – Hypochondrical disorder
$F_{45.3}$ – Somatoform autonomic dysfunction
$F_{45.30}$ – Heart and cardiovascular system
$F_{45.31}$ – Upper gastrointestinal tracts
$F_{45.32}$ – Lower gastrointestinal tracts
$F_{45.33}$ – Respiratory system
$F_{45.34}$ – Genitourinary system
$F_{45.38}$ – Other organ or system
$F_{45.4}$ – Persistent somatoform pain disorder
$F_{45.8}$ – Other somatoform disorders
$F_{45.9}$ – Somatoform disorder, unspecified
F_{48} – Other neurotic disorders
$F_{48.0}$ – Neurasthenia
$F_{48.1}$ – Depersonalization–derealization syndrome
$F_{48.8}$ – Other specified neurotic disorders
$F_{48.9}$ – Neurotic disorder, unspecified.

Causes of Neurosis

- Biological and environmental factors together contribute neurosis, e.g. Faulty socialization, defective role models, low socioeconomic status low educational status
- Psychological factors
  - Maladaptive learning or defective learning
  - Threatening inner desires and impulses
  - Lack of stimulating environment
  - Strained or distorted interpersonal relationship
  - Stressful environment.

Types of Psychoneurosis

Anxiety, Phobia, Hysteria, Obsessive-compulsive neurosis, Dysthymia or reactive depression, Neurasthenia, Depersonalization, Hypochondriasis.

Manifestations

- Neurotic thoughts or behaviours that significantly impair, but do not altogether prevent normal daily living or daily functioning

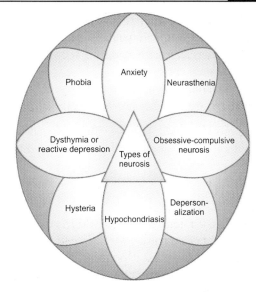

Fig. 13.1: Types of neurosis

- Mental imbalance that causes or results in distress
- Anxiety
- Sadness or depression, mental confusion
- Anger
- Low sense of self-worth
- Behavioural symptoms–phobic avoidance, vigilance, impulsive, compulsive acts, lethargy
- Cognitive problems, e.g. unpleasant or disturbing thoughts, repetition of thoughts and obsession, habitual fantasizing, negativity, cynicism
- Interpersonal problems, e.g. Dependency, aggressiveness, perfectionism, schizoid isolation, socio-culturally inappropriate behaviours.

Treatment

1. Psychotherapy
   - Counselling
   - Individual psychotherapy
   - Group therapy
   - Psychoanalysis
   - Talk therapies
   - Behaviour therapy
   - Family therapy
2. Abreaction therapy

3. Drug therapy
   - Desensitization-cognitive therapy-positive reinforcement
   - Assertiveness therapy
   - Flooding or impulsive therapy.

Prognosis

Good prognosis with adequate family support and favourable socio-cultural environment (see table on next page).

Differences between psychosis and neurosis has been tabulated in page 419.

TYPES OF NEUROSIS
ANXIETY DISORDER
Introduction

Anxiety is an unpleasant state that involves a complex combination of emotions (fear, worry, apprehension) accompanied by physical sensations (palpitations, chest pain, shortness of breath, tension headache etc.) anxiety is having cognitive, conative, affective and behavioural components.

Anxiety is a normative pattern of human emotion, it will be experienced in varying degrees as a state of emotional or physical uneasiness. Every individual in their life time, experiences certain level of anxiety at some moment or other in response to different stressors or varied stimuli or traumatic events within the environment. Certain times anxiety helps for survival, anxiety is designed as a protective mechanism to prevent the organism from engaging in potential harmful behaviours. Anxiety is a part of our natural 'flight or fight' response. It is our body's way of warning us of danger ahead and for the most part anxiety is adaptive. It gears up for the life's challenges and spurs us to action, when we are faced with a threat. However, if anxiety is preventing you from living our life and overwhelmed with fear and worry, you may be suffering from an anxiety disorder.

Definitions

'Anxiety disorder is characterized by recurrent, unwanted thoughts (obsessions) or rituals (compulsions) which feel uncontrollable to the sufferer'.

'A pervasive feeling of dread, apprehension and impending disaster'.

'A response to an undefined or unknown threat which may be due to unconscious conflict or insecurity'.   —*Bimla Kapoor*

Performing the rituals however provides only temporary relief and not performing them markedly increases anxiety. Left untreated, obsessions and the need to perform the rituals can take over a person's life.

Causes

- Traumatic experiences
- Anxiety is a signal to the ego to take defensive action against the 'pressure' from within (Sigmund Freud)
- Stimulation of autonomic nervous system and central nervous system
- Genetic component, e.g. higher frequency of illness was observed in first degree relatives of affected persons than in the relatives of non-affected persons and in monozygotic twins
- Socio-cultural factors, e.g. faulty child rearing practices
- Psychological factors–maladaptive responses, strained interpersonal relationship, stress, unresolved conflicts, disturbing memories, forbidden impulses, conflict between id and ego
- Neurotransmitters and biochemical factors
  - Alpha-adrenergic agonists and alpha-2 adrenergic antagonist can produce frequent and severe panic attacks
  - Serotonergic hallucinogens and stimulants, e.g. lysergic acid diethylamide (LSD) and 3, 4 methylene dioxymethamphetamine (MDMA) are associated with the development of both acute and chronic anxiety disorders
  - Alteration in GABA levels
  - Increased levels of norepinephrine, serotonin
- Behavioural factor: Unconditional inherent response of the organism to painful stimuli

Differences between Psychosis and Neurosis

	Psychosis	*Neurosis*
Introduction	In 1845, Ernst Von Feuchtersleben used the word, 'psychosis' as an alternative to insanity and mania	In 1769, William Cullen used the term for 'disorders of sense and motion'
Causes	Organic causes Functional causes Psychiatric disorders	Biological, Environmental, Psychological
Psychodynamics	Very serious illness, Impairment of ego functioning, Reality testing impaired Signs of grave maladjustment to life	Mild to moderate illness; Ego functioning and reality testing are not affected much Maladjustment to life is limited
Types	Organic psychosis, Functional psychosis Affective psychosis	Anxiety, phobia, hysteria, neurasthenia, Hypochondriasis, obsessive-compulsive reactions, dysthymia, depersonalization
Perceptual disturbances	Hallucinations, delusions, illusions, paranoid behaviour	Perception will not be affected
Behavioural changes	Psychotic behaviour can come and go as a result of various influences Impulsiveness Retardation Withdrawal Do not attempt to socialize Vocational, social, sexual adjustments are markedly impaired Routine activities markedly disturbed Mental functions affected more (though disturbances)	Over activity and impulsiveness Does not have significant affect over normal functioning Difficulties in living Anxiety, neurasthenia, obsessive-compulsive neurosis disorder, phobias, depression, anger, irritability, mental confusion, low sense of self worth Disturbing thoughts Dependency Aggressiveness Perfectionism Socioculturally inappropriate behaviour Cognitive domain will not be affected, but disturbed with neurotic thoughts or behaviour
Defense mechanism used	Denial Regression Introjection Identification	Repression Displacement Isolation Reaction formation Undoing Substitution Conversion
Treatment	Drug therapy Antipsychotic medications Psychotherapy Extreme cases needs hospitalization	Rarely hospitalized Treated in OPD Drug therapy–sedatives, tranquilizers
Prognosis	Recurrences are more Poor prognosis	Good prognosis Recurrence is very less

- Cognitive factor: Cognitive distortions; negative automatic thoughts
- Medications and substances which can induce anxiety are: caffeine and other stimulants, drugs, e.g. heroin, cocaine and amphetamines, decongestants, steroids, e.g. cortisone, weight loss products, hormonal pills, withdrawal from alcohol or benzodiazepines.

Incidence

25 per cent of population in the world is affected with anxiety disorders, it will strike the individual at any point of life; occurs more frequently in women.

Characteristics:
- Free floating anxiety without knowing exactly why you are feeling that way
- Sudden, intense panic attacks that strike without warning
- Unwanted obsessions and compulsions
- Phobia of an object or situation that does not seem to bother other people
- Persistent and often overwhelming fear or worry which may be distressing or immobilizing and disruptive
- Constant anxiety, unrelenting and all consuming
- Self imposed isolation or emotional withdrawal or extreme distress or disrupting daily routine
- Extreme social isolation
- It may interfere with normal activities like going outside or interacting with other people or work or relationships
- Negatively impacts work and personal relationships.

Manifestations

- Cognitive component of anxiety includes expectation of a diffuse and uncertain danger, forgetfulness, blocking or important details, rumination, poor judgement, decreased attention, concentration, creativity and productivity, difficulty in making decisions

Somatically the body prepares the organism to deal with threat (emergency reaction)
- Dyspnoea, sneezing
- Tension headache, fatigue
- Insomnia, sleep disturbances
- Anorexia
- Nausea and vomiting
- Chest pain or tightness in chest
- Hypertension
- Increased heart rate/palpitations
- Increased sweating or perspiration
- Increased blood flow to the major muscle groups
- Immune and digestive system functions are inhibited
- Pale skin
- Trembling, twitching and tremors
- Pupillary dilatation
- Chills or hot flashes
- Tightness of neck or back muscles
- Urinary frequency
- Diarrhoea
- Poor posture
- Frequent minor illness
- Accident proneness
- Headache
- Fatigue
- Cold and clammy hands
- Stomach upset or uneasiness
- Shortness of breath
- Dizziness
- Muscle tension or aches.

Emotional component of anxiety
- A sense of dread or panic
- Nervousness and jumpiness
- Self consciousness
- Insecurity
- Fear of going to die or going crazy
- Strong desire to escape or avoidance, hyper vigilance, confusion
- Angry outburst
- Suspiciousness

- Restlessness
- Social withdrawal
- Decreased motivation
- Crying
- Critical of self or others
- Self depreciation
- Anhedonia
- Persistent apprehension
- Free floating fear (generalized and specific)
- Disturbances in perception of fear
- Irritability, depression
- Worthlessness, helplessness, hopelessness.

Behavioural component: both voluntary and involuntary behaviours may arise at escaping or avoiding the source of anxiety, maladaptive behaviours in extreme anxiety disorder, however, anxiety is not always pathological or maladaptive.

Two factor theory of anxiety:
Sigmund Freud recognized anxiety as a, 'Signal of danger' and a cause of 'defensive behaviour'.

According to Freud, individuals will acquire feelings through classical conditioning and traumatic experiences; maintains anxiety through operant conditioning. When we see or encounter something associated with a previous traumatic experience, anxious feelings resurface. We feel temporarily relieved when we avoid situations which make us anxious, but this only increases anxious feelings, the next time we are in the same situation and we want to avoid that situation again and therefore will not make any progress against the anxiety.

Excessive anxiety occurs in response to an actual or anticipated situation or as a pathological state.

Levels of anxiety (Anxiety Continuum)

- Mild +
- Moderate ++
- Severe +++
- Panic +++++ - Hildegard Peplau
(for description details refer below table)

Levels of anxiety				
Characteristics	*Mild*	*Moderate*	*Severe*	*Panic*
Conditions causes	Exposure to slight stressor or mild stimuli	Repeated exposure to the painful stimuli	Acute stress disorder Medical conditions. For example, Bronchial asthma, Cardiovascular diseases OCD, Social phobia Substance induced Pronounced anxiety	Alteration in neuro-transmitter levels. For example, GABA, epinephrine, norepinephrine, serotonin, Amygdale, hippocampus dys-function Genetics-1st degree relatives, mono-zygotic twins Traumatic or stressful events or life stressors
Physiological changes	Increased heart rate Increased respiratory rate Hypertension Diarrhoea Cold and clammy skin	Increased urinary frequency Poor appetite Not chewing properly	Marked symptoms Hearing impaired Dilated pupil Decreased perception to pain or injury Anorexia	No appetite

contd...

contd...

Characteristics	Mild	Moderate	Severe	Panic
	Dilated pupil Decreased salivation Decreased appetite			
Speech	Volume is appropriate to context	Pitch increases repeatedly by questioning	Demands for help	Not clear
Activity	Increases to meet the demand or need	Restlessness, unable to meet routine, social and vocational demands	Tremors, facial grimaces purposeless	May scream, run about
Muscle tone	Little tightness	Tensed up all time	Tensed and rigid	Poor and lack of motor coordination

Major Anxiety Disorders

- Panic disorder with or without agoraphobia or panic attacks
- Generalized anxiety disorder
- Obsessive compulsive disorder
- Phobias
- Post traumatic stress disorder.

Types of Anxiety

1. Separation Anxiety

It occurs in people who have the fear, the loss of love or even abandonment by their parents, if the child fails to control their impulses in conformity with their parent standards and demands, when a child is separated from parent or away from home.

2. Castration Anxiety

The castration fantasies of oedipal child in relation to childs' developing sexual impulses.

3. Existential Anxiety

Philosophical ruminations are a part of this condition, a part of obsessive compulsive disorder, anxiety is related to sex, religion and death.

4. Test Anxiety

The uneasiness, apprehension or nervousness felt by students who have a fear of failing exam. Students suffering from test anxiety may experience embarrassment by the teacher, fear of alienation from parents or friends, time pressure or feeling a loss of control, emotional cognitive, behavioural and physical components. For example, sweating, dizziness, headache, nausea, etc. are common, an optimal level of anxiety is necessary to complete the task. Many adults share the same experience with regard to their career or profession.

5. Stranger Anxiety

Anxiety while meeting or interacting with unknown people.

6. Anxiety in Palliative Care

Clients with chronic disorders (cancer, heart disease, etc.) will have anxiety about the disease prognosis; to improve the quality of life and to lessen the fear associated with it, the services of counselling, relaxation techniques and drug therapy, e.g. benzodiazepines, etc. will be provided.

7. Generalized Anxiety Disorders/ Free Floating Anxiety

Persistent, chronic generalized anxiety, most common form, experienced mostly by women.

8. Social Anxiety/Social Phobia

A debilitating fear of being seen negatively by others and humiliated in public. Social phobia results, it may be extremely shyness. In severe cases, social situations are avoided all together, e.g. performance anxiety.

Manifestations

Psychological
- Irritability
- Restlessness
- Fear
- Apprehension
- Vigilance
- Sensitivity to noise
- Poor concentration
- Worrying thoughts
- Depression obsession
- Depersonalization.

Physical
- Hyperactivity
- Nervousness
- Tremors
- Trembling
- Muscular tensions
- Sweating
- Palpitation, discomfort in chest
- Dizziness
- Epigastric discomfort
- Dry mouth
- Dysphagia
- Diarrhoea
- Increased respiratory rate
- Frequent, urgency in micturition
- Menstrual discomfort
- Amenorrhoea

- Prickling sensations
- Tinnitus.

Treatment of Anxiety Disorders

A healthy and balanced life style can control and reduce anxiety

- Cognitive behaviour therapy–it focusses on changing both maladaptive thinking patterns or cognitions or behaviours. It helps to identify and challenge the negative and irrational beliefs that are holding back from working through fears. The duration of therapy is 12–20 weeks, it can be given either individually or in groups
  - Cognitive restructuring
  - Jacobson progressive muscle relaxation techniques, e.g. controlled breathing, guided imagery
  - Exposure therapy –systematic desensitization, impulsive therapy, flooding
  - Paradoxical intention
- Other psychotherapies–self hypnosis, supportive psychotherapy
- Other therapies–yoga, meditation.

Exposure Therapies

Paradoxical Intention

It promotes a sense of mastery or control over the threatening situation and enhances tolerance to face the discomfort. The therapist insists the client to hyperventilate to the panic situation.

Systematic desensitization and progressive relaxation technique.

Constructing and anxiety hierarchy, gradual exposure paired with relaxation, inorder of increasing difficulty.

Impulsive Therapy

The anxiety provoking stimuli will be presented through imagery in a vivid manner, while the therapist attempts to prevent the client from fleeing the scene.

Flooding

The individual will be presented with anxiety situation either in imagery or with the environment, without any relaxation or pause upto the anxiety subsides.

Drug Therapy

Anxiolytics: Clomipramine, Buspirone are beneficial.

Benzodiazepines, e.g. Alprazolam, xlonazepam.

Beta blockers to control palpitations, e.g. propronolal.

Bio Feedback

Using sensors that measure physiological arousal brought by anxiety, it will teach the individual to recognize and control these body processes.

Hypnosis

Clinical hypnotherapist will use different therapeutic approaches in a state of deep relaxation.

Acupuncture

Traditional method may be used to reduce anxiety.

Self-Help Tips for Controlling and Reducing Anxiety

- Exercise regularly–yoga and aerobic activities are particularly calming
- Get enough good sleep–lack of sleep can exacerbate anxiety, try to cultivate good sleeping habits, have a calm mind, a warm water bath, having a glass of warm milk before going to bed will facilitate good sleep
- Eat a healthy, adequate nutritious diet, make sure your diet includes plenty of fruits and vegetables
- Meditation
- Practicing relaxation exercises

- Avoiding alcohol and drugs usage to cope-up with anxiety as they can make the problem worse, and eventually will cause problems of their own
- Avoid consuming stimulants like caffeine before going to bed as caffeine can increase anxiety, causes insomnia and even it can provoke panic attacks.

PANIC ATTACKS/ANXIETY ATTACKS/ EPISODIC PAROXYSMAL ANXIETY

Anxiety is not an illness, it is a behavioural condition; not everyone experiences the same panic attack symptoms, every individual is different biologically and therefore react differently to each other as a response to the same or similar stimuli. The varied stressors or stimuli in the environment also held responsible for predispose panic attacks. People who have repeated, unexpected panic attacks and worry about the attacks are said to have panic disorders.

Definition

" Panic attacks or panic disorders are characterized by unexpected or intermittent or sudden severe episodes of intense fear or terror or anxiety of serious consequences unrelated to particular stimuli in which the physical symptoms are more predominate and severe."

Prevalence

In life time 1.5–2 per cent of total population are subjected to panic attacks, females are more prone for panic attacks (2–3 times) than men. Generally begins in the late teens through the mid 30s. Sudden onset occurs without any warning, unprovoked onset of fear, there is no clear cause or fear and lasts for a few minutes or little longer.

Causes

- Genetic factors : It is inherited, run in families, 15 per cent of first degree relatives will be suffering with panic disorders. Monozygotic twins are prone to get, the individuals with genetic abnormalities if subjected to stress and tension may prone for panic disorders. Biological changes that occur during times of stress and tension unconditional inherent response of the organism to a painful stimuli.

- Brain dysfunction: The organs which are responsible for anxiety response, are the amygdala and limbic system, specifically hippocampus dysfunction or imbalance in the functioning pattern leads to panic disorders.
- Brain chemistry: Increased levels of norepinephrine, undefined abnormality in serotonin, abnormalities in stress hormone, i.e. cortisol, alteration in GABA levels.
- Physiological factors: Lactate induced hyper ventilation or chronic hyper ventilation causes oversensitive carbon dioxide resulting into panic attack.
- Psychological factors: Painful or traumatic events, e.g. accidents, divorce or separation, early life abuse, developmental trauma–in early infancy or in early childhood, critical or strict parents, pessimistic personality traits. Life stressors–financial difficulties, marital problems, bereavement, family conflicts, interpersonal difficulties.
- Environmental factors: Poverty, occupational difficulties, alcoholism and drug abuse, e.g. cocaine, marijuana.
- Cognitive factors: Distortion of thoughts, negative automatic thoughts.

Clinical Manifestations

a. Physical symptoms

- Shortness of breath or dyspnoea
- Tachycardia, palpitations, pounding of heart, sometimes these symptoms is so severe, that the person fears he/she is having heart attack
- Chest pain or chest discomfort

- Blurry vision
- Shaking or trembling
- Dizziness or unsteadiness, fainting
- Nausea, bloating, indigestion
- Abdominal discomfort or distress
- Sweating or perspiration
- Choking sensations or suffocating
- Lump in throat
- Feeling light headed
- Pale, cold and clammy skin
- Blushing or skin blotches
- Feels urgency in urination and defecation
- Easily fatigue
- Muscle tension–pain or tightness of body (chest, neck, shoulders)
- Numbness in arms and legs
- Headache or migraine.

b. Behavioural/Emotional Manifestations

- Intense fear or dread which is generally irrational
- Derealization (perceives danger is very real)
- Depersonalization (being detached from one self)
- Often feels as if they are about to die or pass out
- Fear of loosing control or going crazy or mad
- Hot or cold flushes
- Reluctant to discuss their panic attacks with others
- Paraesthesia (numbness or tingling sensations)
- Unnecessary worry, impending sense of doom
- Exaggerated experiences of normal bodily sensations or reactions
- Develops substance abuse problems
- Risk of suicidal attempts
- They may develop 'anticipatory anxiety' related to fear, they may be reluctant to discuss their panic attacks with others.

HYPOCHONDRIASIS

The term, 'hypochondriasis' derives from two Greek words 'hypo' means 'below' and 'chondros' means 'cartilage of breast bone'. The term originally was coined by 'Hippocrates'. In 19th century the term employed to mean, 'illness without a specific cause'. In modern usage, the term, is often used to label for individuals, who hold the belief that they have a serious illness, despite repeated reassurance from physicians that they are perfectly healthy.

Definition

'Excessive preoccupation or worry about having a serious physical illness, despite repeated medical reassurance'.

'Fears that minor bodily symptoms may indicate a serious illness, constant self examination and self diagnosis, and a preoccupation with one's body'.

Factors Contributing to Hypochondriasis

- Cancer–the illusion that they are more likely to develop the disease.
- Multiple sclerosis.
- Signs of serious illness contribute to exacerbating the hypochondriac's fear, that they actually have that illness.
- Death of family members or friends.
- When approaching the age or a parent's premature death from disease, many healthy, happy individuals fall prey to hypochondriasis. These individuals believe that, they are suffering from the same disease that caused their parents' death, sometimes causing panic attacks with corresponding symptoms.
- Following life stress.
- In extreme, majority of people experience physical pain or anxieties over non-existent ailments are not actually 'faking it' but rather, experience the natural results of other emotional issues.
- During recovery from medical illnesses.
- Neurochemical changes, e.g. epinephrine and serotonin.

- Associated with OCD, depression, anxiety, phobias, somatization disorder.

Aetiology

- Psychodynamic theory
  It is an alternate channel to turn sexual, aggressive or oral drives or an ego defense against guilt and low esteem or a sign of excessive self concern. The aggressive feelings towards others are transformed into physical complaints by repression or displacement.
  Withdrawal of sexual libido from external objects transfers into narcissistic libido into actual somatic changes–Freud
  Defense against guilty, low self-esteem, excessive badness.
  Expression of pre-genital wishes for caring, nurturing, sympathy, attention and physical contact.
- Sociocultural theory
  Learned social behaviour–to have attention of caring and secondary gains of sick role to convey their distress and disability.
- Neuropsychological theory
  An underlying perceptual cognitive abnormality Misinterpreting normal bodily functions and emotional arousal by misattributing factor to a serious disease process.

Manifestations

- Many problems with hypochondriasis experience a cycle of intrusive thoughts followed by compulsive checking
- An individual preoccupies himself with a fear or belief that he has a serious disease which persists and interferes with his social and occupational functioning
- Symptoms related to gastrointestinal and cardiovascular systems
- The hypochondriacs are profoundly preoccupied with their body structures, their health status and functional limitations

- Often complain of abnormal bodily sensations, disturbed body functions or anatomical deviations suggesting disease
- Often are not aware that depression and anxiety produce their own physical symptoms that might be mistaken for signs of a serious medical disease
- Clinging, demanding and harbouring unrealistic expectations.

Management

- In preliminary visits, develop rapport with the client, explore the clients' problems and do physical examination to diagnose clients' needs.
- To treat hypochondriasis, one must acknowledge the interplay of body and mind.
- Regular contact with a single primary care physician with whom, the client develops confidence is always helpful.
- Regular scheduled visits and supportive psychotherapeutic approach are beneficial to win the confidence and to have keen observation over clients' problem.
- Diagnostic procedures and medicines are the first-line of treatment for primary hypochondriasis.
- Concentrate for clients' social and interpersonal problems by cognitive behavioural therapy, a psychoeducational 'talk' therapy, helps the worries to address and cope with bothersome physical symptoms and worries, reduces the intensity and frequency of troubling bodily symptoms.
- Selective serotonin reuptake inhibitors (SSRIs), e.g. fluoxetine and paroxetine can reduce obsessional worry through readjusting neuro-transmitter levels.
- Supportive psychotherapy with SSRI or placebo is of helpful.
- Ask the client to maintain a dairy about his symptoms and external events, which may be helpful as a, 'self monitoring and control' a cognitive therapeutic approach is beneficial.

- Restrict self checking behaviour as they tend to increase illness or worries.
- Motivate them to maintain a healthy life style, e.g. good night sleep, well balanced diet, positive outlook, pleasure, exercise, socialization, achievements in daily activities.
- Encourage to practice relaxation exercises, e.g. deep breathing, yoga, meditation to overcome stress and decrease depression or anxiety.
- Teach coping strategies, prepare the client to adjust and adopt to the situations.
- Group psychotherapy may be of helpful for the clients, who has less than 3 years duration of illness.
- When a person is sick with a medical disease (RA, DM) there will be often psychological consequences like depression or anxiety will be experienced physical manifestation of these affective fluctuation, hence if any significant associated symptoms are seen, related drug may be given for symptomatic alleviation.
- Many hypochondriac require constant reassurance, either from doctors, family or friend.

Course: Symptoms may be temporary or persist or recur for many years. Some can adjust to it or even block its impact, others have a difficulty in describing their symptoms and may fear that they are going crazy.

DEPERSONALIZATION

Alteration in the perception or experience of oneself, so that the self is felt to be unreal, sufferers will have persistent or recurring feeling of being detached from reality or one's body or world or mental processes and by a feeling of being an outside observer of one's life.

Depersonalization is most often described as a symptom of emotions. For example, fear, panic, DSM-IV categorizes depersonalization as a 'dissociative disorder'. Depersonalization and 'derealization' are the two terms used interchangeably, however derealization means, 'nothing is real'. It may be an indicative of neurological disorder.

Causes

Depersonalization can happen to anyone, but they are most prominent in people suffering from:
- Psychological trauma
- Panic disorders
- Clinical depression
- Bipolar disorder
- Symptoms of borderline personality disorders
- Some epileptic conditions, e.g. temporal lobe epilepsy
- Side effect of certain drugs, e.g. hallucinogens
- Overdose of stimulants, e.g. caffeine, nicotine, alcoholic beverages etc. can induce depersonalization effect
- Post traumatic stress disorder
- Withdrawal symptom from many drugs
- Hypochondriasis
- Neurological diseases, e.g. Alzheimer's disease, multiple sclerosis, lyme disease (neuro borreliosis)
- Early schizophrenia
- Occurs after life threatening dangers, e.g. accident, assault, serious illness or injury.

Symptoms

- Feels isolated both from their own body and external world
- Sufferers feels like a movie or things seen 'unreal' or 'hazy'
- Recognitions of self breaks down
- Feel as though, life is a dream or an illusion
- Increases the feelings of 'fakeness', 'feedback loop' that amplifies itself or feeling like a 'ghost'
- Clients may have difficulty fully comprehending what they hear and see
- Feeling a sense of vertigo or detachment, anxiety, depression, lack of meaning, lack of joy and general apathy
- Distorted perception of their identity, body and life that makes them uncomfortable.

Diagnosis

- History–special interview will be conducted on basis of symptoms
- Physical examination to rule out any physical disorder
- Carryout psychological tests (to assess intellectual levels and emotional status of an individual).

Treatment

Depersonalization will often disappear without treatment. If disease persists, recurs or causes distress then treatment will be planned.
- Based on underlying cause treatment will be given on individual basis.
- Drug therapy–based on manifestation the following drugs will be prescribed. Antianxiety drugs (benzodiazepine-xanex ; antidepressants (SSRI and TCA, MAOI); antipsychotics (gabapentin or olanzapine or risperidal); sedative
- Psychodynamic psychotherapy
- Behaviour therapy
- Hypnosis
- Drug therapy–sedatives and antidepressants may help some people
- Any stress associated with onset of depersonalization, is treated promptly.

Prognosis

- Relief is achieved through treatment; complete recovery is possible for many people
- A few remain unresponsive for all treatments.

NEURASTHENIA
(ICD-10 $F_{48.0}$; ICD-9 300.5)

The term, 'Neurasthenia' derived from 2 Greek words, 'Neuro' means 'nerve' 'asthenia' means 'weakness', i.e. nervous weakness. The term was coined by George Miller Beard.

Definition

'A clinical condition characterized by symptoms of fatigue, anxiety, headache, impotence, neuralgia and depression'. *—GM Beard, 1869*

Causes

- Result of exhaustion of the central nervous system's energy reserves
- Heredity
- Urbanization
- Competitive environment
- Upper class
- Sedentary environment.

Incidence

- Americans are prone to neurasthenia, which is otherwise called as, 'Americanitis'.

Primary/Essential/Cardinal Symptoms of Neurasthenia

Chronic and persistent fatigue, muscular weakness regard to environment

- Complain of giddiness or dizziness (secondary symptoms)
- Lessened vasomotor tone of the cerebral vessels
- Sensation of pressure tenderness over the spine or constriction
- Backache-referred to small of the back, sometimes to the midscapular regions and at times sacrum
- Spinal hyperaesthesia
- Tenderness constitute the symptoms gave rise to spinal irritation
- Diffuse tenderness/aching of entire head-headache with exaggerated fatigue sensation
- Spontaneous pain or aching
- Rachialgia
- Occasionally-tenderness of teeth or gums
- Localized tenderness of the clavus of hysteria
- Subjective numbness, pricking, formication, velvety sensations or a subjective sense of heat or cold

- Sensory organs- eye weakness and fatigue of intrinsic and extrinsic muscles of the eye, weakness, irritability of retina, cortical exhaustion
- Ear-localized fatigue, auditory hyperaesthesia, tinnitus
- Olfactory hyperaesthesia, inordinately of odours
- Eating-extreme dislike of various wholesome articles of food; dyspepsia
- The sense of weakness-referred to the legs and small of the back
- Tendon reactions-irritability, knee-jerks, lowered muscle tone, ankle clonus
- Pronounced cutaneous reflexes-Babinski sign never present
- Psychic disturbances-a diminished capacity for sustained effort, incapable of long-continued physical effort
- Client find it more and more difficulty to sustain attention (alarms the patient greatly), looses memory, difficulty in concentration, lack of capacity for enjoyment (anhedonia)
- Lack of spontaneity of thought
- Neurasthenia simplex is uncomplicated, never terminates in mental disease
- Insomnia-disturbed especially in morning hours; sleep is interrupted a number of times and often is accompanied by a desire to empty the bladder. Less frequently, the patient has difficulty in falling asleep the oncoming first sleep being delayed for an hour or more
- Patient usually awakens with a feeling of lethargy and depression
- Sexual/genital disturbances. Exhaustion, weakness, irritability, diminished sexual power, premature ejaculation, diminution of secretion normally accompanying the sexual act

Secondary/Teritary/Adventious Symptoms

- Vasomotor changes (chronic fatigue)
- Sensory symptoms-generalized fatigue sensations

- Localized fatigue sensations, e.g. headache (diffuse) pronounced in occipital region, frontal region; backache; limb-ache
- Motor symptoms-muscular fatigue-exaggerated fatigue; muscular weakness; muscular exhaustion; tremors-intension and fine in quality
- Psychic symptoms-diminution in the capacity for sustained mental effort; ready mental exhaustion; diminution in the spontaneity of thought
- Loss of personal force, aggressiveness and will power, hesitation, uncertainty, indecision, markedly increased irritability, loss of self control or inhibition
- Somatic symptoms-atony of digestive tract-constipation, faintness prostration, atony of circulatory apparatus, anomalies of the secretions, disturbances of the sexual functions; signs of weakness, enfeeblement; deficient innervation.

GIDDINESS OR DIZZINESS

Treatment

- Physical exercises, walking for an hour, twice daily
- Adequate rest, to avoid fatigue
- Avoid starchy food and sweets
- Stimulants, alcohol, tobacco, tea and coffee are best withdrawn absolutely
- Advise the patient to increase fluid intake
- Maintain input and output chart
- Advise the patient to have liberal use of baths in evening, shortly before retiring as it relieves fatigue and induces sleep
- Massage therapy may be helpful
- Electrotherapy- pretense treatment
- Family therapy- encourage the family members to provide support to the client
- Psychotherapy
- Americanitis Elixir of Rexall drug company have soother for bouts related to neurasthenia.

OBSESSIVE COMPULSIVE NEUROSIS/ OCD (ICD-10 F$_{42}$; ICD-9 300.3)

OCD is a psychiatric anxiety disorder, characterized by a subject's obsessive, distressing, intrusive thoughts and related compulsions/tasks/rituals attempt to neutralize the obsessions. Obsession and compulsions are source of distress, time consuming and causes impairment in individual's ability socially, occupational and school functioning.

Definitions as per DSM-IV-TR

Obsessions

- Recurrent and persistent ideas, thoughts, impulses or images that are experienced at some time during the disturbance, as intrusive and inappropriate that causes marked distress or anxiety, e.g. thoughts of committing violence.
- Thoughts, impulses or images are not simply excessive worries about real life problems.
- The personal attempts to ignore or suppress such thoughts, impulses or images to neutralize them with some other thought or action.
- The person recognizes that the obsessional thoughts, impulses or images are a product of his or her own mind and are not based in reality.
- The tendency to haggle over small details that the viewer is unable to fix or change in any way. This begins a mental preoccupation which is inevitable.

Compulsions

- Repetitive behaviour or mental acts, that the person feels driven to perform in response to an obsession or according to rules that must be applied rigidly
- Mental acts are aimed at preventing or reducing distress or preventing some dreaded event or situation, however these mental acts either or not connected in a realistic way with what they are designed to neutralize or prevent clearly excessive.

As per ICD-10 ($F_{42.9}$ - unspecified obsessive-compulsive disorder; $F_{42.8}$–other OCD)

- Recurrent obsessional thoughts
  Ideas, images or impulses that enter the individual's mind again and again in a stereo-type form, these are distressing because they are violent/obscene/senseless and the sufferer often tries unsuccessfully to resist them.
- Compulsive acts or rituals
  Stereotype purposeless behaviour (obsessional rituals, e.g. hand washing, counting, checking, touching) repeated again and again that are not enjoyable by an individual.

As per ICD-9

The outstanding syndrome is a feeling of subjective compulsion-which must be resisted to carry out some action, to dwell on an idea, to recall an experience or ruminate on an abstract topic; the unwanted thoughts or ideas perceived by the patient to be inappropriate or nonsensical. Obsession rituals are performed to relieve anxiety.

Classification of OCD as per ICD-10

- Predominantly obsessional thoughts or ruminations ($F_{42.0}$)
  These may be ideas, thoughts, mental images or impulses which are very much distressing to the individual, e.g. a woman getting an idea to kill her child, whom she loves.
- Predominantly compulsive acts/obsessional rituals ($F_{42.1}$)
  For example, washing, checking, counting, etc. the underlying overt behaviour is a fear, the ritual act is a symbolic attempt to avert the danger or fear.
- Mixed obsessional thoughts and acts ($F_{42.2}$)
  Majority of OCD individuals will have both obsessional thoughts and compulsive acts. Thoughts and acts respond differently to treatments
$F_{42.8}$ - Other OCD
$F_{42.9}$ - Unspecified OCD.

Causes

- Autoimmune responses to group A strepto-coccal infection.
- Unconscious conflicts manifested as OCD symptoms (Sigmund Freud).
- Abnormality in the neurotransmitter serotonin or blocked or damaged receptor sites that prevent serotonin from functioning to its full potential.
- Environmental factors.
- Miscommunication between the orbital-frontal cortex, the caudate nucleus and the thalamus may be a factor.
- Familial origin, in monozygotic twins, 1st degree relatives of OCD clients the disease is common.
- Behavioural theories–interplay between classical and operant conditioning paradigms. The external aversive stimuli interact with the organism with previous learning, such stimuli have acquired specific significance; this results in the stimuli gaining more strength resulting in sensitization. Ritual acts produce relief and thus through negative reinforcement increase the possibility of repetition of the phenomena
- Mower's 2 stage theory: Role of exposure and response prevention.
  - A neutral stimulus become associated with fear, as it occurs with an event, which provokes discomfort. Due to this association, various objects, thoughts, images also capable of causing discomfort.
  - Responses that reduce anxiety or discomfort are developed and maintained.

According to Wolpe, compulsions are anxiety elevating and relieving. Obsessions were thought to occur automatically in response to anxiety evoking stimuli, compulsions occur as a reaction to anxiety and the act as aimed at temporarily relieving compulsions.

- Psychodynamic theory
  Freud explained, the anal erotic phase of psychosexual development is responsible for the

evolution of anankastic traits to defend against the unacceptable anal impulses.

- Ego psychological theory

  The conflict was thought to arise due to inadequate mastery of the oedipal conflict, resulted in regression to the anal sadistic stage to avoid anxiety to which the subject was already predisposed due to difficulties in the anal period of development. It stimulates anal and aggressive impulses against which defense mechanisms are used, e.g. isolation, undoing, reaction formation, orderliness, rigidity, magical thinking, regression.

- Psychological factors

  Maladaptive thinking and learning; strained interpersonal relationship, stress.

Clinical Picture

- OCD sufferers performs task or compulsions to seek relief from obsession related anxiety, e.g. repeatedly checking that one's parked car is locked before leaving

- Turning lights on and off a set number of times before exiting the room

- Repeatedly washing hands at regular intervals throughout the day.

  To others these tasks may appear odd and unnecessary. But for the sufferer, such tasks can feel critically important and must be performed in particular ways to ward off dire consequences and to stop the stress from building up

- Rearranging matters rigidly

- Obsessional rituals
  - Repeated hand washing
  - Repeated clearing of the throat, although nothing may need to be cleared
  - Specific counting systems, e.g. counting in groups of 4, arranging objects in groups of 3, grouping objects in odd/even numbered groups etc.
  - Perfectly aligning objects at complete, absolute right angles or parallel

- Having to 'cancel out' bad thoughts with good thoughts; e.g. sexual obsession or unwanted sexual thoughts (fear of being homosexual, fear of being pedophile– sufferers will obsess over whether or not they are genuinely aroused by thoughts)

- A fear of contamination–some sufferers may fear the presence of human body secretions, e.g. saliva, sweat, tears, vomit, mucus or excretions, e.g. urine, faeces

- Some OCD sufferers even fear that the bath soap, which they are using is contaminated

- A need for both sides of the body to feel even

- If one hand gets wet, the sufferer may feel very uncomfortable, if the other is not

- If the sufferer while walking, bumps into something, he/she might hit the object/ person back to feel a sense of evenness. These symptoms also experienced in a reversed manner.

- An obsession with numbers
  - Twisting the head of a toy around, then twisting it all the way back, exactly in the opposite direction
  - OCD sufferers are aware that such thoughts and behaviour are not rational, but feel bound to comply with them the feelings of panic or dread. Sufferers are consciously aware of this irrationality but feel helpless to push it away; due to their insight into the abnormal nature of their compulsions, most OCD sufferers will hide their behaviours, inorder to avoid negative attention
  - The compulsions are purely mental, often called as, the secret illness'
  - Feelings of distress and anxiety
  - Although everyone may experience unpleasant thoughts at one time or another, these are short lived and fade after an adequate time period has lapsed
  - OCD is 'ego dystonic' the disorders is incompatible with the sufferer's self concept

- Persons suffering from OCD are often aware that their behaviour is not rational and are unhappy about their obsession, but nevertheless feel compelled by them.
- Obsessional thoughts: words, ideas and beliefs that intrude forcibly into patient's mind; unpleasant and shocking to the patient.
- Obsessional images: vividly imagined scenes, e.g. violent or disgusting kind.
- Obsessional ruminations: everyday actions are reviewed endlessly.
- Obsessional doubts. Actions not completed adequately, e.g. forgets to turn off the stove; doubting existence of God, etc.
- Obsessional impulses: urges to perform acts, e.g. violent or embarrassing type of activities.
- Obsessional slowness: in performing daily activities.

Treatment

Combination of therapies is helpful than single option.

Behaviour Therapy

- Systematic desensitization
- Flooding
- Modeling
- Implosion
- Shaping
- Aversion therapy
- Reinforcement
    - Positive–suggestive measures, emotional education
    - Negative practice–time out, aversive training
- Emotional education.

Cognitive Therapy

- Self monitoring and control
- Thought stopping–control the obsessive thoughts by producing a strong stimuli which interferes the ongoing thought process, e.g. shouting, 'stop' or a loud bang. The procedure can be modified to result in replacement of neutral thoughts in the place of original obsessions.
- Exposure and ritual/response prevention: gradually learning to tolerate the anxiety associated with OCN, by not performing the ritual behaviour.
- Exposure involves deliberately facing the feared or avoided object, thought, situation or place.
- Response prevention involves delaying, diminishing the anxiety reducing rituals.
- The combination leads to gradual decrease in anxiety, e.g. while going out checking the lock only once (exposure); without going back and checking again (ritual prevention)
- Self monitoring and control.
- Psychodynamic psychotherapy–supportive insight-oriented.
- Drug therapy.
- Selective serotonin reuptake inhibitors (SSRI), e.g. paroxetine (paxil, aropax), Sertraline (Zoloft), Fluoxetine (Prozac, 80mg/day), Fluvoxamine (luvox).

  Action of SSRI: Prevents excess serotonin from being pumped back into the original neuron that released it. Instead, the serotonin can bind to the receptor sites of nearby neurons and send chemical messages or signals that can help and regulate the excessive anxiety and obsessive compulsive thoughts.
- Tricyclic antidepressants, e.g. Clomipramine (anafranil)
- Atypical antipsychotics, e.g. olanzapine (zyprexa)
- Sugar inositol (natural source)–modulates the serotonin action reverses desensitization of the neurotransmitter's receptors
- Psycho-surgery–for some client neither medication nor psychological treatment are helpful, hence as a last resort, a surgical lesion is made in cingulated frontal bundle pathway to alleviate obsessive-compulsive symptoms, e.g. anterior

cingulotomy is done to reduce the intrusiveness of thoughts and distress
- Deep brain stimulation and vagus nerve stimulation, surgical procedures are performed, which do not require the destruction of brain tissue (experimental basis).
- Electroconvulsive therapy
Refractory patients may benefit from a trial of 8-10 ECTs. Improvement is noticed in clients with agitation, but usage of ECT for OCD clients is controversial.

Prognosis

A good prognosis is observed with treatment among the clients who has precipitating event and an episodic nature of symptoms by improvement in personal, social and occupational functioning.

Poor prognosis was noticed when OCD onset is in childhood and if major depressive disorder is coexisting.

Nursing Management

- Assessment: thorough history has to be collected regarding physical functioning and health status, social system, supportive network, social functioning, compulsive activities
- Mental status examination to observe obsessional thoughts, mood pattern, self-esteem
- Pattern of utilization of coping abilities and defense mechanisms.

1. Nursing Diagnosis

Exhaustion related to anxiety and obsessional thoughts.

Goal

Reduces anxiety and performs productive acts.

Interventions

- Identify stressor/root cause for anxiety
- Administer the drugs as per doctor's prescription

- Observe action, side effects of drugs
- Record and report the observations made
- Provide psychotherapy, behaviour therapy based on symptoms.

2. Nursing Diagnosis

Altered physical functioning related to ritualistic behaviour.

Goal

Enhances physical health by maintaining adequate nutrition, rest, sleep, hygiene; controls ritualistic behaviour and obsessive thoughts.

Interventions

- Monitor the clients' anxiety levels due to ritualistic acts
- Ask the client to do ritualistic behaviour in comfortable timings, e.g. early morning, before going to bed
- Serve the food in clients' utensils, ask them to wash hands and cultivate the use of spoon or fork to eat the food (to avoid the feeling of dirty)
- Encourage the client to take high protein and high caloric diet to meet his needs
- Motivate the client to maintain personal hygiene
- Never punish the client for ritualistic behaviour, slowly explain them the effects' of ritualistic acts
- Provide safe and clean environment like bath, washing facilities etc.
- Encourage the client to use moisturiser skin creams based on seasons.

3. Nursing Diagnosis

Social isolation related to anxiety and obsessional thoughts.

Goal

Enhances socialization thereby controls Obsessional thoughts, reduces anxiety.

Interventions

- Provide psychotherapeutic comfortable environment
- Promote social interaction, facilitate socialization process
- Utilize relaxation approach, motivate the client to set limits for ritualistic acts and give sufficient time
- If the client is able to follow non-compulsive behaviour appreciate it
- Never hurry the client, to do the activities in a particular fashion, explain them the effects of having ritualistic behaviour with obsessive thoughts
- Promote supportive system, e.g. family and friends in rendering care and meeting the needs of clients
- Divert the clients' mind, and develop concentration and attention in promoting activities, e.g. reading the literature.

4. Nursing Diagnosis

Ineffective utilization of coping strategies due to obsessional thoughts and compulsive behaviour.

Goal

Learns adequate/alternate coping strategies to overcome obsessive compulsive behaviour.

Interventions

- Observe the anxiety provoking situations, resulting in ritualistic behaviour
- Never argue with the client, approach the client in a friendly manner
- Accept the clients' feelings
- Make the client to understand the effect of ritualistic behaviour, do not disapprove
- Teach the client the new coping strategies, relaxation approach, behaviour modification techniques, therapeutic activities to resolve his problems

- Give positive reinforcement for non-ritualistic behaviour
- Encourage the client to utilize adaptive coping strategies to decrease ritualistic behaviour and to control obsessive thoughts.

5. Nursing Diagnosis

Alteration in role performance related to ritualistic behaviour.

Goal

Performs effectively social roles.

Interventions

- Provide comfortable environment to the client
- Observe the clients' functioning abilities and difficulties within the social, working and family environment
- Motivate the client to discuss the internal conflicts and associated behaviour
- Identify the stressors and adapt suitable strategies to overcome ritualistic behaviour/ compulsive acts
- Motivate the client to participate in social activities and interact with others
- Instruct the family members to provide support to the client in anxiety relieving measures
- Promote humour and inform the client to accept either constructive criticism or compliments
- Encourage the client to perform the activities of his choice in a productive manner
- Inform the client to maintain a record of activities performed successfully in a socially desirable manner to promote self confidence
- If the client is interested in spiritual activities, arrange for spiritual meetings.

PHOBIA

The term 'Phobia' is derived from Greek 'φόβος' means 'fear', phobia is also used in a non-medical sense for 'aversions of all sorts'. It describes negative attitudes or prejudices towards the named subjects.

Definition

'Irrational, persistent, fear of certain situations, objects, activities or persons'.

'Exaggerated pathological fear of a specific type of stimuli or situation'.   —*Bimla Kapoor, 2002*

'Persistent avoidance behaviour secondary to irrational fear of a specific object, activity or situation'.   —*Lalitha, K 2007*

Criteria to define phobia:

* Fear is out of proportion to the demands of the situation
* Cannot be explained or reasoned away
* Beyond voluntary control
* Fear leads to an avoidance of the feared situation–Marks.

Prevalence

* Phobias are the most common form of anxiety disorders. 8–18 per cent of Americans suffer from phobias
* Most common mental illness among women in all age groups and the second most common illness among men, older than 25 years
* Severe fears are present in 10–15 per cent of children
* Specific phobias are found in 5 per cent of children
* Onset of phobia is late second decade or early onset of third decade
* Sometimes onset is sudden without any cause, and spontaneous remittance are observed.

Classification

* Agora phobia (with or without panic disorder)
* Specific phobia (isolated phobias; simple phobia)
* Social phobia–DSM-IV, 4th edition
* Phobic anxiety disorders (specified and unspecified)–ICD-10 (F_{40}).

Causes

* Brain chemistry combine with life experiences play a major role in the development of anxiety disorder and phobia
* Arises from a combination of external events and internal predispositions
* Certain objects may have a genetic predisposition/heredity being associated with fear
* Specific triggering event, e.g. traumatic experiences in early age
* Psychodynamic theory.

  Anxiety is usually dealt with regression, when repression fails to function adequately, other secondary defense mechanism of ego come into action, i.e. displacement. Anxiety is transferred from a really dangerous or frightening object to a neutral object. These two objects are connected by symbolic associations. The neutral object, chosen unconsciously that can be easily avoided in day-to-day activities in contrast to frightening object.

* Learning theory/Behavioural theory

  According to classical conditioning, a stressful stimuli produce an unconditioned response-fear. When the stressful stimuli is repeatedly paired with a harmless object, eventually the harmless object alone produces fear as a conditioned response. If the person avoids the harmless object to prevent fear becomes into phobia.

  According to Operant Conditioning theory, anxiety is a drive that motivates the organism to do what it can, to obviate the painful affect, in the course of its random behaviour, the organism learns that certain actions will enable it to avoid the anxiety-provoking stimuli. Those avoidance patterns remain stable for long period of time, as result of the reinforcement they receive from their capacity to diminish activity.

Stimulus Response Model

Anxiety is aroused by a naturally frightening stimulus that occurs in continuity with a second inherently neutral stimulus. As a result of continuity, especially when the two stimuli are paired on several occasions the originally neutral stimuli take the capacity to arouse anxiety by itself. The neutral stimuli therefore become conditioned stimuli for anxiety production.

Psychoanalytical Theory

The major function of anxiety is a signal to the ego, that a forbidden unconscious drive is pushing for conscious expression, thus altering the ego to strengthen and marshal its defense against the threatening instinctual force. For example, In castration anxiety–the conflict is regarding sexual arousal, ego must call on auxiliary defenses, these are in social and specific phobia is of displacement, symbolization and avoidance. In agoraphobia, it is the separation anxiety playing a central role.

CLINICAL PHOBIAS

1. Social Phobias

Fears involving with other people or social situations, e.g. Performance anxiety or fears of embarrassment by scrutiny of others, (eating in public places).

A marked and persistent fear of one or more social or performance situations in which the person is exposed to unfamiliar people or to possible scrutiny by others. The individual fears that he or she will act in a way that will be humiliating or embarrassing. Exposure to the feared social situation invariably provokes anxiety, which may take the form of a situational predisposed panic attack. The avoidance, anxious, anticipation or distress in the feared situation interferes significantly with the person's normal occupational, social or interpersonal functioning or there is marked distress about having phobia.

Types

a. General Social Phobia (Social anxiety disorder)
b. Specific Social Phobia (Anxiety triggered only in specific situations)

In general social phobia the symptoms may extend to psychosomatic manifestations of physical problems, and suffer full-fledged panic attacks with all the associated disabling symptoms.

In specific phobias fear of single specific panic trigger, e.g. spiders, dogs are common in childhood. People with these phobias specifically have mild anxiety over that fear. Most individual understand that they are suffering with an irrational fear, but are powerless to override their initial panic reaction. Phobias interfere with children participation in and enjoyment of various activities. It may also interferes with their education, family life or their social life. For example, claustrophobia–fear of closed spaces; hemotophobia–fear of sight of blood.

2. Agoraphobia

A generalized fear of leaving home or a familiar 'safe' area, followed by possible panic attacks. As agoraphobia increases in severity, there is a gradual restriction in normal day-to-day activities, certain times restriction will be more, the person will reside in home only. These persons prefer to be accompanied by a family member or friend whenever they are leaving home. Majority of phobic clients will not have any problem related to social functioning.

3. Non-psychological Conditions

Phobia may also signify conditions other than fear, e.g. hydrophobia–fear of water or inability to drink water due to illness. Certain times the term, phobia is used in an analogy with the medical usage of the term. Phobias are described as fear, dislike, disapproval, prejudice, hatred, discrimination or hostility towards the object or 'phobia'.

Treatment

*   Systematic desensitization therapy–some therapist will use virtual reality or imagery exercise gradually to desensitize patients to the feared entity.
*   Cognitive behavioural therapy: Therapist will make the client to understand the cycle of

negative thought pattern and ways to change these patterns. Cognitive behaviour therapy will be conducted in group settings. The techniques include imaginal exposure, performance based exposure, cognitive restricting, home-work assignments, flooding, relaxation techniques.
- Drug therapy: Antidepressants or anxiolytics, serotonin reuptake inhibitors.
- Insight oriented psychotherapy, supportive psychotherapy: The client will understand the origin of phobia, phenomena of secondary gain, role of resistance and healthy way of dealing with anxiety provoking stimuli.
- Social skill training: Role modelling and role playing.

POST TRAUMATIC STRESS DISORDER (PTSD)

Introduction

PTSD is described in ICD-10 ($F_{43.1}$), ICD-9 (309.81). In DSM it is mentioned that traumatic stress without manifesting PTSD. Occasionally PTSD is called as 'post traumatic stress reaction' to emphasize that it is a result of traumatic experience rather than a manifestation of preexisting psychological condition.

Definition

'Certain severe psychological consequences of exposure to or confrontation with stressful events that the person experiences as highly traumatic'.

Incidence

- Women (10.4%) experience more than men (5%); children, disabled, elderly, orphans are more prone for PSTD.

Predisposing Factors

- Comorbid psychiatric disorders–clinical depression or bipolar disorder; general anxiety disorders; abuse (physical, sexual, psychological); addiction, neurotic illness, childhood trauma; recent stressful life situations
- Certain personality traits–compulsive, asthenic, personality disorders-borderline, paranoid, dependent, antisocial traits
- Traumatic painful experiences
- Witnessing abuse inflicted on another child or an adult; kidnapping, robbery
- Inadequate system
- Genetic or constitutional vulnerability
- Automobile accidents
- Serious injury or death of loved one.

Causes

- Actual or threatened death or traumatic memories or experiences related to death
- Serious physical injury or threat
- Threat to psychological integrity
- Childhood physical, emotional or sexual abuse including prolonged or extreme neglect
- Experiencing an event perceived as life threatening, e.g. a serious accident, complications of disease, violent physical assaults or torture (sexual assault or rape), warfare, life threatening, natural disasters, incarceration.

Neurochemical or Neuroendocrinal Factors

- Biochemical changes in the brain and body; chemical imbalance in the neurotransmitters
- Increased sensitivity of the hypothalamic-pituitary-adrenal axis, with a strong negative feedback of cortisol, due to a generally increased sensitivity of cortisol receptors PTSD individuals will show decreased cortisol output
- Traumatic events or emotional experiences triggers a release of stress hormones like adrenaline, which acts on amygdala and the memory is stored or consolidated
- Amygdala, prefrontal cortex, hippocampus are shown to be strongly involved in the formation of memories, especially fear related

- Hyper function of sympathetic nervous system
- Extreme stress has lethal effect on brain development and particularly reduces hippocampus size and abnormalities in the limbic system; frontal and temporal lobes
- Psychodynamic factors: Psychological upsets-trauma, reactivate unresolved psychological conflict instrumental learning
- Biological factor: functioning of neurotransmitters like dopamine, norepinephrine, etc. produces alteration in emotional reactions; serotonin level will be decreased in depression
- Cycle of violence: witnessing childhood abuse may tend to have abuse tendency in adulthood. It will be repeated over generations.

Clinical Manifestations

- Restlessness
- Insomnia
- Aggressiveness
- Clinical depression
- Nightmares
- Memory loss about an aspect of traumatic event
- Intrusion: sufferers are unable to process the extreme emotions brought about by the trauma, plagued by symptoms of cluster triad recurrent nightmares or day time flashbacks during which they graphically re-experience the trauma, characterized by higher anxiety level.
- Hyper arousal: a state of nervousness characterized by 'fight or flight'. Startle reaction, jumpiness in connection with high sounds or fast motions, incomplete processing of thoughts.
- Avoidance: with intrusion and hyper arousal symptoms are too much distressing, the individual strives to avoid contact with everything and to everyone, even with their own thoughts may arouse memories of trauma and thus provoke the intrusive and hyper arousal states.
- Sufferers isolate themselves becoming detached in their feelings with a restricted range of emotional response and can experience emotional detachment 'numbing' or emotional self-mortification.
- Dissociation: Disconnection between depersonalization and derealization; disconnection between memory and affect so that the person is 'in another world'.
- In extreme forms can involve apparent multiple personalities and acting without any memory 'loosing time'.
- Hyper vigilance–close attention to and anticipation of approaching danger.
- Avoidance of reminders, extreme distress when exposed to stressors.
- Anorexia.
- Irritability, memory loss.
- Excessive startle response.
- Anxiety.

Types

- Acute PTSD–subsides after a duration of few weeks to 3 months
- Chronic PTSD–if the symptoms persist, the diagnosis is called as 'chronic'
- Delayed PTSD–it may progress to months, years and decades after the event; endures personality changes.

Diagnosis Criteria

According to DSM-IV-TR
- A_1–the person experienced, witnessed or was confronted with an event that involved actual or threatened death or serious injury or a threat to the physical integrity of self or others
- A_2–the person's response involved intense, fear, hopelessness or horror
- A–significant symptoms of distress in almost anyone and the event was 'outside the range of usual human experience'.

According to ICD-10 $F_{43.1}$
- Significant evidence of trauma
- Onset within 6 months of a traumatic event

- Repetitive, intrusive recollection or reenactment of the event in memories
- Daytime imagery or dreams
- Conspicuous emotional detachment
- Numbness of feelings
- Avoidance of stimuli that might arouse recollection of the trauma.

Management

A multi model approach will be used

- Critical incident stress management–early intervention after a traumatic incident to reduce traumatic effects of an incident and potentially prevents a full blown PTSD
- Eye movement desensitization and reprocessing
- Relationship based treatment
- Emotionally focussed couples therapy with trauma survivors
- Dyadic developmental psychotherapy, cognitive behavioural therapy, group therapy, exposure therapy, talk therapy are helpful to reduce isolation and stigma
- Basic counselling includes education about the condition and provision of safety and support
- Drug therapy–based on clinical manifestation; antidepressants or atypical antipsychotics, e.g. prozac, effexor, zoloft, remeron, zyoreza, seroquel etc. will be given to reduce manifestations of PTSD
- Safe environment will reduce stress and move to reality
- Mood stabilizers, e.g. lithium carbonate/carbamazepine or valproic acid may be effective to reduce clinical manifestations of disease like dissociation, numbness, intrusion etc.
- Antihypertensive, e.g. propranolol or clonidine which helps the heart to relax, relieves HTN and prevents heart attacks, reduces sleep disturbances, hyper arousal, startle response and aggression
- Anxiolytics, e.g. benzodiazepine is given to reduce startle response, anxiety and hyper arousal symptoms.

Nursing Management

- Empathetic, consistency, sincerity, honesty in explanation or clarification, trust-worthy relationship, effective communication, interaction skills, etc. are essential qualities for managing PTSD clients
- Provide calm and quiet, non-stimulating environment
- Therapeutic nurse client relationship is established
- Accept the client as he is, i.e. his distress and emotional reactions
- Supportive sympathetic approach is required, show love and concern, let the client understand that nurses are caretakers and well wishers, who looks after them
- Reorient the client to the present situation
- Never probe details of the trauma in the initial phase after establishing therapeutic-nurse patient relationship and winning the confidence of the client, then try to explore the events related to trauma
- Utilize the psychological processes and direct the client in counselling process, allow the client to ventilate his feelings outwardly, motivate to discuss goals and methods (plan of activities) to attain it
- Enhance the functioning levels, independence level of achievement
- Promote clients' interaction with group members to decrease isolation and enhances alternative coping strategies
- Assess the situational supportive system and strengthen the supportive system; train up the activity levels and help him to attain mastery over it
- Identifies community resources and guide the client to utilize them for maximum efficiency
- Assists the client to divert the mind from traumatic memory to useful activities
- Train up the client in deep breathing, relaxation exercises, healthy life style, e.g. adequate nutrition, avoiding stressors, activity pattern, exercise, sleep promoting measures

- Avoid emotional blaming of the client, for the events occurred
- Never give false hopes and false reassurances, ambiguous statements to the client
- Enquire whether the client is having any suicidal tendency or hints, monitor his behaviour; assure the client to prevent suicidal attempts
- Assist the client to manage by themselves in daily living activities
- If any history of abuse, refer them to appropriate self help groups for addiction purposes
- Assist the client to attain adequate independent skills in dealing with activities
- Educate the client in the utilization of alternative coping strategies and its effectiveness, assist in implementation of the same
- Support the client in rehabilitation activities.

NURSING MANAGEMENT OF THE CLIENT WITH ANXIETY DISORDERS

1. Nursing Diagnosis

Inadequate cooing strategy related to fear for specific stimuli.

Goal

Utilizes adequate coping strategies to overcome fear and faces the stimuli without fear or phobia.

Interventions

- Approach the client in a friendly manner, establish and maintain therapeutic nurse-patient relationship.
- Be brief and firm.
- Motivate the client to ventilate his feelings openly, during ventilation process nurse will act as an active listener, and try to explore the stressor; observe the clients' covert anxiety.
- Clarify the doubts of the client.
- Demonstrate the adequate coping strategies, assist the client to utilize them successfully and appreciate the client, if he does so. If the client is unable to use the coping strategies, suggest

alternative strategies, give freedom to the client to choose coping strategy based on his ability.

- Encourage the client to use behaviour modification techniques to cope up the situation, e.g. systematic desensitization, flooding, implosion, therapy, modelling, positive reinforcement etc.
- Assist the client to improve thinking process in a realistic manner and able to tolerate the anxiety provoking stimuli, let the client to develop control over situation, e.g. cognitive techniques.
- Promote relaxing environment and utilize stress management technique, assertiveness techniques.
- Help the client to utilize problem solving techniques.

2. Nursing Diagnosis

Perceptual disturbances related to anxiety.

Goal

Improves perception, attention and concentration.

Interventions

- Orient the client to the environment
- Encourage the client to perform some interested activities by paying attention and interest in completing the activity, motivate to get efficiency in it
- Ask the client to observe for any distractions or hearing any sounds and ask them to inform to the health professional
- Motivate the client to concentrate in diversional activities
- Educate the client along with written material viz., self help skills, relaxation skills, which promotes the clients' mind to have clear mind
- If the client does approved behaviour, reinforce him to perform it efficiently
- Ask the client to practice deep breathing exercise and have awareness on anxiety provoking stimuli

- Motivate the client to discuss freely their anxieties to the family members and to the health care professionals
- Observe and protect the client from self harm or harming others through aggressive behaviour
- Mobilize family support.

3. Nursing Diagnosis

Impaired communication related to anxiety associated feelings.

Goal

Enhances communication and achieves good socialization skills.

Interventions

- Provide psychological support and reassurance to the client
- Provide calm and quiet (non stimulating/non-disturbing/non-threatening) environment
- Motivate the client to utilize communication techniques
- Clear the doubts and provide necessary information
- Encourage the family members to provide support to the clients in need of hour, accept the clients' feelings
- Promote safety and security of client, explain the client that they should not disturb others
- Be brief, use simple language
- Assist the client to establish good relationship with family members, friends and relatives
- Allow the client to perform the group activities
- Educate the client to have patience/tolerance in communicating
- Reduce the distraction in the environment
- Motivate the client to communicate with other group members in society to develop socialization skills
- Advise the client to utilize cognitive, behavioural techniques.

4. Nursing Diagnosis

Alternation in physiological functioning of an individual due to anxiety.

Goal

Enhances physiological functioning.

Interventions

- Provide comfortable environment to the client
- Permit the family members to stay with the client to provide support, whenever the client is in disturbed mood
- Promote 6–8 hours of sleep, motivate to have warm-water bath and warm milk before sleep; in afternoons, atleast half-hour rest is necessary
- Identify the covert anxiety feelings of the client and teach him to interrupt the responses
- Monitor and record vital signs and weight of the client
- Maintain intake and output chart
- Observe the clinical manifestation of client, identify the stressors (anxiety provoking situations and its grade)
- Provide symptomatic care, e.g. apply glycerine for dry lips
- Administer the drugs as per prescription
- Advise the client to take small and frequent feeds of their choice (among the rich sources)
- Motivate the client to develop interest in eating and offer more fruits to eat
- Some clients with anxiety will eat more; ask them to reduce carbohydrates in diet
- Protect the client from injury by providing safe environment, e.g. non-slippery floor, closed electric circuit
- Encourage the client to cultivate relaxation habits like painting, drawing, etc. to divert the mind
- Teach and assist the client to perform relaxation exercises
- If the client is interested in spiritual activities, provide opportunity for offering prayers and arrange for spiritual meetings

- Educate the client about the physiological changes of the body when experiencing stress
- Use simple language while communicating
- Provide positive feedback to the client and encourage the client to make realistic goals and work for it
- Encourage the client to understand the life situations and measures to adopt to it happily.

5. Nursing Diagnosis

Experiences post traumatic experiences.

Goal

Accepts, understands and adopts to the situation.

Interventions

- Encourage the client to ventilate the traumatic events openly
- Provide supportive, trusting environment
- Assist the client to explore the stressors
- Demonstrate deep breathing, relaxation exercises, adequate coping strategies and encourage them to utilize it, and thereby handles the anxiety provoking situations
- Motivate the client to develop healthy habits, e.g. adequate nutrition, regular sleep and rest, exercises, utilization of adequate coping strategies, etc.

REVIEW QUESTIONS

1. Obsessive Compulsive Neurosis. (5M, RGUHS, 98, 00, 04; 15M, MGRU, 91, 5M, RGUHS, Oct, 07).
2. Agoraphobia. (2M, RGUHS, 04).
3. Name four types of Phobia. (2M, RGUHS, 00, 01, 04).
4. Anxiety state. (5M, RGUHS, 02, 03, 07).
5. Phobia. (5M, MGRU, 99; 2 M, RGUHS, 03, 5M, 02, 03, 04, 07).
6. Obsession. (2M, RGUHS, 02, 03).
7. Differentiate between Psychosis and Neurosis. (5M, RGUHS, 00, 01; 06, 07, 5M, MGRU, 03).
8. Obsessions and Compulsions. (2M, RGUHS, 00; 5M, MGRU, 96,97).
9. Explain the Nursing Problems and Interventions in the Management of patients in Anxiety state. (10M, RGUHS, 99).
10. How does Anxiety lead to Maladoption. What is the role of Nurses in relieving Anxiety and promote Mental Health. (15M, GULB, 94).
11. Anxiety Neurosis. (5M, MGRU, 97, 99, 00, 01, 02, 03, 04, 00, RGUHS).
12. Compulsive behaviour. (5M, MGRU, 90).
13. Types of Phobia. (2M, RGUHS, 00, 01).
14. Neurotic disorders of Childhood. (2M, RGUHS, 03).
15. Psycho-Neurotic disorder. (10M, RGUHS, 05).
16. What are the characteristics of Anxiety? How will you help the patient to cope up with Anxiety. (3+4m, IGNOU, 99).
17. What do you mean by Neurosis? Write types of Neurosis and its Nursing Interventions. (2+7M, IGNOU, 99).
18. Define Hysterical Neurosis. Discuss the symptoms and psychodynamics of Hysterical Neurosis. Describe its Nursing Management. (2+3+5M, IGNOU, 05).
19. Post Traumatic Stress Disorder. (2M, RGUHS, 05).
20. School phobia. (5M, RGUHS, 00).
21. Manic Depressive Psychosis. (5M, NTRU, 96,97; RGUHS 05).
22. Hypochondriasis. (2M, RGUHS, 04).
23. What is Neurosis? Write the Psychodynamics of Neurosis? Explain the treatment and Nursing Management of Depressive Neurosis. (10M, KSDNEB, 2007).
24. Classification of Neurotic disorders. (5M, 2002, 2005).
25. Neurotic disorders. (5M, 2002, 05).
26. Panic disorder. (5M, 2006).
27. Panic Attack. (2M, RGUHS, Oct, 2007).
28. Obsessive Compulsive disorders. (5M, 2000, 02, 03, 05). Describe the definition, clinical manifestations, Medical and Nursing Management of Obsessive Compulsive Neurosis. (10M, KSDNEB, 2007).
29. Mrs. Anitha aged 50 years got admitted to psychiatric ward with Depression, explain in briefly the signs and symptoms of Depression, out line the management of a case of Depression. (10M, KSDNEB, Aug, 2007).

14 Personality Disorder/Characterological Disorder

INTRODUCTION

Individual's characteristics are combined product of heredity, early life experiences and environmental influences. Healthy individual will be able to adjust and adopt/accommodate to the changes which are occurring in the life and its environmental situations. When personality disorder occurs, individual will have fixed fantasies, rigid and ongoing patterns of thought and action; the inflexibility and alteration in behavioural patterns causes serious personal and social difficulties; in socially distressing ways, which often limit their ability and function in relationships and at work.

DEFINITIONS

'An enduring pattern of inner experience and behaviour that deviates markedly from the expectations of the culture of the individual who exhibits it'.

—American Psychiatric Association

'When personality traits are inflexible maladaptive and can cause either significant functional impairment or subjective distress'.

—DSM-IV

'A morbid perversion of natural feelings, afflictions, inclinations, temper, habits, moral disposition and natural impulses without any remarkable disorder or intellect defects or knowing and reasoning faculties and particularly without any insane illusion or hallucination'.

—James Pritchard (father of personality disorder)

CLASSIFICATION

DSM-IV classified personality disorders into
1. Cluster A (odd or eccentric disorders)
   - Paranoid personality disorder
   - Schizoid personality disorder
   - Schizotypal personality disorder
2. Cluster B (dramatic, emotional, erratic disorders)
   - Antisocial personality disorder
   - Histrionic personality disorder
   - Narcissistic personality disorder
3. Cluster C (anxious and fearful disorder)
   - Avoidant personality disorder
   - Dependent personality disorder
   - Obsessive compulsive personality disorder.

ICD-10 (F_{60}–F_{69}) classified personality disorders as

- Paranoid personality disorders
- Schizoid personality disorders
- Dissocial personality disorders
- Emotionally unstable personality disorders
  - Impulsive type
  - Borderline type
- Histrionic personality disorders
- Anakastic personality disorders
- Anxious, avoidant personality disorders (avoidant)
- Dependent personality disorders
- Other personality disorders (narcissistic personality disorders).

Incidence

- 5–15 per cent of adults have one or more personality disorders.

Risk Factors

- Women may develop borderline personality disorder; men are more likely to develop antisocial personality disorder and obsessive-compulsive personality disorder
- History of childhood (verbal, physical or emotional) abuse
- Family history of schizophrenia, personality disorders
- Childhood head injury
- Unstable family life.

Causes

- Genetics or heredity, e.g. Obsessive compulsive personality disorders; paranoid personality disorders; schizoid personality disorders and antisocial personality disorders
- Family history, e.g. Borderline personality disorders and antisocial personality disorders are common among first degree relatives
- Brain dysfunction. (frontal lobe and amygdala part), abnormal brain processing of emotionally charged; low threshold of excitability of the limbic system
- Alteration in levels of neurotransmitters, e.g. decreased level of serotonin and dopamine and increased level of norepinephrine will cause borderline personality disorders
- Release of toxic chemical substances
- Post-traumatic stress disorder, e.g. borderline personality disorders
- Developmental factors, e.g. extreme parental rage or humiliation defect in parental role, loss of a loved person, child abuse-physical, emotional and sexual abuse, etc. are prone for borderline personality disorder
- Child neglect
- Childhood trauma, adverse or painful experience or head injury prone for cluster B personality disorder, borderline personality disorder, histrionic personality disorder and cluster C personality disorder
- Children with alcoholic and drug abuse parents
- Parental failures in early childhood prone for borderline personality disorders
- Childhood pathology, e.g. antisocial and impulsive behaviour
- Parental rejection, peer group rejection, etc. develop an intense fear of relationship and discomfort in social interactions and are prone for avoidant personality disorders
- Neglecting experiences or critical traumatic experiences in early childhood, e.g. narcissistic and dependant personality disorders
- Chronic psychiatric illnesses, e.g. maladaptive disorders or responses
- Excessive parental control and criticism leads child to respond in part with perfectionism, control and orderliness
- Socio-cultural factors, e.g. involuntary isolation, divorce
- Broken families or chaotic home, hospitalization, prolonged separation, relationship difficulties, deprivation, frustration, internal conflicts,

disappointments, assault, maladaptive cooing responses, exposure to loss, death, grievance.

Screening and Diagnosis

• Enquire about personal history and emotional wellbeing with client's friends and relatives
• Rule out any substance abuse problem.

Treatment

• Approach the client in a friendly manner, combination of therapies will be recommended. Provide supportive environment.
• *Psychodynamic psychotherapy*: Educate the client about his condition and related issues. It makes them to understand or to identify their responsibility for the turmoil in their lives.
• Teach healthier coping techniques, to modify the behaviour and to socialize the client.
• Individual, family and group psychotherapy are of helpful in reducing rejection, sensitivity, individual psychotherapy is focussed on motivation and behaviour.
• *Cognitive behaviour therapy*: It involves actively retraining the way to think about problems which in turn improves emotional environment of the client.
• *Dialectical behaviour therapy*: Teach coping skills which are helpful to control behaviour, especially useful in borderline personality disorders.
• Group therapy and behaviour therapy (e.g. self control techniques) are contraindicated in paranoid personality disorders and schizotypal personality disorders.
• Supportive psychotherapy is helpful in schizoid personality disorders.
• Drug therapy
 – Antidepressants–selective serotonin reuptake inhibitors, e.g. fluoxetine (prozac, sarafem, sertraline)
 – Anticonvulsants–suppress impulsive and aggressive behaviour, e.g. Carbamazepine (tegretol), Valproic acid (depakote)

– Antipsychotics–to have touch with reality, improves thinking process, e.g. Resperidone (risperidal), olanzapine (zyprexa), haloperidol (haldol)
– Anxiolytics–Alprazolam (Xanax), Clonazepam (klonopin)
– Mood stabilizers–to relieve symptoms associated with personality disorders, e.g. lithium (eskalith, lithiobid).
• Self-help group and therapeutic community approaches are of helpful
• Dynamic therapy is used to externalize the patient's inner emotions and to reduce anxiety and learn coping skills in histrionic personality disorders, dependent personality disorders.
• Assertiveness techniques (behavioural therapy) are helpful in improving patient's self-esteem in avoidant personality disorders cases.
• Dialectical behavioural therapy (a comprehensive long term treatment) is helpful to decrease destructive behaviour, improves interpersonal relationship, reduces suicidal tendency.

Complications

• Social isolation
• Substance abuse
• Depression, anxiety and eating disorders
• Self destructive behaviour, e.g. Suicidal tendencies
• Violence and homicide
• Incarceration (committing serious crimes).

TYPES OF PERSONALITY DISORDERS

PSYCHOPATHY

The term 'psychopathy' is derived from the Greek words, 'psyche' means 'soul', mind and 'pathos' means 'to suffer'. It is a unique disorder. It is correlated with 'antisocial personality disorders and dissocial personality disorders'. It is described in ICD-10 $F_{60.2}$, ICD-9-301.7, DSM-IV-TR.

ICD-10 referred psychopathy, antisocial personality, asocial personality, amoral personality as synonyms for dissocial personality disorder. It results when gross disparity occurs between the behaviour and prevailing social norms.

Definitions

'The existence in any person of such hereditary, congenital or acquired condition affecting the emotional volitional rather than the intellectual field and manifested by anomalies of such character as to render satisfactory social adjustment of such person difficult or impossible'.

—*Washington State Legislature*

'A persistent disorder or disability of mind (whether or not including impairment of intelligence) which results in abnormally aggressive or seriously irresponsible conduct on the part of the person concerned'.

—*The Mental Health Act, UK*

'A condition characterized by lack of empathy or conscience and poor impulse control or manipulative behaviours'.

Causes

- A combination of psychological, biological, genetic and environmental factors
- Heredity.

Manifestations

- Manipulative
- Deceitful
- Abusive
- Cortical under arousal
- Fraudulent behaviour
- Intimidation
- Violence to control others and to satisfy their own selfish needs, fearlessness, risk seeking behaviour, inability to internalize social norms
- Lacking in or devoid conscience and in feelings for others
- Violating social norms and expectations without guilt or remorse

- Causes social disharmony
- No concern for the feeling of others
- Gives disregard for any sense of social obligation
- Egocentric
- Lacks insight of any sense or responsibility or consequences
- Superficial and shallow emotions
- Callous, incapable of forming lasting relationships, unresponsiveness in general interpersonal relations
- Typically never perform any action unless they determine it can be beneficial for themselves
- Causes harm through their actions, hence they are not emotionally attached to the people they harm
- Carelessness and failure in treating themselves
- Inability to process contextual cues
- Impulsive, grandiosity
- Considerably anger, anxious, distress, commits violent acts as a reaction to negative emotions (crimes of passion)
- Risk seeking behaviour
- A low tolerance for frustration and aggression
- No empathy, remorse, anxiety or guilt in relation to their behaviour
- Marked proneness to blame others or to offer reasonable rationalization
- They mimic conscientious manner, when it suits their needs
- Failure to sustain relationship
- Superficially charm and above average intelligence
- Unreliable, untruthful, insincere, lack of remorse or shame, guilt
- Poor judgement and failure to learn from experience
- Incapacity to love
- Poverty in major affective reactions impersonal, trivial, poor integration
- Failure to follow any life plan.

Types of Psychopathy

- Primary psychopathy–root disorder, biological in origin. Characteristics are: arrogance, callousness, manipulativeness, lying, grandiosity, interpersonal aggression
- Secondary psychopathy–an aspect of another psychiatric disorder or social circumstances, results from a combination of genetic and environmental influences, impulsivity, boredom proneness, need for stimulation, parasitic life style, early onset of behavioural problems, irresponsible, lack of long term goals, reactive aggression, anxious, trouble toleration, depressive, weak behavioural controls, juvenile delinquency, breaking probation, lack of realistic long term goals, may commit suicide.

Diagnosis Criteria

- Clinical rating scale/check list
  Fctor-1 scale is associated with extroversion and positive effect.
  Factor-2 scale is associated with reactive anger, anxiety, risk of suicide, criminality and impulsive violence.
  Pseudo-psychopathy personality disorders or Frontal Lobe disorder.
  Causes: Childhood or conduct disorder.
  Signs and symptoms: Abusive, aggressive, deceitful, irresponsible, incapable of insight and planning.

SOCIOPATHY

It occurs due to social conflicts; both psychopath and sociopath are two distinct kinds of 'antisocial personality'.

Causes.

Parental neglect
    An interaction between genetic predisposition and environmental factors.
    Negative social factors

Parental neglect
Poverty
Delinquent peers.

Manifestations

- Normal temperaments
  Low or high intelligence
- Alleged drunken behaviour
- Deceitfulness
- Social coarsening
- Loutish behaviour
- Lacks justification or social skills
- Undesirable behaviour
- Bed wetting
- Fire setting
- Cruelty to animals
- Anger outbursts
- Frequent lying
- Aggression to peers
- Impulsivity
- Weak behavioural control
- Irresponsibility
- Lack of realistic long term goals
- Proneness to boredom/need for stimulation
- Parasitic life style
- Early behavioural problems
- Juvenile delinquency
- Revocation of conditional release (breaking probation).

ANTISOCIAL PERSONALITY DISORDERS

Definition

'A condition in which individuals exhibit a pervasive disregard for the law and the rights of others'.

'Sociopath' and 'Psychopath' describes 'antisocial personality disorder'. It affects in men three times more and prevalent in prison population. Early adolescence is a critical time for antisocial personality disorder and it is a chronic disorder. Intensity of symptoms tends to peak during the teenage years and early 20s and then may decrease over time.

Risk Factors

- History of child abuse, deprived environment, neglect, antisocial environment in home, having an antisocial parents, alcoholic parent, being involved in a group of peers, attention deficit disorder and reading disorders.

Causes

- Idiopathic
- Hereditary factors/genetics
- Environmental influence–chaotic home, punitive school, community and improper working environment, family conflicts, lack of control, abusive alcoholic parents, drug addicts
- Difficulty in developing emotional bonds
- Few healthy role models for behaviour
- No rewards for socially acceptable actions
- Conduct problem
- Abusive or neglectful childhood environment.

Manifestations

- Indifferent to the needs of others
- Manipulate through deceit or intimidation may have trouble holding down a job
- Fails to pay debts or fails to fulfill parenting or work responsibilities
- Usually loners
- Aggressive, violent, involves in fight
- Frequent encounters with the law
- May also possess a considerable amount of charm and wit
- Persistent lying or stealing
- Tendency to violate the rights of others (property, physical, sexual, emotional, legal)
- Inability in keeping jobs
- A persistent agitated or depressed feeling (dysphoria)
- Inability to tolerate boredom
- Disregard for hurting others
- Impulsiveness

- A sense of extreme entitle
- Inability to make or keep friends
- Reckless behaviour
- Provoking arguments with a sibling or fellow being student
- No acceptable behaviour.

Treatment

Approach has to be adopted to alleviate symptoms
- Medicines based on symptoms, e.g. if depression, antidepressant will be administered
- Antipsychotic drugs
- Psychotherapy–to develop appropriate interpersonal skills and instill moral codes
- Develop and maintain strong therapeutic nurse-patient relationship
- Group therapy and family therapy
- Individual psychotherapy.

Complications

Increased risk for
- Physical trauma, injury, accidents
- Drug and alcohol abuse
- Suicide, homicide
- Depression, bipolar disorder, anxiety
- Committing crimes and then goes to prison.

Prevention

- Encourage social interaction, nonpunitive techniques, set definitive rules
- Decrease the development of problemmatic behaviour
- Reduce negative methods of behaviour modification technique
- Formulate and inform rules for discipline and conduct
- Encourage study habits, minimize failures
- Guidance and counselling services
- Motivate the client to develop social interaction consistent approach, provide respect for others.

Nursing Management

- Observe the behaviour, set limits which are not acceptable
- Provide congenial, safe and calm environment to express their feelings
- Explain in slow tone, the ways of unacceptable behaviour, which is harmful to both, self and to others
- Teach relaxation exercises and motivate them practice
- Encourage the individual to participate in diversional activities, where he can express his feelings in an acceptable manner like drawing, music, writing
- Teach self control behaviour modification techniques, allow him to practice
- Administer the drugs as per orders
- Assign some responsibilities and observe how he is able to do
- Provide healthy support, explore the under lying feelings related to shame, guilt, anxiety and fear
- Maintain non-stimulating or non-threatening environment to lessen aggressive feelings, keep away all dangerous objects within reach to prevent self injury or to others
- Teach coping strategies, provide opportunities to practice
- If aggressive behaviour is noticed, mechanical restraints may be necessary
- All staff in the unit has to follow the same techniques, if the client's behaviour crosses the limits
- Promote acceptable behaviour; make the client to gain insight into his own and develop positive attitude and consistency
- Provide positive feedback for healthy independent behaviour
- Enhance problem-solving skills, client's strengths, coping skills
- Explain the importance of behavioural change
- Enhance the client's interaction with others and teach him the importance of group support and development of social skills, encourage the client to have small group interactions and utilize the community resources for their development
- Involve the client in non-competitive activities and tasks first and then allow him to progress into competitive activities
- Encourage the client to maintain consistent relationship and establish behavioural goals
- Win the client's confidence and maintain healthier relationship
- Provide positive feedback to the client whenever appropriate behaviour has exhibited
- Teach the client how to adjust themselves in difficult situations.

PARANOID PERSONALITY DISORDER

It is a long term, wide spread disorder and people with paranoid personality disorder are unwarranted suspicious and mistrustful that other people are hostile, threatening and demeaning. These beliefs are maintained in the absence of any real supporting evidence. Patients with paranoid personality disorder are not delusional, most of the time they are in touch with reality; misinterprets others' motives and intentions. They feel that others are trying to humiliate them, hostile and they like to live socially isolated manner. They will not formulate and maintain intimate relationship with others.

Causes

Familial Factors

- Chronic schizophrenia, delusional disorder, psychotic disorder
- Interpersonal causes
- Childhood traumatic experiences
- Stressful environment
- Genetics, e.g. twins may prone to get.

Incidence

- The disorder is more common in men than in women.

Manifestations

- Suspiciousness carry over in all realms of life, mistrustful
- Difficulty in maintaining jobs
- Have fewer close relationships, as they feel others will hurt them, like to be isolated avoiding social relationship
- Angry, aggressive, hostile, unfriendly, argumentative
- Generalized distrust of other people
- Full of insults and threats
- Feel insecure
- Violent
- Frequently convinced that their sexual partners are unfaithful
- Hidden criticisms
- Never inclined to share intimacy
- Sometimes they like to be aloof or isolated, unsuccessful or negative interaction with others
- Little no sense of humour
- Excessive sensitiveness; grudging persistently
- Lacks justification in sexual fidelity of spouse
- Gives more importance to 'self'
- Stubborn, self important.

Diagnosis

- By interview with the client
- In DSM-IV-TR it was mentioned to diagnose the client should have atleast 4 symptoms listed below:
  - Unfounded suspiciousness that people want to deceive, exploit or harm the patient
  - Pervasive belief that others are not worthy of trust or that they are not inclined to or capable of offering loyalty
  - Fear that others will use information against the patient with the intention of harming them. Reluctant to share even harmless personal information with others
  - Interpreting others remarks as insulting or demeaning

- Tendency not to forgive real or imagined sights and insults
- An angry and aggressive response in reply to imagined attacks by others. The counter attacks for a perceived insult is often rapid
- Suspicious in the absence of real evidence, that a spouse or sexual partner is not sexually faithful, resulting in such repeated questions, e.g. where have you been? 'whom did you see'?

Treatment

- Psychotherapy–After establishing professional relationship, developing trust, winning confidence, demonstrate nonjudgemental attitude and a professional desire to assist the patient psychotherapy is initiated.
- Group therapy–Include family members, encourage them to meet the 'self help groups' dedicated to recover from this disorder.
- Supportive psychotherapy–Analyse the problem in dealing with other people, the patient's motivations and possible sources of paranoid traits, never challenge the patients' thoughts too directly.
- Medication–If the client is anxious, anti-anxiety drugs may be prescribed, during high stress and extreme agitation, low dose of antipsychotic, neuroleptics can be given. Selective serotonin reuptake inhibitors, e.g. Prozac, for the clients with angry, irritable and suspicious.
- To reduce symptoms, antidepressants can be given.

Prognosis

- Chronic, life-long condition.

Nursing Management

- Develop and maintain therapeutic nurse patient relationship
- Encourage the client for effective communication

- Monitor the client's behaviour
- Provide safe and conducive environment to protect self and others
- Teach alternative ways of coping strategies and problem solving techniques in overcoming the problematic situations
- Family education activities are carried out to assist the client in dealing with the sensitive situation
- Encourage for healthy interactions and identify the stressors for the frustration
- Never whisper or criticize in front of the client
- Encourage the client not to have inhibitions, heitation, support the client in stressful time
- Provide support and guidance to the client, when he is performing the activities in a desirable manner
- Motivate the client to express his feelings openly, outwardly
- Sincerity, honesty, concern to the clients feelings is required, be consistent and firm, provide positive feedback for the acceptable behaviour exhibited by the client
- Be nonjudgemental, avoid any discussions about the rules or requirements, counsel the client, teach the alternative strategies to cope-up.

BORDERLINE PERSONALITY DISORDER/EMOTIONALLY UNSTABLE PERSONALITY DISORDER

Definitions

'A mental illness is characterized by emotional dysregulation, extreme 'black and white' thinking or splitting and chaotic relationships'.

'A pervasive pattern of instability of interpersonal relationship, self image and marked impulsivity, beginning in early adulthood and present in a variety of contexts'.

Profile

A pervasive instability in
- Mood

- Interpersonal relations
- Self image
- Identity
- Behaviour
- Disturbance in the individual's sense of self; in extreme cases it can lead to 'periods of dissociations'
- Negative impact on many or all of the psychosocial facets of life including employability and relationship in home, work and social settings
- Co-morbidity is common.

Causes

- Traumatic childhood
- Vulnerable temperament
- Stressful maturational events in adolescence and adulthood
- Failing in accomplishing developmental tasks
- Childhood abuse or trauma or neglect
- Abuse (emotional, sexual, physical) by the care takers
- Affective disorders
- Substance abuse disorder
- Reactive attachment disorder
- Ill treatment by parents
- Post traumatic stress disorder
- Defective family environment
- Genetics
- Chronic stress
- Neuro-dynamics–serotonin, norepinephrine acetylcholine and GABA neurotransmitters alterations
- Enhanced amygdala activation and prefrontal cortical area dysfunctions
- Low level stressors
- Unresolved life events
- Over involvement or under involvement of parents.

Manifestations

- Avoid real or imagined abandonment
- Unstable and intense interpersonal relationships
- Extremes of idealization and devaluation

- Identity disturbance, unstable self image or sense of self
- Recurrent suicidal behaviour, gestures, threats or self mutilating
- Affective instability due to marked reactivity of mood behaviour (dysphoria, irritability, anxiety)
- Emptiness feelings, difficulty in controlling anger
- Severe dissociative symptoms
- Frequent, strong and long-lasting states of aversive tension, often triggered by perceived rejection, being alone or perceived failure
- Lability (changeability) between anger and anxiety or between depression and anxiety and temperamental sensitivity to emotive stimuli
- Negative emotional states–extreme feelings in general
  - Feelings of destructiveness or self destructiveness
  - Feelings of fragmentation or lack of identity
  - Feelings of victimization
- Sensitive to the way, how others treat them
- Reacting strongly to perceived criticism or hurtfulness
- Shifts from positive to negative, generally after a disappointment or perceived threat of losing someone
- Self image rapid change from extreme positive to negative
- Impulsive behaviour are common, e.g. alcohol or drug abuse, unsafe sex, gambling, recklessness
- Insecure
- Ambivalent
- Preoccupied or fearful attitudes towards relationships
- Manipulative or difficult, inner pain and turmoil
- Powerlessness, defensive reactions
- Limited coping and communication skills
- Paranoid ideas
- Relationship instability

- Angry out bursts, abundant fears
- Disturbances in identity
- Suicidal behaviour
- Emptiness.

Co-morbidity

- Anxiety disorder
- Mood disorder
- Eating disorder.

Diagnosis

- Self reported experiences of the client
- A comprehensive personal and family history
- A physical examination
- Blood tests to exclude HIV or syphilis
- EEG, CT scan to exclude epilepsy and brain lesions.

Treatment

Psychotherapy

- Dialectical behaviour therapy–cognitive behavioural techniques; emphasizes an exchange and negotiation between therapist and client, between the rational and the emotional and between acceptance and change (hence dialectic). The learning of new skills–interpersonal effectiveness, assertiveness technique, social skills coping adaptability.
- Transference focussed psychotherapy–a form of psychoanalysis therapy, the therapist works on the relationship between the patient and the therapist and he will try to explore and clarify the aspects of this relationship
  - Medications: Antidepressants–selective serotonin reuptake inhibitors to relieve anxiety and depression
  - Antipsychotics–to treat distortions in thinking or false perceptions
  - Therapeutic community and psychiatric rehabilitation services–to avoid stigma and social exclusion associated.

- Psycho-education and skill training.
- Marital and family therapy: useful in stabilizing the relationship, to resolve stress and conflicts to improve family communication and problem solving provides support to family members.
- Schema focussed therapy–integrative approach based on cognitive behavioural skills based techniques with object relations and gestalt approaches. It targets deeper aspects of emotion, personality and schemas. It focusses on relationship with the client.

Nursing Management

- Place the client near to the nurses station
- Have a keen insight into client's behaviour in all the means, e.g. communications, performing activities
- Based on client's need one-to-one relationship has to be maintained
- Identify the stressors which promote undesirable behaviour of the client, try to avoid them
- If the client is developing destructive behavioural tendency, observe closely, never allow the client to keep potentially dangerous objects
- Remove sharp or dangerous objects in the client's environment
- Encourage the client to interact and share his past experiences, review the events, explore the feelings related to these episodes
- Allow the client to participate in small group discussions, where he can exchange his feelings
- Set clear and realistic goals for client's activities
- Set limitations for client's inappropriate behaviour like destructive behaviour, e.g. mutiliation behaviour, fears related leaving alone or verbal or physical threats
- Rotate the staff for client's care, so that he will not develop any dependency
- Motivate the client to establish and maintain effective communication skills and relationship with significant members
- Avoid labelling the client by his activities

- Never show sympathy or empathy to the client's humiliation attitude or activities
- Give positive reinforcement for client's appropriate behaviour
- Promote consistency
- A written contract has to be established for acceptable and appropriate behaviour
- Encourage the client to participate actively in assertiveness techniques, problem solving techniques
- Never do argument or criticism for client's activities
- Provide consistent feedback for acceptable or unacceptable social behaviour.

HISTRIONIC PERSONALITY DISORDER (ICD-10 F$_{60.4}$; ICD-9 301.50)

Definition

'Characterized by a pattern of excessive emotionality and attention seeking including an excessive need for approval and inappropriate seductiveness'.

It begins in early adulthood.

Causes

- Genetics
- Childhood experiences
- Environmental influences.

Incidence

- More Common in Women than in Men.

Manifestation

- Pervasive and excessive pattern of emotionality and attention seeking, i.e. constant seeking of reassurance or approval
- Individuals are lively, excessive dramatics with exaggerated display of emotions
- Enthusiastic and flirtatious
- Inappropriately seductive appearance or behaviour

- Excessive concern with physical appearance
- Self centeredness, self indulgent and intensely dependent on others
- Low tolerance of frustration or delayed gratification
- Rapidly shifting emotional states that may appear shallow to others
- Opinions are easily influenced by other people, but difficult to back-up details
- Tendency to believe that relationships are more intimate than they actually are
- Makes rash decisions
- Threaten or attempts suicide to get attention
- Inappropriately sexually provocative express strong emotions with an impressionistic style
- Project their own unrealistic fantasized intentions onto people with whom they are involved
- Selection of marital or sexual partners is highly inappropriate
- Women may have inappropriate and intense anger, may engage in manipulative suicide threats by manipulating interpersonal behaviour
- Male show identity diffusion, disturbed relationships, lack of impulse control, antisocial tendency are inclined to exploit physical symptoms
- Engage in uninhibited behaviour
- Able to function at a high level and can be successful socially and at work
- Affects person's social and romantic relationships or their ability to cope with losses or failures
- Often fails to see their own situation realistically, tends to dramatize and exaggerate
- Failure or disappointment is usually blamed on others
- Go through frequent change in job, easily bored, have trouble in dealing with frustration as they crave for novelty, competitiveness and excitement, they may place themselves in risky situations, ends up in depression
- A style of speech, i.e. excessively impressionistic and lacking in detail
- Shows self dramatization, exaggerated expression of emotions
- Over-involvement (superficial resonance with others)
- Aggressiveness
- Over-concern with physical attractiveness
- Egocentricity
- Self indulgence
- Persistent manipulative behaviour in achieving the needs.

Diagnosis

- Observation of appearance, behaviour
- Collection of history
- Psychological evaluation.

Treatment

- Psychotherapy based on the case report method aimed at self development through resolution of conflict
- Family therapy based on manifestations.

Nursing Management

- Establish and maintain therapeutic nurse-patient relationship
- Promote effective communication strategies and healthy interactions
- Provide safe and calm (non-stimulating) environment
- Provide immediate/positive feedback for acceptable behaviour
- Try alternatives of socially and legally acceptable methods of dealing in handling frustration
- Provide emotional support and counsel the client, prepare schedule of activities and ask the client to stick on it
- Assist the client to understand the relationships realistically
- Encourage to take sufficient time in taking decisions
- Observe the client's behaviour, watch for suicidal tendency, explain to them the harmful

effects of such tendency, make him to understand and not to commit or execute the plan of action

- Advice him to the privacy and healthy manner to express the feelings related to sex appropriately
- Encourage the client to share their emotional feelings appropriately with the people who exhibit concern
- Motivate him to involve in socially approved activities
- Enhance realistic thinking
- Set limitations for behavioural activities or tendencies
- Teach adaptive coping strategies to overcome aggression.

OBSESSIVE-COMPULSIVE PERSONALITY DISORDER (ICD-10 F$_{42}$; ICD-9 300.3)

'An anxiety disorder, characterized by a subject's obsessive, distressing, intrusive thoughts and related compulsions (tasks or rituals) which attempt to neutralize the obsessions'.

Definitions

'Obsession is a 'recurrent, persistent thoughts, impulses that are experienced at some time during the disturbances as intrusive and inappropriate which causes marked anxiety or distress'.

'Compulsion is a repetitive behaviour or mental acts that the person feels driven to perform in response to an obsession or according to rules that must be applied rigidly to reduce or neutralize the distress or dreaded situation'.

Causes

- Abnormalities in the brain and, serotonin, neurotransmitter function alteration
- Psychological factors–unconscious conflicts, repression of feelings

- Autoimmune response to group A streptococcal infection.

Manifestation

- Performs tasks or compulsions to seek relief from obsession related anxiety, e.g. repeatedly washing hands at regular intervals throughout the day
- Rearranging matters rigidly
- Repeated clearing of throat
- 'Counting steps'
- Aligning objects perfectly
- 'Cancel out' bad thoughts with good thoughts
- Unwanted sexual thoughts
- A fear of contamination
- Obsession with numbers
- Thought avoidance paradox
- Ego syntonic
- Not aware of anything abnormal about themselves; they will readily explain why their actions are rational and it is impossible to convince them otherwise
- Twisting the head of a toy around, then twisting it all the way back exactly in the opposite direction
- OCD sufferers are aware that such thoughts and behaviours are not rational, but feel bound to comply with them to fend off feelings of panic or dread
- Tends to drive pleasure from their obsessions or compulsions
- Individuals are 'perfectionistic' 'overly organized' and pay extreme attention to detail in an exaggerated and unhealthy way; that interferes with task completion
- Experience difficulty in work situations and intimate relationships
- Unable to throw out worthless items
- Stubbornness
- Unwelcome thoughts or ideas.

Treatment

- Behaviour therapy–'exposure and ritual prevention' technique. It involves gradually learning to tolerate the anxiety associated with not performing the ritual behaviour.
- Cognitive therapy.
- Medications, e.g. selective serotonin reuptake inhibitors–paroxetine (paxil) sertaline (Zoloft).
- Psychodynamic psychotherapy.

Nursing Management

- Guidance and counselling plays a significant role. Explain the situation and encourage the client to substitute maladaptive behaviour and energies into adaptive or coping strategies to overcome the problem.
- Individual psychotherapy also plays vital role. Teach how their behaviour has to be modified.
- Encourage them to constantly observe their behaviour and teach them to utilize 'self control' technique to overcome ritualistic behaviour and ask them to divert their mind and energies into useful activities.

DEPENDENT PERSONALITY DISORDER

Dependent personality disorder is described as "a pervasive and excessive need to be taken care of that leads to a submissive and clinging behaviour as well as fears of separation. The dependent and submissive behaviours are designed to elicit caregiving and arise from a self perception of being unable to function adequately without the help of others."

Incidence

- Common in women than in men, it begins in early adulthood is present in a variety of contexts.

Manifestations

- Experiences great difficulty in making everyday decisions
- Tends to be passive and allow other people to take the initiative and assumes responsibility for most major areas of their lives
- Depends on a parent or spouse to decide where they should live; what kind of job they should have and who are their friends, how to spend their free time, which school they have to attend
- Assumes responsibility, goes beyond age appropriate and situation–appropriate requests for assistance from others
- Difficulty in initiating projects or doing things independently
- Obtains nurturance and support from others
- Feels discomfort or helpless when alone due to exaggerated fears of being unable to care for themselves
- When a close relationship ends, devastation or helplessness occurs; they seek another relation to provide the care and support which they need
- Do not trust their own abilities to make decisions and feel that others have better ideas
- Avoiding personal responsibility
- Unable to meet ordinary demands of life
- Preoccupied with fears of being abandoned
- Easily hurt by criticism or disapproval
- Low self-esteem and self-doubt
- Subordination of one's own needs.

Treatment

- Psychotherapy
- Drug therapy –antidepressants, sedatives and tranquilizers
- Cognitive behavioural therapy.

Nursing Management

- Assess the behaviour pattern of an individual
- Provide guidance and counselling, individual psychotherapy may be of helpful
- Identify the abilities, strengths and motivate them to utilize it in overcoming or handling stressful situations
- Encourage them to solve their problems on their own efforts and lead an independent life

- Motivate the family members to provide situational support, concern, love in the time of need
- Certain behaviour modification techniques can be used to substitute maladaptive behaviour into adaptive strategies and assertiveness techniques
- Family members have to help to raise the self confidence of the client
- Encourage the significant personalities to give supporting hand by making the client to be assertive and independent
- Modify the goals and make the client to understand in a better manner
- Develop a sense of optimism about the client's strengths
- Promote healthy, appropriate expression of feelings
- Make the client to understand the deficiencies and provide assistance to over come that
- Never criticize or hurt the inner feelings of the client, as they are sensitive; slowly help them to overcome their problems.

NARCISSISTIC PERSONALITY DISORDER

Definitions

'Enduring patterns of inner experience and behaviour that are sufficiently rigid and deep seated to bring a person into repeated conflicts with his/her social and occupational environment'.

'A pattern of grandiosity in the patient's private fantasies or outward behaviour, a need for constant admiration from others and lack of empathy or others'.

Incidence

- Common in late adolescence and early adulthood.

Causes

- Arrested psychological development
- Young child's defense against psychological pain

- Problems or unsatisfactory relationships in parent-child relationship or interaction
- Harsh and punishing super ego.

Sub-types

- Craving narcissists–People who feel emotionally need and undernourished; clingy or demanding to those around them
- Paranoid narcissists–Intense contempt for themselves, but projects outward onto others; drives other people away from them by hypercritical and jealous comments and behaviours
- Manipulative narcissists–Enjoys 'putting something over' on others, obtaining their superiority feelings by lying to and manipulating them
- Phallic narcissists–Tend to be aggressive, athletic, exhibitionistic, enjoys by showing off their bodies, clothes and overall 'manliness'.

Manifestations

- Significant emotional pain or difficulties in relationships and occupational performance
- Grandiose sense of self-importance, e.g. demanding special favours from others or choosing friends and associates on the basis of prestige and high status rather than personal qualities
- Lives in a dream world of exceptional success, power, beauty, genius, perfect love
- Thinks themselves as 'special' 'privileged' only can understand by higher status people
- Demands excessive amounts of praise or admiration from others
- Feels entitled to automatic deference, compliance or favourable treatment from others
- Exploitative towards others and takes advantages of them
- Lacks empathy and does not identify with other's feelings
- Frequently envious of others
- History of intense but short term relationships with others
- Inability to make or sustain genuinely intimate relationships

- Tendency to be attracted to leadership or high profile positions or occupations
- A pattern of alternating between unrealistic idealization of others and equally unrealistic devaluation of them
- Assessment of others in terms of usefulness
- Center of attention or admiration in a working group or social situation
- Hypersensitivity to criticism, however, mild or rejection from others
- Unstable view of the self that fluctuates between extremes of self-praise and self contempt
- Preoccupation with outward appearance, image or public opinion rather than inner reality
- Painful emotions based on shame
- Impairment.

Diagnosis

- Collection of client's history, both from the client and family members.

Treatment

- Drug therapy–antidepressants to relieve narcissistic grandiosity
- Psychotherapy–psychoanalysis–Gestalt therapy
- Hospitalization–low functioning patients with NPD may require hospitalization
- Parents must be able to show empathy in their interaction with their children.

Nursing Management

- Develop and maintain therapeutic nurse-patient relationship
- Encourage the family members to have healthier interaction and relationship with their children
- Promote 'emotional bondage' among family members
- Enhance 'parent-child relationship'
- Set clear realistic goals, where the child can achieve it
- Set limitations for unacceptable behaviour

- Provide interpersonal support and safe environment
- Family education has to be given for fulfillment of needs of children
- Teach adaptive, appropriate coping strategies to handle the difficult situations
- Encourage the client to build-up a support system to meet client's needs
- Adopt consistent approach.

AVOIDANT/ANXIOUS PERSONALITY DISORDER (ICD-10 $F_{60.6}$; ICD-9 301.82)

Definition

'Personality disorder characterized by a pervasive pattern of social inhibition, feelings of inadequacy, extreme sensitivity to negative evaluation and avoiding social interaction'.

'A pervasive pattern of social inhibition, feelings of inadequacy and hypersensitivity to negative evaluation, begins by early adulthood and present in a variety of contexts'.

—American Psychiatric Association

Causes

- Perceived or actual criticism or repeated rejection by parent or peers in childhood
- Interpersonal difficulties
- A combination of social, genetic and biological factors
- Temperamental factors characterized by behavioural inhibition.

Characteristics

- People with avoidant personality disorder consider themselves to be socially inept or personally unappealing and avoid social interaction for fear of being ridiculed, humiliated or disliked
- They typically present themselves as loners and report feeling themselves as loners due to fear of being shamed or ridiculed

- Feels a sense of alienation from society (self imposed social isolation)
- Exaggerates the potential difficulties, physical dangers or risks involved in doing something ordinary, but outside their usual routines
- Avoids activities that involve significant inter-personal contact, because of fears of criticism, disapproval or rejection
- Will not possess any close friends
- Easily hurts by criticism or disapproval or rejected (hyper-sensitive)
- Embarrasses by blushing, crying or showing signs of anxiety in front of other people
- Uncommunicative in social situations because of a fear of saying something inappropriate or foolish or of being unable to answer a question
- Low self-esteem
- Tends to be underachievers and finds it difficult on job activities
- Mistrust of others; extreme feelings of anxiety, tension and apprehension
- Avoids occupational activities
- Emotional distancing related to intimacy
- Unwilling to get involved with people unless, certain of being liked
- Highly self conscious
- Preoccupied with being criticized or rejected in social situations
- Feelings of inadequacy inhibits new inter-personal situations
- Chronic substance abuse/dependence
- Inferiority feelings, extreme shy, fearful and withdrawn in new situations
- Reluctant to take personal risks or engage in any new activities as they feel always embar-rassed
- Fixed fantasies.

Comorbidity

- Social phobias, anxiety disorder, panic disorder, obsessive compulsive disorder.

Treatment

- Social skills training
- Cognitive therapy
- Group therapy.

SCHIZOID PERSONALITY DISORDER (ICD-10 $F_{60.1}$) AND ICD-9 (301.20)

Definition

'Schizoid Personality disorder is a personality disorder characterized by lack of interest in social relationships, a tendency towards a solitary lifestyle, secretiveness and emotional coldness'.

Prevalence: Less than 1 per cent of the general population will be affected with Schizoid Persona-lity disorder.

History: In 1908, Eugen Bleuler coined the term, 'schizoid' to designate a natural human tendency to direct attention towards one's inner life and away from the external world. Bleuler labeled the morbid, but non-psychotic exaggeration of this tendency as, 'schizoid personality'.

ICD-10: Criteria to diagnose Schizoid Personality disorder:

- Emotional coldness, detachment or reduced affection
- Limited capacity to express either positive or negative emotions towards others
- Consistent preference for solitary activities
- Very few friends or relationships and a lack of desire for such
- Indifference to either praise or criticism
- Taking pleasure in few activities
- Indifference in social norms and conventions
- Preoccupation with fantasy and introspections
- Lack of desire for sexual experiences with another person.

DSM-IV-TR manual for diagnosing mental dis-orders, defines Schizoid Personality disorder as:

A pervasive pattern of detachment from social relationships and a restricted range of expression of emotions in interpersonal settings, beginning by early adulthood and present in a variety of contexts, as indicated by 4 (or more) of the followings
- Neither desires nor enjoys close relationships, including being part of a family
- Almost always chooses solitary activities
- Has little interest in having sexual experiences with another person
- Takes pleasure in few activities
- Lacks close friends or confidants other than first-degree relatives
- Appears indifferent to the praise or criticism of others
- Shows emotional coldness, detachment, or flattened affectivity.

Does not occur exclusively during the course of schizophrenia, a mood disorder with psychotic features, another psychotic disorder, or pervasive development disorder and is not due to the direct physiological effects of a general medical condition.

Manifestations

Schizoid behaviour, explained by Emile Kretchmer in 1925:
- Unsociability, quietness, reserved, seriousness and eccentricity
- Timidity, shyness with feelings sensitivity, nervousness, excitability and fondness of nature and books
- Pliability, kindliness, honesty, indifference, silence and cold emotional attitudes, over sensitive and cold (refer below table for description.)

Clinical features of schizoid personality disorder		
Area	*Overt*	*Covert*
Self concept	1. Compliant 2. Stoic 3. Non-competitive 4. Self-sufficient 5. Lacking assertiveness 6. Feeling inferior and an outsider in life	1. Cynical 2. Inauthentic 3. Depersonalized 4. Alternately feeling empty 5. Robot-like and full of omnipotent, vengeful fantasies 6. Hidden grandiosity
Interpersonal relations	1. Withdrawn 2. Aloof 3. Have a few close friends 4. Impervious to others' emotions 5. Afraid of intimacy	1. Exquisitely sensitive 2. Deeply curious about others 3. Envious of others' spontaneity 4. Intensely needy of involvement with others 5. Capable of excitement with carefully selected intimates
Social adaptation	1. Prefer solitary occupational and recreational activities 2. Marginal or eclectically sociable in groups 3. Vulnerable to esoteric movements owing to a strong need to belong 4. Tend to be lazy and indolent	1. Lack of clarity of goals 2. Weak ethnic affiliation 3. Usually capable of steady work 4. Sometimes quite creative and may make unique and original contributions 5. Capable of passionate endurance in certain spheres of interest
Love and Sexuality	1. Asexual, sometimes celibate 2. Free of romantic interests 3. Averse to sexual gossip and innuendo	1. Secret voyeuristic and pornographic interests 2. Vulnerable to erotomania 3. Tendency towards compulsive 4. Masturbation and perversions

contd...

contd...

Area	Overt	Covert
Ethics, Standards and Ideals	1. Idiosyncratic moral and political beliefs 2. Tendency towards spiritual, mystical and para-psychological interests	1. Moral unevenness 2. Occasionally strikingly amoral and vulnerable at odd times, at others times altruistically self sacrificing
Cognitive style	1. Absent-minded 2. Engrossed in fantasy 3. Vague and stilted speech 4. Alterations between eloquence and inarticulateness	1. Autistic thinking 2. Fluctuations between sharp contact with external reality and hyper-reflectiveness about the self 3. Autocentric use of language

Treatment

Fairbaim delineated 4 central schizoid themes:

1. The need to regulate interpersonal distance as a central focus of concern
2. The ability to mobilize self preservative defenses and self reliance
3. A pervasive tension between the anxiety laden need for attachment and the defensive need for distance which manifests in observable behaviour as indifference
4. Over valuation of the inner world at the expense of the outer world

- Drug therapy: Antipsychotics may have efficacy in alleviating them; Resperidone-to treat negative symptoms
- TCAS, MAOIS, SSRIs, low dose benzodiazepines and
- ß-blockers may help social anxiety in the Schizoid Personality disorder
- Closer compromise- The Schizoid Personality disorder may be encouraged to experience intermediate positions between the extremes of emotional closeness and permanent exile
- Long term therapy: working through
  - to change fundamentally the old ways of feeling and thinking
  - to rid oneself of the vulnerability to experiencing those emotions associated with old feelings and thoughts
  - adequate support for the emergence of the real self.

IMPULSIVE AGGRESSIVE PERSONALITY DISORDER (ICD-10 $F_{60.30A}$)

Aggression is a response to a potential threat or provocation across a variety of species, seems to be an inborn response tendency. It is a cluster B personality disorder, where impulsive aggression in couples with a highly reactive and unstable affect modulation. Patients with border personality disorder will respond to disappointment and frustrations with intense emotions like rage, fear of abandonment and dysphoria. These will trigger the generation of an impulsive, often aggressive response to provocation.

Clients with narcissistic personality disorder may also act aggressively in an impulsive manner when feeling humiliated or narcissistically injured. Patients with antisocial personality disorder may also act aggressively with little apparent remorse about their aggressive and antisocial behaviour, which may result in criminal activities.

Causes

- Frustration or provoked
- Interpersonal conflicts
- Disruptive relationships
- Familial abuse
- Occupational failure
- Neurobiological and psychosocial underpinnings

- Higher order cortical centres that serve to suppress the emergence or more primitive forms of aggression, when it is inappropriate
- The cortical inhibitory mechanisms and the limbic systems, prefrontal cortex involved in the generation and modulation of aggression is required
- The amygdala responds to threat and provocative stimuli
- Sub-cortical regions may then serve to signal other critical nodes, e.g. Hypothalamus that modulate the body's hormonal internal milieu and cortical regions initiating motor action
- Release of serotonin, a neurotransmitter or blockades the reuptake and direct agonism of 5-HT$_2$ receptors, resulted in blunted hormone responses in personality disorder clients with impulsive aggression
- The serotonin system modulates the activity of inhibitors areas in the prefrontal cortex and other related areas, e.g. anterior cingulated cortex
- Postnatal lesions of the prefrontal cortex, particularly in orbital regions, early in development may result in antisocial and aggressive behaviour in adulthood
- Temporal lobe tumors or lesions
- Impairment or reduction in prefrontal cortical inhibition of subcortex capacity or exaggerated responsiveness in excitatory circuits of subcortical areas, e.g. amygdala may be associated with aggression
- Reduced prefrontal gray matter has been associated with autonomic deficits and aggression in clients with antisocial personality disorder
- Disconnection between inhibitory centres and limbic centres involved in the generation of aggression may be responsible for the disinhibition of aggression. The dysjunction may be related to under-activation of serotonin activity modulating the prefrontal

cortex and or over-activation of the limbic cortex
- Aggression is moderated by a variety of neuromodulators, e.g. Monoamines, neuro-peptides and neuro-steroids
- *Catecholamine*: Increased reactivity of the nor-adrenergic and dopaminergic system may facilitate aggressive behaviour in humans. Reduced presynaptic concentrations of catecholamine, e.g. Norepinephrine, coupled with supersensitive post-synaptic receptors may be responsible for exaggerated irritability in response to stress

- *Peptides*: Vasopressin plays an important role in modulating memory and behaviour
- *Steroids*: Testosterone was correlated with aggression and suicidal tendencies
- *Genetics*: Polymorphisms in genes that regulate the activity of neuro-modulators, e.g. Serotonin or genes for structural components of critical brain regions regulating aggression.

Manifestation

- Emotional instability
- Lack of impulse control
- Outbursts of violence or threatening behaviour, 'behavioural explosions' specially in response to criticism by others
- Acts impulsively without consideration of the consequences
- Lack of self control
- Often accompanies psychopathy or emotional 'agnosia'.

Treatment

- Cognitive behaviour therapies: To validate and understand the intense affects experienced by people with these personality disorder; provides alternative ways of channelizing the impulses generated by these intense feelings away from self-injurious or aggressive behaviour toward more interpersonally effective coping strategies

- Psychoanalytic therapies–Uses exploration of unconscious conflict in here and now distortions of the transference to help shift deeply ingrained assumptions and strategies
- Drug therapy–Used to reduce the diathesis to impulsive aggression may facilitate the inter-apsychic shifts, e.g. Selective serotonin reuptake inhibitors –may reduce irritability and aggression consistent
- Mood stabilizers that dampen limbic irritability, reduces the susceptibility to react to provocation or threatening stimuli by overt action of limbic system, e.g. amygdala
- Carbamazepine (Tegretol), diphenylhydantoin (dilantin) can be used.

REVIEW QUESTIONS

1. Character disorder. (2M, GULB, 94).
2. State Personality disorders. Write the aetiology and clinical manifestations. (5M, MGRU, 03).
3. Antisocial Personality disorder. (2M, RGUHS, 04).
4. Psychopathic Personality. (5M, RGUHS, 00, 03).
5. Sociopath. (2M, 5M, RGUHS, 03).
6. Define Psychopath. List the different types of Psychopathology in human behaviour. Explain different types of Personality disorder with illustrations. (2+5+8M, IGNOU, 01).
7. Four characteristics of Psychopathic Personality. (2M, RGUHS, 00).
8. Define abnormal personality. Classify personality disorders. (5+2M, NIMS, 99).
9. Paranoid personalty disorder. (5M, GUHS, 00).
10. Schizoid personality disorder. (5M, GUHS, 01).
11. Borderline personality disorder. (5M, MGRU, 01).
12. Histrionic Personality disorder. (5M, RGUHS, Oct, 07).
13. Aeitiology of personality disorder. (5M, RGUHS, 00).
14. Nursing management of personality disorders. (5M, RGUHS, 00).
15. Personality disorders. (5M, KSDNEB, 2007).
16. Passive Aggressive Personality disorder. (5M, RGUHS, Oct, 2007).
17. Self concept. (2M, RGUHS, Oct, 2007).

15

Childhood Disorders

INTRODUCTION

The practice of child psychiatry differs from adult psychiatry; when child has any behavioural deviation, it results into disturbance in other family members also, specifically the primary care givers. Evidence of disturbance in child's behaviour is based on observations of behaviour made by parents, teachers and other well-wishers. They too have sound knowledge related to growth and developmental aspects of children in specific age. Professionals has to have the ability/skills to change the attitude by enriching the knowledge of care-takers and other family members on Child Psychology, Growth and Development of children, working with family, coordinating the efforts of others, who involved in child care. Multidisciplinary approach plays a vital role in dealing child with behavioural problems.

DEFINITION

'Behavioural abnormalities pertaining to the child in cognitive, conative and affective domains ranging from mild to severe and persistent, altering child's functioning levels causing distress to the child, his/her parents, their families and to the people in the community'.

CLASSIFICATION OF CHILDHOOD DISORDERS

As per ICD-10

Mental retardation F_{70}–F_{79}

F_{70} – Mild mental retardation

F_{71} – Moderate mental retardation

F_{72} – Severe mental retardation

F_{73} – Profound mental retardation

F_{78} – Other mental retardation

F_{79} – Unspecified mental retardation

Disorders of psychological development F_{80}–F_{89}

$F_{80.0}$ – Specific speech articulation disorder

$F_{80.1}$ – Expressive language disorder

$F_{80.2}$ – Receptive language disorder

$F_{80.3}$ – Acquired aphasia with epilepsy

$F_{80.8}$ – Other developmental disorders of speech and language

$F_{80.9}$ – Developmental disorder of speech and language, unspecified

F_{81} – Specific developmental disorders of scholastic skills

$F_{81.0}$ – Specific reading disorder

$F_{81.1}$ – Specific spelling disorder

$F_{81.2}$ – Specified disorder of arithmetical skills

$F_{81.3}$ – Mixed disorder of scholastic skills

$F_{81.8}$ – Other developmental disorders of scholastic skills

$F_{81.9}$ – Other developmental disorders of scholastic skills, unspecified

F_{82} – Specific developmental disorder of motor Function

F_{83} – Mixed Specific Developmental disorder

F_{84} – Pervasive developmental disorders

$F_{84.0}$ – Childhood autism

$F_{84.1}$ – Atypical autism

$F_{84.2}$ – Rett's syndrome

$F_{84.3}$ – Other childhood disintegrative disorder

$F_{84.4}$ – Overactive disorder associated with mental retardation and stereotyped movements

$F_{84.5}$ – Asperger's syndrome

$F_{84.8}$ – Other pervasive developmental disorders

$F_{84.9}$ – Pervasive developmental disorder, unspecified

F_{88} – Other disorders of psychological development

F_{89} – Unspecified disorder of psychological development

F_{90} – F_{98} Behavioural and Emotional Disorder with onset usually occurring in Childhood and Adolescence

F_{90} – Hyper kinetic disorders

$F_{90.0}$ – Disturbance of activity and attention

$F_{90.1}$ – Hyperkinetic conduct disorder

$F_{90.8}$ – Other Hyperkinetic disorders

$F_{90.9}$ – Hyperkinetic disorder, unspecified

F_{91} – Conduct Disorders

$F_{91.0}$ – Conduct disorder confined to the family context

$F_{91.1}$ – Unsocialized conduct disorder

$F_{91.2}$ – Socialized conduct disorder

$F_{91.3}$ – Oppositional defiant disorder

$F_{91.8}$ – Other conduct disorder

$F_{91.9}$ – Conduct disorder, unspecified

F_{92} – Mixed Disorders of Conduct and Emotions

$F_{92.0}$ – Depressive conduct disorder

$F_{92.8}$ – Other mixed disorders of conduct and emotions

$F_{92.9}$ – Mixed disorder of conduct and emotions, unspecified

F_{93} – Emotional Disorders with onset Specific to Childhood

$F_{93.0}$ – Separation anxiety disorder of childhood

$F_{93.1}$ – Phobic anxiety disorder of childhood

$F_{93.2}$ – Social anxiety disorder of childhood

$F_{93.3}$ – Sibling rivalry disorder

$F_{93.8}$ – Other childhood emotional disorders

$F_{93.9}$ – Childhood emotional disorder, unspecified

F_{94} – Disorders of Social Functioning with Asset Specific to Childhood and Adolescence

$F_{94.0}$ – Elective mutism

$F_{94.1}$ – Reactive attachment disorder of childhood

$F_{94.2}$ – Disinhibited attachment disorder of childhood

$F_{94.8}$ – Other childhood disorders of social functioning

$F_{94.9}$ – Childhood disorders of social functioning, unspecified

F_{95} – Tic disorders

$F_{95.0}$ – Transient disorders

$F_{95.1}$ – Chronic motor or vocal tic disorder

$F_{95.2}$ – Combined vocal and multiple motor tic disorder (de la Tourettis syndrome)

$F_{95.8}$ – Other tic disorders

$F_{95.9}$ – Tic disorders, unspecified

F_{98} – Other behavioural and emotional disorders with onset usually occurring in childhood and adolescence

$F_{98.0}$ – Nonorganic enuresis

$F_{98.1}$ – Nonorganic encopresis

$F_{98.2}$ – Feeding disorder of infancy and childhood

$F_{98.3}$ – Pica of infancy and childhood

$F_{98.4}$ – Stereotyped movement disorders

$F_{98.5}$ – Stuttering

$F_{98.6}$ – Cluttering

$F_{98.8}$ – Other specified behavioural and emotional disorders with onset usually

$F_{98.9}$ – Unspecified behavioural and emotional disorders with onset usually occurring in childhood and adolescence.

Classification of Childhood Disorders based on Clinical Course

DSM-III-R classified the disorders in infancy, childhood and adolescence as follows:

Development Disorders

Such as mental retardation, pervasive developmental disorders and specific developmental disorders.

Disruptive Behaviour Disorders

Such as hyperactive and conduct disorders.

Anxiety Disorders of Childhood or Adolescence

Such as separation anxiety, avoidant behaviour and overanxious disorders.

Eating Disorders

Anorexia nervosa, Bulimia nervosa, pica and rumination disorders of infancy.

General Identity Disorders of Childhood

Such as transsexualism, gender identity disorders of adolescence or adulthood
- Tic disorders
- Elimination disorders
- Speech disorders
- Other disorders.

MENTAL RETARDATION (MR)

Mental Retardation is the common developmental disorder, the synonyms used for Mental Retardation are: 'Mental Deficiency/Mental Defectiveness/ Developmental Disabilities/Mental Handicap (UK)/Mental Sub-normality (Scotland)/ Mental Deficiency (England and Wales).

Definitions

'Significantly sub average general intellectual functioning resulting in or associated with current impairments in adaptive behaviour manifested during developmental period'.
– American Association on
Mental Deficiency (1983)

'A condition where intelligence is low and sub average learning and low performance'
—N Kesaree, S Kolli

'Persistent slow learning of basic motor and language skills (mile stones) and a significantly below normal global intellectual capacity as an adult'

'A condition of arrested or incomplete development of the mind, characterized by impairment of skills manifested during developmental period that contribute to cognitive, language, motor and social abilities.'
– ICD -10

Thus 'Mental Retardation is a developmental disorder (occurs below 18 years of age), characterized by impairment in cognitive ability (intellectual capacity), language, conative, social and personal adaptation'.

Incidence and Prevalence

- Three per cent of the world population is estimated to be mentally retarded. In India, more than 20 million children are suffering with mental retardation
- Boys are more suffering with mental retardation than girls
- Mortality is high in severe or profound mental retardation due to associated physical conditions
- Common in the age group of 2–3 years. Peak in 10–12 years of age.

Classification

Mental retardation can be measured by Intelligent Quotient levels (IQ) or Developmental Quotient levels (DQ), which denotes cognitive and functional ability.

$$IQ = \frac{\text{Mental age}}{\text{Chronological age}} \times 100$$

Types of mental retardation	
Degree of Mental Retardation	*IQ range in Mental Retardation*
Borderline (Feeble-minded)	70-90
Mild (Moron)	51-70
Moderate (Imbecile)	36-50
Severe (Imbecile)	21-35
Profound (Idiot)	0-20
Cretin-MR due to Hypothyroidism	—

(*Source*: Wechsler Adult Intelligence Scale)

'Adaptive Behaviour or Adaptive Functioning' is the skills needed to live independently. Structured interviews, scales, quality of behaviour needed skills, e.g. living skills, communication skills, etc. will also be used to measure the extent of Mental Retardation.

Types

Borderline Mental Retardation (Feeble–Minded) (70–90 IQ levels)

Early development is normal, low achievers, many of them belong to low socio-economic groups, history of drop outs from school, are able to lead independent life.

Mild Mental Retardation (Moron) (51–70 IQ levels)

Eighty five to Ninety per cent of total mental retardation cases belong to mild mental retardation. Environmental influences, psycho social deprivation, restrictive child rearing practices, malnutrition, low socio- economic class are the causes for mild mental retardation.

They have deficits in intellectual skills, studies upto 6–8th standard, problem in reading and writing; difficult in academic school work, normative living skills, walking, talking, toilet training, language abilities, development of domestic skills, behaviour, social and emotional adjustments like a normal person. Can fully adjust, educable, can learn motor skills better than verbal skills, finds difficulty in complex ideas, drawing generalization, can learn motor skills better than verbal skills and writing, emotionally they are stable, overactive, temper tantrum is common at times, can understand simple terms, they can be trained in special schools. Poor ability to abstract and ego centric thinking. In adult life most of them lead independent life in normal surroundings.

Moderate Mental Retardation (35–50 IQ levels, Imbecile)

Ten per cent of mental retardation cases belong to moderate mental retardation. Children can be 'trainable' aimed at 'self help skills', they can speak and support themselves, able to perform 'semi-skilled or unskilled work' under supervision, can learn few basic skills. Communication skills develops much slowly, limited progress in scholastic work, studies upto 2nd grade, unaware of needs, have less neuro pathological complications, partially dependent on others for their care.

Severe Mental Retardation (Imbecile, 21–35 IQ levels)

Seven per cent of total mental retardation cases, belongs to severe MR, slow motor development in preschool years, trainable for normal living activities, allow them to do daily living activities under supervision, contributes partially to self maintenance, some children may learn social behaviour, able to communicate in simple way, engaged in limited activities, delayed speech and communication skills.

Profound Mental Retardation (Idiot 0–20)

One-two per cent of all mental retardation cases are profound type. Considerable organic pathology, nervous system damage is noticed, associated conditions are: blindness, deafness, seizures are common, delayed mile stones, motor impairment, totally dependent, can not do anything on their own, death may occur due to variety of problems or complications.

Predisposing Factors

- Low socioeconomic strata or poverty
- Low birth weight of the child
- Advanced maternal age
- Consanguinity
- Extreme malnutrition
- Lack of stimulating environment
- Poor sensory experience
- Influence of bad role models
- Defective/low standard education due to defective scholastic environment
- Psychosocial disadvantage, e.g. poor health practices, poor housing, disuse of language, etc.
- Parental deprivation
- Exposure to under privileged environment
- Child abuse
- Prolonged isolation of care takers during developmental period
- Sensory deprivation and social deprivation.

Causes

Genetic Conditions

Abnormal genes will be inheriting from parents, errors when genes combine or for other reasons, e.g. Down syndrome, Fragile x syndrome, Phelan Mc Dermid syndrome, Mowat Wilson syndrome, Phenyl ketonuria, Trisomy x syndrome, Turner's syndrome, Cat's cry syndrome, Deletion syndromes, e.g. Prader Willi syndrome, Klinefelter's syndrome.

Biochemical Factors or Metabolic Disorders

Amino acids, e.g. Phenyl ketonuria, Maple's syrup urine disease, Hyperammonemia, Hartnup's disease, Homo-cystinuria; Glucose, e.g. Galactosemia, glycogen storage disease, Mucopolysaccharidosis, Gargoylism; Lipids, e.g. Taysach's Gaucher's, Niemann- Picks diseases; Purines, e.g. Lesch-Nyan syndrome; Mucopolysaccharides. For example, Hurler's syndrome; Miscellaneous. For example, Wilson's disease (copper), crystallinuria; Vitamin deficiency disorders.

Prenatal Causes

Physical damage. For example, injury, hypoxia, radiation, lead poisoning, placental dysfunctions, endocrinal disorders. For example, hypothyroidism, hypo parathyroidism, diabetes mellitus, malnutrition, anemia, hypertension, Rh incompatability, toxemias of pregnancy, abuse-smoking, alcohol, drugs.

Problem During Birth

Prematurity, low birth weight, hypoxia, problems during labour and birth. For example, not getting enough oxygen, brain damage results in developmental disability, prolonged or difficult birth, instrumental delivery, head injury, intraventricular haemorrhage, cord prolapse, growth retardation.

Perinatal Insults

Hypoxia, hypoglycaemia, hyper bilirubinaemia, meningitis, trauma, dehydration, encephalitis poisoning, drowning, status epilepticus.

Health Problems of Young Child

Whooping cough, measles, mercury and lead poisoning, post vaccinal encephalitis, bilirubin encephalopathy.

Sensory Deprivation

Environmental restrictions, isolation for long time, deprived parent-child interaction, deprivation of socio-cultural stimulation.

Miscellaneous Conditions

CNS malformation, neurogenetic syndromes, migration defects.

Brain Diseases

Tuberous sclerosis, neurofibromatosis, epilepsy, head injury, stroke, meningitis, congenital brain malformations, brain tissue damage, under-development of the brain.

    Cranial malformations

    Hydrocephalus, microcephaly

    Psychiatric condition

    Autism, Rett's syndrome, childhood schizophrenia, asperger's syndrome.

Altered Physiology/Clinical Manifestations

Limitations in adaptive capacity or ability, in self care, communication, self use, self direction, social skills, community use, health and safety, functional academics, leisure and work, deformities in hand or feet, failure to achieve age appropriate skills (developmental delays) to some degree in almost all areas.

In Infancy

- Poor feeding lead to poor weight gain, evidenced by uncoordinated sucking either breast or bottle
- Delayed visual alertness and curiosity
- Decreased or lack of auditory response
- Decreased spontaneous activity
- Delayed head and trunk control; delayed milestones
- Floppy or spastic muscle tone (hypotonic)
- Abnormalities in physical and neurological–unusual facial features (head too small or too large)
- Delayed development in motor skills–crawling, sitting, standing.

In Toddler

- Delayed independent living skills, sitting and ambulation
- Delayed communication failure to develop receptive and expressive language, delayed speech, slower to use words

- Disinterested or slow to learn, self care (feeding, dressing)
- Cognitive impairment–shorter attention span and distractibility
- Behavioural disturbance, clumsiness
- Impaired ability to communicate to others and control impulses.

Other Manifestations

- Seizures
- Lethargy
- Vomiting
- Abnormal urine odour
- Failure to feed and grow normally
- Behavioural problems, e.g. explosive out bursts, temper tantrums, aggressive behaviour, anxiety, depression.

Diagnosis

Multidisciplinary evaluation should be individually tailored to the child. A team of professionals like pediatric neurologist, developmental pediatrician, psychologist, social scientist, speech therapist, physical therapist, special educator, social worker and nurse, will evaluate the child.

- Complete history is collected from family members and care takers
- Mental history
- Physical examination to exclude physical illness
- Neurological assessment
- Assessment of mile stones like intellectual levels, cognitive ability, language pattern and communication skills, hearing, conative behaviour
- Urine and blood for metabolic products
- Hormonal studies–T3, T4, TSH
- Culture for biochemical studies
- EEG to exclude seizures, MRI, CT scan to study the structural abnormality of brain
- Antibodies for diagnosing infections, liver function tests in Wilson's disease
- Sensory test–assessment for vision, hearing

- Amniocentesis for pregnant mothers to detect chromosomal abnormalities, chronic villi sampling, chromosomal analysis
- Bayley scales (motor, language, visions) for 2 month–3 years; McCarthy scale (cognitive index), Stanford-Binet intelligence tests (mental abilities, 2 years and more; Wechsler intelligence scale for children (above 6 years); Vineland scale tests for social adaptive abilities (self help skills, self control, interaction with others, cooperation); child development inventories– to evaluate child's cognitive, verbal and motor skills
- Education evaluation–reading, writing, regularity in schooling, living-learning skills, daily living skills, social abilities
- Psychological investigation– personality assessment
- Parents also involved in answering developmental status observation tests.

Management

Multidisciplinary team will formulate treatment strategies. Team consists of psychiatrist, neurologist, developmental pediatricians, occupational and physical therapists, speech therapists, social workers, nurse, nutrition expert, educators and others (family).

Goals

- Develops a comprehensive, individualized programme for the child
- Provision of emotional support and counselling for parents and sibling of MR child
- Involve family as an integral part of the programme
- Provision of guidance, counselling services to the MR child and to the family
- Meet the needs of severe and profound MR child.

Overall Measures/Interventions

- If treatable cause is identified, treat the cause first
- Associated medical problem also has to be paid attention.

Institutionalization/Hospitalization

- 1/4 to 1/3 of severe and profound mentally retarded children may be in need of hospita-lization
- *Indications*: Behavioural difficulties like destructive, assaultive behaviour, psychosis, social factors, e.g. no one to look after, single parenthood, incompetent parents
- Consider the strengths, abilities and weaknesses of the mentally retarded child in determining what kind of support is needed
- Behavioural Modification Techniques, needed manipulation of environment, special schooling, etc. were developed to increase the adaptive behaviour to develop new skills and to provide guidance for parents and teachers
  Residential care: According to National Planning for mentally handicapped in India, 1979, New Delhi envisaged that, residential units are meant for profound MR cases with IQ levels below 25 or total dependents, functions of residential units are: to provide total personal care from birth to death, to provide comprehensive health care and recreational facilities, to render care for asso-ciated physical handicaps and other behavioural abnormalities, to provide vocational training through occupational therapy by engaging the child in productive work, to prevent secondary disabilities and prolonged institutionalization, sufficient training will be given to obtain productive or remunerative jobs, to foster the job satisfaction
- *Types and facilities of residential units for trainable (IQ 25-50)*: (a) Large institutions– dormitory type for accommodating the clients, useful for research purpose, more economical,

easy to look after (b) Cottage systems or colony of cottages: residential facility, provision of home like atmosphere (c) Day care homes : located in cities for looking after the children during day time

- *Staffing pattern in residential units:-* Psychiatrist (to assess and treat psychiatric and behavioural problems of the child), Clinical Psychologist (to assess potentialities and abilities of the child and to provide guidance and counselling), Pediatrician (to assess and treat clinical conditions of the child), Occupational Therapist (to train up the child occupational or vocational skills), Psychiatric Medico Social worker (to mobilize and help the child to utilize community resources and agencies), Psychiatric Nurse (to render care and to meet the total needs of the child) and other Para Medical Staff on full time basis

- *Services*: (1) Assessment: the abilities/potentialities, needs, weaknesses, developmental level, physical health, etc. of children will be assessed (2) Training: based on needs and requirements of children teaching, guidance, vocational training, speech training, needs fulfillment training, etc. will be planned and provided (3) Vocational services: boys–binding of books, printing, weaving, carpentry, chair canning, hair dressing, basket and mat making, poultry, gardening, leather work, candle making, hotel servers, drawing and art; for girls–cooking, laundry, home arrangement and management, knitting, craft work, dress making, home economics, etc. (4) Medical services: Treatment of minor ailments (5) Social services: identifying links between home and families, institutions, community and co-children (6) extra curricular activities: accompanying and taking care of the children in outing, picnics, tours

- *Programmes for the educable (IQ 50–75)*: A significant change can be made with proper education and vocational training to the mild

mentally retarded children, certain rehabilitation programmes are carried out to engage the child in useful activities, thereby he/she will be of helpful to the community by attaining productive status within the society

Sheltered work shops: Work oriented rehabilitative facilities, where mild mentally retarded children, who are capable of holding unskilled, semi skilled jobs will be trained up in controlled working environment.

Purposes

- Child will attain individualized vocational goals and become productive citizen whereby child can be able to lead normative living
- Potential behavioural problems can be prevented, as the child is engaged in work
- Care takers will be free from stress
- Child will be happy, as he can have free hand to spend money from his own earnings
- Expertise guidance and work experience can be provided
- Permits the child to develop work attitudes and acceptable occupational skills
- Provides self support by earning themselves by gaining working skills.

The Day Care Hospitals and Day Hospitals: Complete medical supervised treatment will be provided for mentally retarded child, where the child can travel and placed in day care centre in day time, free transportation facilities, with escorts will be provided to bring and leave the child from day care centres to house vice versa., the MR child continuous presence in home will not be there, thereby reduces more stress on family, allows the child to rest with family members in night time, the child activities can be supervised in day time by care takers, they can guide the child in therapeutic activities, excessive dependence over the hospital staff will slowly reduces, provides clarification and counselling services to the client and his family in rendering care for MR child.

Child Guidance Clinics: These clinics will be attached to paediatric and Psychiatric out patient departments in Medical Care Institutions; the services are: diagnoses and evaluates the condition of MR children, provides Counselling for parents and care takers, Disseminates knowledge and clinical training to the Health Care Professionals.

Mobile teams: Health Care Professional in teams visits the schools and screen the children for Mental Retardation, after identifying, grade them into categories, if needed refer them to the specialized services, Clinical Psychologist will provide counselling services to the children on developmental aspects, Health Educational Sessions will be conducted in schools, the topics like: behavioural problems among children and its prevention, early identification and seeking medical services and Advises, mile stones of children–common developmental aspects to be observed, care of mentally handicapped children and available rehabilitative services and needed interested topics also will be discussed.

Recreational therapeutic activities: Provide physical training, e.g. gymnastics, athletics and entertainment activities like music, dancing, reading, in door games, etc. socializes the client by engaging the child to participate in play and stimulates sensory and motor responses, promotes new interests suiting the needs and abilities of the client, healthy ambitions and trust will be developed.

Rehabilitation of mentally retarded children: It plays a vital role, based on level of intelligence, aptitude and abilities of the child rehabilitation activities will be planned. The child needs warmth, protection, love, affection, appreciation and occupational or vocational skills. Several rehabilitation centres were working to meet the total needs of MR children. In rehabilitation centres, the restoration and conservation of human resources can be made. The child will learn occupational skills in specific areas, based on the skills and achievement

in suitable job, child will be placed, after discharging into the community, the client will learn the regular working habits, sense of readiness, responsibility and confidence, etc. if he can works out, he can get pocket money to meet his/her needs on their own, remaining money will be kept in bank for future expenses. Adequate guidance and counselling services will be provided during training in rehabilitation centres.

Long leave: There is a provision for long leave up to 6 months, client can go from hospital to home and to the community, if the client exhibits controlled behaviour, care takers has to give consent stating that they will look after clients' welfare and can supervise clients' activities. When the client is on long leave, the Medico–Social Worker will visit the child and recommend either for continuity of trail or for total discharge from hospital or back to hospitalization.

Patient clubs: It provides a sense of loyalty and responsibility, sense of belonging to the organization stimulates and plans for future activities, attachment to fellow beings, motivates for good ideas, encourages to participate with other groups, provides an opportunity or media through which the MR children can interact other members in the community. In specific hours, clients are free either to attend or to leave the club. Weekly membership will be collected, refreshments will be served for the participants.

Industrial centres: Limited number of clients will be selected based on their abilities and potentialities the training, guidance, supervision of activities (semi skilled or skilled), will be done under controlled environment and these are regularized for 3–4 months. Clients will be helped to adjust to the new type of environment, later based on skills attained, the client will be recommended for suitable job.

Educational guidance: Characteristics of MR children, who needs special education are: slower rate of development, restlessness and easily distracted in the class room, not having interest in the material, lacks motivation, resulting in repeated failures, less mature, less proficient in motor skills, clumsy in fine motor coordination, can not enjoy crayons at preschool level, have language difficulties, shorter attention span, socially less adaptable, more self centred, less aware of other people, vigilant needs individual attention, difficulty in understanding, remembering and following the rules for the simplest games, etc.

Schooling: Education must be provided in the least restrictive, most inclusive settings, where the children have every opportunity to interact with non-disabled peers and have equal access to community resources.

- Observe the requirement of skills needed for the child in schooling, help the child to apply those skills even at home
- Teachers can identify the abilities and interests of the child, create opportunities for success
- Plan for Individualized Educational Programme, if necessary, talk to the specialists, identify effective methods of teaching, adapt suitable curriculum to reach the goal or higher end
- Be concrete and demonstrate as early as possible, provide hands on materials and experiences, opportunities to try the things out
- Teach the child to practice all steps one by one, if needed provide assistance
- Provide immediate feed back, appreciation, teach the child the Daily Living Activities, Social Skills, Occupational Awareness, Vocational Skills based on IQ levels of the child
- To meet the needs of the child talk with parents and to the child too.

Approaches: Academic force feeding drill is useful for the children older than 10 years, where the child will have difficulty in adjustment and developmental progress, posting of special teachers who has been trained up in taking care of MR children.

- Emphasizes the child development and adjustment; teacher has to be sensitive to the clients' needs, interested, well adjusted, dedicated, spends more time in child welfare, works for child's' improvement, have self control, tailoring of needs for individualized child, provides learning opportunities, life experi-ences, physical training, speech training, works for total development of the child, meeting hygienic needs of the MR children by "3R" principle, i.e. Repetition, Reinforcement, Rehearsal.
- Step wise training programmes will be conducted like: prevocational and vocational training, Home Bound employment, employment in sheltered work shops, complete employment
- In 1977, in Mumbai a one year training programme, for training graduate teachers in the education of physically handicapped children was started
- In India , many Rehabilitation Centres in various parts of the nation were launched to identify and provide rehabilitative services for mentally retarded children, e.g. CADABAMS, Association for Mentally Handicapped, Spastic Society, etc. in Bangalore were located.
- Library facilities: the MR child will be allowed to go to the library and read interested materials. Some times on the specific days, librarian will take the books on trolley to the wards, where the children will have the opportunity to pick up and choose the books of their own interest and read it.
- Scouts and Games: it inculcates the idea of providing service to the community, child will develop moral codes, controls their temperament, child will get an opportunity to participate in camps and get companionship, guidance from others, chance to move and stay for few days away from hospital.

Role of Parents and Family

- Family assessment is necessary, identify the family stressors, family coping abilities, suppor-

tive system and agencies, available recreational programmes, community agencies
- Having a child with severe disabilities at home requires dedicated care by the parents. Family involvement is essential in rendering care to the child. Provide good psychological support for both (to the family and to the child)
- Family has to meet the total needs of MR children, e.g. hygiene, counselling, support, etc.
- An individualized family service care plan has to be devised and the case manager has to be appointed to ensure that the interventions have been implemented, review discussions will be planned and revised periodically
- Medico Social worker can organize the services and assists the family, e.g. day care centres, house keepers, child care givers, etc.
- Motivate the child for independence for example, allow the child to perform Daily Living Activities, i.e. dressing, feeding, bathing, grooming, etc.
- Give child chores, e.g. keep in mind child's age, attention span, abilities, etc. break down the tasks into simple activities and motivate the child to do the activities one by one, assistance can be provided, if child needs help, give positive feed back, appreciate the child's abilities and efforts
- Help the parents to develop right attitude towards MR child, handle the guilty feelings of parents with due care
- Find the opportunity for the child in social activities, e.g. recreational activities, sports and games, etc. help the child to develop social skills, assist the child to develop the ability to make fun
- Educate the parents about the child's condition and discuss its prognosis good interaction, good interpersonal relationship and good social network
- Show other family who has MR children to share practical advice and emotional support (role modelling)

- Provide habit training for MR children to carry out essential activities, e.g. ADL.

Complications of Mental Retardation

- Seizures
- Cerebral palsy
- Sensory deficits
- Communication disorders (speech and language)
- Neuron degenerative disorders
- Psychiatric illnesses.

Prevention of Mental Retardation

Primary Prevention (Health Promotion and Specific Protection)

Good obstetric care–Meticulous Antenatal Care includes regular antenatal checkups, immunization against specific vaccines, e.g. Rubella, TT, if elderly pregnant woman (more than 35 years of age), advice the mother to have investigations like Amniocentesis, HIV testing, Ultra sound, Chorionic villi sampling, etc. to detect any chromosomal abnormalities or genetic defects of the foetus, Genetic Counselling, blood test for identification of venereal diseases if anything is identified advice the mother to go for termination of pregnancy or to follow medical advice, avoidance of alcoholism, smoking, drug abuse, exposure for teratogenic substances and radiation, adequate monitoring of mother and child, protection of pregnant mother and child from Rh incompatibility, promote institutionalized deliveries, utilizing advanced technology in delivery practices, good child maternal and child rearing practices, premature baby care, prevention of accidents and injuries, adequate feeding and supplementation of nutrients to the child to prevent metabolic disorders, educate the parents regarding the growth and developmental pattern of children for easy monitoring, better housing and living conditions for children, needed dietary restriction against identified diseases, utilization of Family Planning services.

Secondary Prevention (Early Diagnosis and Prompt Treatment)

Early recognition of diseases like metabolic, hormonal disorders and providing prompt treatment, prepare the parents and allow them to consider the option of abortion if needed, early intervention and training of the child by physiotherapy, training of the child for self help skills, compulsory usage of iodised salts, specialized schooling, provision of family support, plan for vocational training: work preparation, selective placement, post placement and follow-up, following protection measures against accidents and injuries, e.g. wearing seat belt, adequate treatment for emotional and behavioural difficulties, training of Behaviour Modification Techniques both for the child and his parents, e.g. positive reinforcement, shaping, prompting, role modelling, extinction, etc. teach innovative techniques for the child to enhance communication and language, implementation of varied therapeutic techniques as per medical advice.

Tertiary Prevention (Disability Limitation and Prevention of Complications)

Vocational training are given to develop vocational or occupational skills and social skills to the child to reduce the disability and provide optimal functioning. Utilizes rehabilitation measures adequately by the parents to prevent disability limitation.

Nursing Management of the Child with Mental Retardation

- Child has to be brought regularly to the clinic to assess developmental levels or mile stones, IQ levels, abilities, strengths, weaknesses, limitations/disabilities, concomitant psychological problems and needed guidance have to be provided based on their level of mental retardation
- Clarify the doubts of parents

- Provide moral support to accept the child and to involve actively in provision of care
- Handle gently the guilty feelings of the parents, explain the need of provision of affection, security, approval, positive attitude and concern to the child
- If any medical condition is associated, treat them adequately.

For Profound MR Children

- As they are totally dependent, teach or train-up them the basic survival skills very patiently
- Make the child to unlearn old habits and replace it by new one
- Provide habit training, e.g. hygienic care, sensory training for example, handling different textures, identifying colours and motor skill training, e.g. dressing, feeding
- If the child does any single task effectively, appreciate them for accomplished achievements
- Safe guard the child from physical dangers by keeping away the hazardous material
- Behaviour modification techniques has to be utilized
- Explain the parents not to over protect the child.

For Moderate MR Children

- Train the child for satisfactory living skills, e.g. ADL, routine procedures like following table manners, norms, gardening, cleaning, etc. protective measures against fire, traffic, water, assaults, etc.
- Encourage the child to speak simple phrases, rhymes, songs, etc. as he can cope up with short sentences
- Extensive attention, coaching has to be given for education, they can be able to perform minor educational activities under supervision
- The care takers has to allow their children to develop at their own rate without any rejection, or over protection or forcing them to achieve beyond their potential, encourage them to do the activities in their own pace

- Based on their capacities or the abilities needed vocational skill training has to be given, e.g. blacksmith, laundry, scrubbing, polishing, brushing, etc.

For Mild MR Children

- Training has to be given in socialization, vocational skills, social living skills, disciplinary principles, etc. which the child has to follow in future for their productive life
- Provide small jobs like cooking, cleaning, painting, gardening, printing, etc.
- 'Token economy' is of helpful for improvement among MR children
- If any problem arises, refer the child to 'Child Guidance Clinic' for further consultation and advice
- Protect the children from infections and environmental dangers like keeping hazardous material out of reach
- Make the child to learn and follow the social norms, practices, cultural norms, e.g. greeting others, modification of habits, hygienic way of handling or dealing with the things
- Meet the needs of children specifically psychological needs
- Teach the child only one aspect at a time, if possible demonstrate it, always advice them to practice it by following Maxims of Teaching like simple to complex, etc.
- Allow the child to participate group or social activities
- Develop necessary virtues to teach MR children, e.g. patience, repetition, modesty, genuine, positive attitude
- Organize guidance and counselling programmes to the parents of MR children, which are of great help to them
- Protect the MR children from teasing and taunting by other children
- Allow the child to perform uncomplicated productive tasks, if he /she does well, appreciate for accomplished outstanding performance.

Prognosis

A Multi Dimensional Therapeutic Approach is implemented in treating MR children. A vast improvement in Therapeutic Technology is in force throughout Globally. No longer MR children need hospitalization, except profound MR cases. By considering their developmental aspects (physical, psychological, social, cognitive, etc.) these children are brought into main stream along with other normative children. Presently various community agencies, rehabilitation centres (Nationally, Internationally) where specialized multidisciplinary team members are working for the welfare and better prognosis of MR children globally.

AUTISM

WHO, American Psychological Association classified 'Autism' as a developmental disability that results from central nervous system disorder. In 1943, Dr Leo Kanner labeled 'the autistic disturbances of affective contact' and early infantile autism. WHO in ICD-10, DSM 1V 290.00 section described autism, which manifests itself, 'before the age of 3 years', children are marked by delay in their social interaction, communication, symbolic or imaginative play, exhibits lack of interest in other people.

The word 'Autism' is derived from Greek word 'autos' means 'self'. In 1911, Swiss Psychiatrist, Eugene Bleuler first used the word, 'Autism' in American Journal of Insanity.

Definitions

'Qualitative impairment in social interaction, communication, restricted repetitive and stereo typed patterns of behaviour, interests and activities, delays in abnormal functioning'

—DSM 1V, 299.00 section

'A pervasive developmental disorder characterized by a total lack of responsiveness to people, gross language developmental deficits or distortions, bizarre responses to environmental aspects, e.g. resistance to change or peculiar interest in an animate or inanimate object'.

—*American Psychiatric Association, (1980)*

Incidence

It is a rare disorder (2–4 cases/1000), long term illness with a poor prognosis.
- Common in boys than in girls, in first born male
- Onset occurs before 30 months of age.

Predisposing Factors

- History of perinatal complications- maternal bleeding, meconium in the amniotic fluid, etc.
- Anoxia during pregnancy and delivery
- Drug abuse in pregnancy
- Maternal rubella infection, congenital rubella
- Phenyl ketonuria
- Encephalitis
- Meningitis
- Tuberous sclerosis
- Familial interpersonal factors
- Rett's syndrome and Fragile x syndrome.

Causes

- *Abnormalities in brain functioning,* e.g. Defects in temporal lobe and lateral lobe of brain, limbic system, purkinji cells in cerebellum, 3rd ventricle of brain and brain stem
- *Genetic component*: Monozygotic and dizygotic twins autism cases were observed, siblings of autistic children show a prevalence of autistic disorder
- *Biochemical factors*: Elevated plasma serotonin levels
- *Psychosocial factors*: Parental rejection, deviated personality, broken families, family stress, improper stimulation, defective communication pattern, lack of warmth and affection, aloofness, obsessive in nature, emotionally cold, parental deprivation, sibling conflicts.

Manifestations

- *Behavioural manifestations*: No reaction to physical contact, more ritualistic behaviour, preoccupied with one or more stereo typed behaviour, repetitive mannerisms related to parts of objects, intense or violent tantrums, aggressive or explosive behaviour, over active, uncooperative or resistant in nature, feels difficulty in regulating their behaviour resulting in crying, verbal out bursts, prone for self injurious, inappropriate behaviour poorly modulated behaviour, anxious, always feels stress, reacts negatively to the changes in their surroundings, extensive withdrawal in overwhelming situations, depressed, obsessions, compulsions, routines around foods, co morbid mood, dislikes being touched or kissed, no separation anxiety when kept in unfamiliar environment with strangers, empathy will not develop, spends a lot of time stacking objects, lining things up, putting things in a certain order.
- *Communication pattern*: Does not use speech to convey the message, delay in spoken language, lacks conversational skills, does not respond to his/her name, impairment in the use of multiple non-verbal behaviour, e.g. eye to eye contact, facial expression, body posture, gestures, stereo typed, idiosyncratic language, absence of imaginative activity, e.g. adult roles, story telling abnormality in the production and content of speech, impairment in the ability to initiate or sustain conversation with others.
- *Social behaviour*: Social smile remains as a reflex, non-responsive and disinterested in others, delay in social interaction, absence of social cues, doesn't smile when smiled at, little social alienation, feels difficulty in establishing friendship, poor peer interpersonal relationships, lacks communication and interpretation skills, poor in sharing enjoyment, interests or achievements with other people, lives in their own world, likes to live alone, passively accepts

cuddling, hugging, extensive withdrawal in overwhelming situations likes being in a well known place.

- *Sensory development*: Has poor eye contact, stares into open areas, doesn't focus on anything specific, doesn't follow directions, doesn't point or wave good bye; doesn't understand the concept of pointing, will look at the pointing hand rather than the object being pointed at. Some times seems to be deaf, tunes other people out, hands cover the ears often, unable to filter out sounds in certain situations, over sensitivity or under reactivity to touch, movement, sights or sounds. Physical clumsiness or carelessness, poor body awareness, easily distracted, impulsive physical or verbal behaviour, difficulty in learning new movements, difficulty in making transition from one situation to another, over responsive or unresponsive to sensory stimuli, difficulty in sensory integration.
- *Play activities*: Use toys in place of words, in a repetitive manner, flushes toilet over and over again, turn the light on and off, watch a toy spin for hours, lack of varied, spontaneous lay, social initiative play appropriate to developmental level, prefers to play alone, delay in symbolic or imaginative play, does not know how to play with others, attachments to toys, objects or schedules, pretends dislike in playing, shows unusual attachments to toys, objects or schedule.
- *Intellectual levels*: IQ levels are below 50 (40%), 70 or more (30%) resistant to transition and change.
- *Motor aspects*: Odd movement patterns, likes to spin around in a circle, walks on his toes, delay in motor skills, unusual repetitive motions or stemming, spends lot of time repeatedly flapping their arms or wriggling their toes, others suddenly freeze in position, perseveration, restricted activities, attachment to unusual objects, heightened pain threshold.

- *Effects on education*: Delay in academic achievement, learning difficulties.

Treatment

- Drug therapy, e.g. lithi , resperidone
- Behaviour therapy, e.g. contingency management, positive reinforcement, self care skills, role modelling
- Psychotherapy, e.g. counselling, supportive therapy
- Special schooling includes vocational training
- Residential treatment
- Cognitive therapy: patient education, self monitoring and self control method
- Social therapy: to enhance peer interaction, to make the child to be integrated in mainstream of social environment
- Teacher training–developing skills in handling autistic children.

Complications: Epileptic seizures.

Nursing Management

Assessment

Assess the intellectual ability, cognitive levels, communication skills, interaction pattern, social skills, language skills, motor skills, behaviour pattern, sensory development, ritualistic behaviour, play activities, etc. of autistic child. Family perception, emotional condition of care takers, interaction pattern among family members.

Goals

- To meet the total needs of children
- To promote and establish good interpersonal relationship
- To develop social skills, communication skills, interpersonal skills
- To protect the children from harming themselves and to others
- To provide emotional support to the entire family.

Interventions

- Serve the child one to one basis
- Meet the child's basic human needs, as the child may not be able to verbalize, nurse has to be aware of those needs and set up routine and meet them, e.g. hydration, nutrition, elimination and rest, etc.
- Utilizes and teaches certain "behaviour modification techniques", formulates schedule and fix up the activities
- Encourage the child to do the activities on his own, e.g. dressing, hygienic needs
- Educates the 'self care techniques' to the child
- Provide moral support to the parents as they were very anxious, depressed and feeling guilty, clarify their doubts and try to involve them in meting child's needs, as they play an integral and vital role in providing care to the child
- Permit limited number of caregivers to ensure warmth, acceptance, affection and availability to the child
- Teaches the parents about the disease and it's prognosis, so that they will be able to work with him at the appropriate developmental level
- Teach the child the signs, symbols, eye contact (non-verbal)
- Demonstrate 'communication skills', 'social skills'. Teach the importance of establishing and maintaining good interpersonal relationship
- Encourages, appreciates the child, ensures positive and social reinforcement to the child for the exhibition of desirable behaviour, e.g. touching, cuddling, hugging
- Motivates the child to express or to communicate his needs verbally
- Clarifies and makes the child to interpret his behaviour
- Provide the 'language training' to the child, e.g. verbs, objects and show action or motion what it means, then he will follow it easily
- Help the child to learn creative activities, e.g. drawing, art, mirroring
- Ensure security and diversion to the child

- Give familiar objects to the child, e.g. blanket, toy, etc. to feel comfortable
- Assist the child to learn their own body parts
- Protect the child from injuries and hurting others
- Administer the medications as prescribed
- Make the child to adjust socially to the environment.

SELECTIVE MUTISM
(ICD-10 F94.0, ICD-9 309.83, 313.23)

Selective Mutism is a social anxiety disorder to reflect the involuntary nature of this disorder, in 1994 the former name 'Elective Mutism' has been changed into 'Selective Mutism'. It is a rare psychological disorder, children are totally capable of speaking and understanding the language, but fail to speak in certain social situations, when it is expected of them. They are able to function normally in other areas of behaviour and learning, appear to be severely withdrawn and unwilling to participate in group activities. Some times it denotes extreme form of shyness; but intensity and duration will distinguish in other areas. For example, a child who may be silent in school for years or with strangers but speaks excessively and freely at home or with close friends.

Incidence

Seven in 1000 children, common in girls than in boys.

Causes

- Hereditary
- Pervasive developmental disorder
- Psychotic disorder.

Frequency: The duration of disturbance is atleast one month.

Characteristics

- Consistent failure to speak in specific social situations not due to lack of knowledge or comfort with, the spoken language required in social situations

- Disturbance interferes with educational or occupational achievement or with social communication
- Results in higher anxiety levels
- The behaviour is often viewed externally as willful or controlling, as the child usually shuts down all communication and body language in such situations
- Find it difficult to maintain eye contact
- Often will not smile and have blank expression
- Move stiffly and awkwardly
- The child find situations where talk is normally expected to handle, e.g. saying hello, good bye, thank you, etc.
- They tend to worry about things more than others
- Sensitive to noise and crowds
- Find it difficult to talk about themselves or express their feelings, and their body language perceived as, 'rudeness'
- They have good intelligence, perception, inquisitiveness, sensitive to others' thoughts and feelings, i.e. empathy
- Possess justice skills (able to differentiate right and wrong, good/bad/fairness
- Able to concentrate, focussed.

Treatment

Based on age of the child and other factors.
- A change of environment, e.g. changing schools, where the condition of the child not known will make the difference
- *Stimulus fading*: Used in children, the suffering child is brought into a controlled environment with someone, whom they are at ease with and can communicate, gradually another person is introduced into the situation involving a number of small steps
- Sliding technique is used, where a new person is slide into the tackling group, which can take a long time for the first one or two faded

- *Desensitization*: The child is allowed to communicate via non-direct means, e.g. phone, web chat
- Drug therapy: Antidepressants, e.g. fluxetine (prozac) may be effective
- Behaviour therapy, family therapy, demonstration of effective communication behaviour, individual psychotherapy and counselling technique are of helpful.

SPEECH DISORDERS

Signs of Problems in Language and Speech Development

6 months: Will not respond to sounds coming from side or behind (does not turn eye and head)

10 months: Will not respond for his name

15 months: Will not understand and respond for 'bye-bye' or 'no-no'

18 months: Does not have a vocabulary of 10 words

21 months: Does not respond to direction or instruction

24 months: Will not use 2-word phrases repeats spoken word incorrectly

30 months: Has speech, i.e. not intelligible to any family member

36 months: Has not started to ask any simple question or unable to use simple sentences

Has speech that is not intelligible to strangers.

42 months: Consistently falls to produce final consonants

After 4 years: Stutters/dysfluent

After 7 years: Has speech sound errors

At any age: Monotonous voice, inappropriate pitch, loud or not audible
- Quality of voice should be assessed, e.g hoarseness or whispered
- Is the pitch of the voice is normal for that age or not

- Articulation of voice; child's speech should be intelligible by three years of age
- *Fluency*: Between 2–6 years of age, majority of children will have dysfluent speech, e.g. repeating the beginning of words or whole words or syllables slow
- If bilingual household, usually slow in speech occurs
- Certain times children will follow their elders way of communicating
- Usually eating difficulties will be associated with speech difficulties.

Management

- Counselling and reassurance of parents is essential as the parents were emotionally disturbed and worried for child stuttering problem
- Ask the parents to avoid competition with other children of same age group and undue comparison frequently
- Primary stuttering and non-fluent speech of a young child (between 2–5 years of age) can be neglected as it may pass off as the childs' age is progressing. Parents should be advised, not to show undue attention, concern, pressurize the child to repeat or to correct or to become conscious of his problem
- The children with secondary stuttering should be given emotional support and to seek professional guidance, i.e. speech-language therapist or language pathologist for achieving adequate communication skills
- Educate the parents about:
  - The factors stressors predisposing for communication disorders
  - Signs of delay in language and speech development
  - The child with stuttering problem will not have any defect in their intelligence levels and stuttering is reversible
  - Encourage the family to have prompt follow-up care for any voice changes or ear infections, early interventions are required

- Child should be supplemented with proper nutrition and rest
- The child should be helped to lead normal life
- Encourage the child to expand sentences which aids in language acquisition
- Promote personal growth, self esteem and confidence among child
- Help the parents to resolve conflicts and recognize the need for consistent discipline as it can decrease the child's emotional stress
- Encourage the parents to speak, act and proceed the family activities in a relaxed manner and to avoid stress
- Promote slow, quiet rhythmic physical activities, e.g. listening to music will calm up the excitement of child
- Answer to the childs' questions honestly, never talk to the child sarcastically
- Prevention of communication disorders begins with effective prenatal care, prompt follow-up care and stimulating child's speech will decreases delay in language development.

CLUTTERING
(ICD-10, $F_{98.6}$; ICD-9, 307.0)

It is a language and communication disorder. In 1960, the term, 'cluttering' has been changed 'Tachyphemia', derived from Greek word, means 'fast speech'. It is outward manifestation of central language imbalance.

Characteristics

- Speech, i.e. difficult for listeners to understand due to rapid speaking rate, erratic rhythm, poor grammar and words or groups of words unrelated to sentence
- Shorter attention span, poor concentration
- Poor organized thinking
- Inability to listen, lack of awareness
- No problem for putting thoughts into words, but those thoughts become disorganized during speaking

- Most clear at the start of utterances, but their speaking rate increases and intelligibility decreases towards the end of utterances, e.g. I want to go for shopping to buy flowers, the clutters will say, I want to go for shopping to buy a…….. bunch of fl…..owers
- Shared speech, especially dropped or distorted sounds and monotonous speech that starts loud and trails off into a murmur
- Disorderly/messy hand writing, hasty, repetitions, uninhilated poorly integrate in ideas and space
- Unaware of the disorder
- Performs better when speaking under stress
- Gives long answers
- Careless in speech, effortless, no fear to speak, do not know exactly what they want to say it any way
- Typically outgoing or extroverted
- Not fluent in speech
- Disorganized, tangential, grammatically incorrect speech with word substitutions
- Impatient listeners, frequently interrupt and have poor turn taking skills in conversation.

Treatment

- 'Delayed auditory feed back' is used to produce a more deliberate, exaggerated oral-motor response pattern
- Story telling: to improve narrative structure, to relieve distress, to teach new coping skills, appropriate problem solving techniques and moral values, as children will not separate imaginary experiences from real experiences, and correlates everything to the real life, this technique is of helpful. Story should have illustrations and content that tend to explore, how to cope-up with everyday situation
- Showing picture books
- Language therapy, turn taking practice, pausing practice, etc. may be of helpful.

FLUENCY DISORDERS

Speech is a complex process which requires perfect coordination between various neuromuscular factors. Clarity of speech gradually improves and complete development of speech occurs by four years of age. If neuromuscular coordination is disturbed, an abnormal flow of speech results with impaired rate and rhythm in speech pattern.

Unclear Speech

If the child have a major disorder of language, cognitive development or hearing, it develops unclear speech and language based on learning disabilities later in school years.

Stuttering/Stammering

It is a communicative/speech disorder, occurs in 1 per cent of total children. The flow of speech is disrupted by involuntary repetitions and prolongation of sounds, syllable, words or phrases, involuntary, silent pauses or blocks in which the stutter is unable to produce sounds.

Causes

- Genetic
- Neuro pathology
- Neural schizophrenia
- Less blood flow to the broca's and Wernicke's area
- Anxiety or stress situations.

Onset and Development (refer below table)

Phase	Description	Age
I	• Disfluencies tend to be single syllable, whole word or phrase repetitions, interjections, pauses and revisions • The child will not exhibit visible tension, frustration or anxiety, when speaking disfluently	2-6 years

contd...

contd...

Phase	Description	Age
	• Normal disfluency will occur when the child is learning to walk or refining motor skills • Periods (days or weeks) of fluency and disfluency • Changes in the child's environment can cause normal disfluency	
II	• Disfluencies tend to be repetitions and sound prolongations • More than two disfluencies put together ('chaatu s-g-go there') and periods of fluency and disfluency come and go in cycles • The child demonstrates little awareness or concern about his/her Disfluencies but may express frustration	2-6 years
III	• Disfluency most commonly occurs at the beginning of words or phrases • The child tends to be more dysfluent when excited or upset • Repetitions are usually part word as opposed to whole word • The stuttering comes and goes in cycles, sometimes triggered by events and stressors • The child may show awareness that speech is difficult in addition to the frustration	2-6 years
IV	• Types of Disfluencies include repetitions, prolongations and blocks • Stuttering becomes chronic, without periods of fluency • Secondary behaviours appear (eye blinking, limb movements, lip movements, etc.) • Stuttering tends to increase when excited, upset or under some type of pressure • Fear and avoidance of sounds, words, people or speaking situations may develop • The person may feel embarrassment or shame surrounding stuttering	6-13 years

contd...

contd...

Phase	Description	Age
V	• Speech is characterized by frequent and noticeable interruptions • The person may have poor eye contact and use various tricks to disguise the stuttering • Person anticipates stuttering, fears and avoids speaking • The person identifies him/herself as a stutterer and experiences frustration, embarrassment or shame • The person may attempt to choose a lifestyle where speaking can often be avoided	14 +

Characteristics

• Frequent repetition or prolongation of sounds, syllables or words with hesitation and pauses that interrupts speech. They usually disfluent on initial sounds, when beginning to speak and become more fluent towards the end of utterances, struggle in their behaviour, e.g. over tense speech production, in the beginning of sentences, they have difficulty, e.g. I wa.... Wa..... want to go for shop.

• These children are aware of the disorder, performs better, when speaking under stress

• Have a hard time, fluently giving short answers, inhibited, neat hand writing

• Fearful of their own speech, abnormal hesitation or pausing before, typically withdrawn, shy, introvert

• Feeling loss of control during speech

• Know exactly what they want to say, but can not say it

• Organized speech, effective listening skills

• Stuttering will not have any impact over intelligence

• Stuttering is variable, e.g. some times to talk in certain situation they may face severe difficulty, in other time, they may have fluency in speaking

• A stutter is exacerbated when the child is excited, upset or under some type of pressure

- Disfluency in speech includes repetitions, prolongations, blocks, pauses
- Secondary motor behaviours, e.g. eye blinking, lip movements, etc. may be used during moments of frustration or stuttering
- Child will feel shame, embarrassment, fear, avoidance of sounds, words, people
- By 14 years, the stutter is classified as 'Advanced Stutter' characterized by frequent, noticeable interruptions, poor eye contact and uses various tricks to disguise the stuttering
- If people are identifying them as 'stutters', they will develop deeper frustration, embarrassment and shame
- Core stuttering behaviours include disordered breathing, phonation, articulation (lips, jaw, tongue), these muscles are over tensed, making speech difficult or not possible
- Avoidance behaviour.

Types

- Mild stuttering or non-chronic stutter or situational stuttering: difficulty in speaking in isolated situations or stressful conditions, 10 per cent disfluency in speaking, spontaneously recovers
- Chronic or severe stuttering: frequent and long in duration, visible signs of struggle and avoidance behaviour often they are accompanied by strong feelings and emotions in reaction to the emotional problems, e.g. hatred, shame, fear, 15 per cent disfluency in speech, experiences difficulty when communication is required, muscle tensing up, facial and neck tics, excessive eye blinking, lip and tongue tremors, body movements, inability to maintain eye contact with the listener.

Treatment

An integrated approach to stuttering and tailor therapy to each individual's needs

- Fluency shaping therapy: trains stutterers to speak fluently by relaxing their breathing, vocal folds and articulation (lips, jaw and tongue) in speech clinics first, then transferred to daily life outside
- Stuttering modification therapy: to modify one's moments of stuttering
  - Identification of core behaviours, secondary behaviours, feelings and attitudes that characterizes stuttering
  - Desensitization: freezes core behaviour, tells people that he is a stutter
  - Modification/easy stuttering–cancellations– stopping in a disfluency, pausing few moments and saying the word again
  - Stabilization: the stutterer prepares practice assignments makes preparatory sets and pull outs automatic, changes his self concept by speaking fluently
- Drug therapy- anti-stuttering medications: Haloperidol, as it has severe side effects, not in use, Risperidone and Olanzapine reduces stuttering (33–50%) with less side effects, Dopamine agonists, e.g. Ritalin, selective serotonin reuptake inhibitors, e.g. Prozac, Zoloft, etc. increases stuttering, hence contraindicated
- Anti-stuttering Devices: speaking in chorus with another person or hearing one's voice echo in a well. Common types of altered auditory feedback are:
  - Delayed auditory feedback- delays the user's voice in his ear, a fraction of a second
  - Frequency shifted auditory feedback- changes the pitch of the user's voice in his ear
  - Masking auditory feedback - Produces a synthesized sine wave in the user's ear at the frequency at which the user's vocal folds are vibrating.

MOVEMENT DISORDERS

Mannerisms

The children after completing 3 years of age, curious, to be independent, curious to learn and this is the time, we have to teach them the manners, ethical codes and behaviour, which has to be exhibited. Children are always happy and living in their own world, content with their life and the things around them, at times children will have mood swings, they feel that they do not get enough attention from their parents. Certain times child exhibits voluntary, repetitive, stereo typed, rhythmic movements without any underlying organic pathology or any other psychiatric condition. The movements like body rocking, hair pulling, twisting, mannerisms, temper tantrums, etc. will be performed when his emotional needs were not fulfilled or to catch hold the attention of parents.

Methods to deal with children in their mood swings and mannerisms

- Parents has to be flexible to a certain extent.
- Give them various choices of handling things, teach various ways, in which they can do their tasks and behave well.
- Identify the stressor, divert the child from painful stimuli, e.g. change the environment to improve his mood or divert his mind by involving him in play activities, offer some toys to play.
- If the child cribs meaninglessly, parents has to pretend that it never happened, so that the child will understand, his behaviour has no effect on the parent and ultimately he will give up the cribbling behaviour.
- When the child is 3–6 years of age, he will be extremely keen observant and receptive, grasps everything very fast. This is the age, the parents have to foster good behaviour and thoughts in child's mind, the child will maintain it through-out or the rest of the life.
- Based on the child's temperamental level, provide guidance to the children to learn etiquette behaviour; parents has to show love, support and concern for the child at all times.
- Provide stimulation to the child, cut jokes, share attention and love to them, to enhance trust and with the parents.

- Try to understand child's needs and encourage him to enjoy the life. Never force the children into unnecessary hobbies and interests.
- Make the child to understand his own strengths and weaknesses, if it is desirable or acceptable behaviour, parents have to enforce or promote their interest.
- Encourage the children to develop new hobbies and interests, let them divert their mind by playing with toys.
- Parents have to set themselves as role models, children will learn through imitation and practice.

TIC DISORDER

Definition

'Sudden, abnormal, involuntary, rapid, repetitive and purposeless contraction of a small group of muscles involving face, throat and shoulder'.

Incidence and Prevalence

Tic disorders are transcient or chronic in nature, they may appear as early as 2 years to 21 years of age, more common in males about 3 times, prevalence rate is 0.5/1000 population.

Causes

- Psychogenic, e.g. tension producing behaviour, stress
- Neurogenic, e.g. complication of encephalitis
- Familial, e.g. Tourette's disorder
- Substance abuse
- Physiological, e.g. fatigue due to illnesses
- Medical conditions, e.g. Huntington's disease.

Classification

Tic disorder
1. Motor tics
   a. Simple Motor tics. For example, Eye blinking, eye twitching, grimace.

b. Complex Motor tics. For example, Gesture, obscene acts.
2. Vocal tics
   a. Simple Vocal tics, e.g. Coughing, Barking, throat clearing.
   b. Complex Vocal tics. For example, Echholalia, Coprolalia (Uttering obscene words and phrases).
   Chronic/complex tics. For example, Gilles De La Tourette's syndrome.

Causes: Idiopathic, autosomal dominant disorder

Incidence: Occurs before the age of 13 years.

Manifestations

- Vocal tics, e.g. grunts, barks, sniffs, echolalia, coprolalia
- Complex vocal tics have more organized pattern
- Multiple motor tics
- Learning difficulties
- Neurological signs: hyperactivity

Diagnosis: EEG- abnormal evoked potentials
Abnormal CT brain findings.

Treatment

Drug therapy: Haloperidol 0.5–6 mg OD or Pimozide 1–10 mg OD or Cloridine 0.05–0.25 mg OD.
Behaviour modification therapy as adjunct therapy.
Individual and family counselling as adjunct therapy.

Prognosis: Transient tics have better prognosis, chronic tics have prolonging in nature, continues up to adulthood.

Nursing Management

- Provide supportive and empathetic environment
- Improve social relationship, enhance situational support
- Client education and counselling
- Promote self esteem, self confidence of the client by implementing positive behaviour modification techniques and comprehensive nursing process.

ATTENTION DEFICIT HYPERACTIVITY DISORDER (ADHD)

ADHD is the most common disorder of childhood is characterized by 'deficits in attention, concentration, activity level and impulse control'. ADHD children frequently experience peer rejection and engage in a broad array of impulsive and disruptive behaviour with negative consequences on self esteem and adaptive coping. Morbidity and disability often persist into adult life.

Aetiology

- Genetic predisposition–It is believed that ADHD results from the combined effects of several genes and interactions with the environment. In the genes the neurotransmitter levels, e.g. dopamine, norepinephrine (catecho-lamine) which are helpful for modulation of attentional circuits will impaired results in impaired attention regulation.
- Prefrontal, parietal and temporal association cortices and their projections to the striatum have core ability to focus attention and motor ability. In extreme stress cases alteration in neuro transmitter levels impairs prefrontal cortical functioning.
- Behaviour dis-inhibition results in problems with memory, self regulation of affect, motivation, arousal, capacity for reasoning and reflection. Goal directed behaviour.
- Neuro developmental difficulties related to activation, focus, sustaining effort, modulating emotions, utilizing working memory and regulating behaviours.
- Early neuro developmental problems, e.g. obstetric complications, prematurity, foetal distress, genetic abnormalities.

- Intrauterine exposure to toxic substances, e.g. alcohol, cocaine, smoking, etc. foetal insults may cause subtle functional abnormalities in the frontal cortex and other brain structures.
- Neuronal environmental interactions affects efficiency of brain functioning.
- Psychosocial adversity in infancy.
- Disorganized or chaotic environment disruption in family equilibrium.
- Disruption in bonding during the first three years of life.

Clinical Features

Inattention

- Makes careless mistakes in school work
- Difficulty in organizing tasks or play activities
- Not listen when spoken to directly
- Does not follow instructions, fails to finish school work
- Reluctant to engage in tasks that require sustained mental effort
- Easily distracted by extraneous stimuli
- Forgets in daily activities.

Hyperactivity/Impulsivity

- Runs about or climbs excessively in situations, in which it is inappropriate
- Feelings of restlessness
- Difficulty in playing or engaging in leisure activities
- Often talks excessively
- Often gives answers before questions have been completed
- Has difficulty in awaiting turn
- Interrupts others
- Impairment in cognitive tasks can be observed before 7 years
- Impairment in social, academic or occupational functioning.

Clinical Course

- ADHD is a chronic disorder leads to a negative impact on child's functioning throughout the life cycle
- ADHD children exhibits impaired academic functioning, poorly performs cognitive tasks, lower self esteem and poor social functioning
- High School drop outs or less education levels
- Lower occupation rankings at 25 years of age
- Increased risk for developing antisocial personality disorder and substance abuse disorders in adulthood.

Diagnosis

- Collect history from parents, teachers and other children
- Physical examination
- Assist in investigative procedures
- Identify the causative factors, assess comor bid patterns.

Treatment

Goals

- To improve attention span and learning ability
- To control hyperactive behaviour
- ADHD is a complex disorder affecting every area of functioning and there by requires a comprehensive treatment programme.

Treatment Includes Psychosocial Treatments
- Parental guidance
- Counselling.

Intensive support
- Psycho education includes:
  1. Intensive support and
  2. Education of the family
- Class room interventions
- Contingency management
- Social skills training
- Cognitive behaviour therapy
- Individual psychotherapy

- Ongoing therapeutic alliance between the therapist, the child and family to ensure collaboration in the complex task of helping child to achieve optimal functioning
- School interventions, ensure appropriate learning needs; teacher guidance; provision of conducive environment to optimize child's learning
- Behavioural management plan–Positive reinforcement on desired work habits, social skills groups
- Special educational services.

Medications

- Principles of pharmacotherapy–begin with one medication slowly titrating medications dosages up as needed until optimal effectiveness is achieved with minimal side effects
- Monitor and record vital signs, height and weight
- Central nervous system stimulants: stimulant medications successfully treat ADHD, but to relieve comorbid symptoms (depression), this, antidepresent drugs will be given
- First line, e.g. dexadrine 2.5 mg/day Ritalin–5–10 ml/day (methylphenidate).

Dextroamphetamine

Second line
- *Atomoxetine*: Bupropion; ventafaxine (to decrease suicidal tendency among adolescents)
- TCAS: Nortriptyline, desipramine, imipramine Clonidine at HS to produce sleep (catapres), Guanfacine (Tenex) (enhance cognitive functioning in the prefrontal cortex) considered when most other medications are ineffective:
- MAOIS: Pheneizine, selegine, pemoline (cyclert)
- Atypical antipsychotics: Risperidone, olanzapine
- Typical antipsychotics: haloperidol, thorazine. Antipsychotics are helpful in treating the agitation and aggression of ADHD children.

EATING DISORDERS

Introduction

Eating is controlled by several factors like physical health, voluntary control, appetite, habits, family cultural pattern, peer group influence and food availability. Eating disorders are treatable medical illnesses in which certain maladaptive patterns of eating observed and involves serious disturbances in eating behaviour includes extreme and unhealthy reduction of food intake or severe or over eating; as well as distress feelings or extreme concern about body shapes, weight and body image. Many affected individual initially appear to function normally but it can cause significant physical and emotional turmoil. Eating disorders frequently occur with other psychiatric disorders such as depression, substance abuse and anxiety disorders. However, eating disorder includes alteration in eating pattern, dieting (skipping the meals, fasting) perfectionism, etc.

Eating disorders frequently develop during adolescence or early adulthood. Cases were reported even during childhood or later in adulthood also. Females are much likely to develop the eating disorder than males.

Classification (ICD-10; $F_{50-50.9}$)

$F_{50.0}$– Anorexia nervosa
$F_{50.1}$– Atypical Anorexia Nervosa
$F_{50.2}$– Bulimia Nervosa
$F_{50.3}$– Atypical Bulimia Nervosa
$F_{50.4}$– Overeating associated with other psychological disturbances
$F_{50.5}$– Vomiting associated with other psychological disturbances
$F_{50.8}$– Other eating disorders
$F_{50.9}$– Eating disorder unspecified.

Causes

- Genetic
- Biological
- Psychological
- Socio-cultural factors

- Altered functioning pattern of an individual
- Secondary to medical disorders–endocrinal metabolic disturbances, electrolyte imbalances.

Specific disorders and its causes, clinical manifestations, investigations, treatments is described accordingly.

GENERAL TREATMENT MODALITIES OF EATING DISORDERS

Eating disorders are treatable and restoration of weight can be possible. Early diagnosis and prompt treatment has shown good prognosis or better outcomes. Eating disorder requires a comprehensive treatment plan includes monitoring, psychosocial interventions, medical care, nutritional counselling and drug therapy. At a time of diagnosis, the clinician must determine whether the person requires immediate hospitalization or can overcome difficulty or can be treated as out patient cases.

People with eating disorders often do not recognize or admit that they are ill. As a result, they may strongly resist getting and staying in hospital for treatment. Family members can be of helpful in ensuring that the person with an eating disorder receives needed care and rehabilitation.

- Effective communication techniques are used to win the confidence and to establish and maintain effective therapeutic nurse patient relationship
- Nurses have to provide conducive environment in dealing with the client, always nurses have to be judgemental, non-threatening and non-punitive manner, so that the client will be at ease while communication; Encourage the client to express their views freely without any inhibitions or hesitation
- Nurses have to show positive role models to the client
- Explain the client about treatment plan, orient them to unit staff, policies and procedures to be followed, what the unit expects from them, what they can obtain from the unit

- Prepare structured schedules and make a contract with the client about behavioural agreement
- Provide consistent communication with the client
- Manipulate the clients' environment to have desirable behaviour (Milieu therapy)
- Nutritionist will prepare the 'specific menu plans' and discusses with the client and to the unit staff. Encourage the client to keep dietary log noting the type and amount of food consumed, associated thoughts and feelings related to food
- Unit activities includes–community meetings, family therapy, group therapy, stress management, recreational therapy, interpersonal therapy, etc.
- Privilege systems will be planned and implemented when his condition improves and regains the normal eating pattern. For example, for bulimia nervosa cases–unsupervised bathroom visits, unrestricted activities, unsupervised eating meals, etc.
- Cognitive approaches (e.g. problem solving techniques client education dietary logs; self monitoring and self control, assertiveness techniques, etc.) will be used to modify psychopathology; to regulate the feeding pattern, to correct the misbelieves and preconceptions or myth related to body image, body structure and food, etc.
- Behavioural approaches like role modeling, shaping, reinforcement, etc. techniques will be used to modify the eating pattern or habits
- Interpersonal therapies will be used to modify the eating pattern or habits
- Interpersonal therapies will be used to correct the strained interpersonal relationships
- Individual psychotherapy, in which guidance and counselling services will be provided to the client to alter the thinking processes and to practice healthy eating pattern.

Family Therapy

- Family therapist will focusses the family to develop good family interactions and assists the client to adopt to the family environment and resolves the conflicts if any.

Group Therapy

- It provides deeper insight into the feelings and behaviour supportive groups or self help groups will be of helpful in providing constructive/ moral support and positive feedback.

Drug Therapy

- Based on behavioural manifestations, appropriate medications will be used to modify symptomatology and to regain healthy life style.

NURSING MANAGEMENT OF THE CLIENT WITH EATING DISORDERS

1. Nursing Diagnosis

Altered nutritional balance related to eating practices and food consumption.

Goal

To maintain weight and nutritional status of the client.

Interventions

- Check and record the weight of the client
- As per nutritionist guidance explain the specific menu, nutrients requirements, benefits, consumption pattern to the client
- Prepare therapeutic contract and schedule
- Set realistic goals related to weight (either to reduce or to regain)
- Counsel the client on healthy eating habits.

2. Nursing Diagnosis

Anxiety related to body image, structure, myths and pseudo-beliefs associated with it.

Goal

Relief from anxiety, participates actively in the treatment regimen.

Interventions

- Encourage the client to develop compensatory behaviour which has to be adopted
- Guidance and counselling services has to be planned for modifying the eating pattern, and to overcome the myths and beliefs associated with it
- Teach factual information to the client related to food practices, exercises, coping strategies and behaviour modification techniques.

3. Nursing Diagnosis

Inadequate cooing strategies related to eating behaviour.

Goal

The client will be able to express his feelings overtly.

Interventions

- Identify the stressors predisposing the altered behavioural pattern
- Teach problem solving techniques, strategies to overcome maladaptive eating behaviour
- Teach relaxation techniques, diversional activities, activity therapeutic measures, clarify the boundaries and doubts related to it
- Encourage the client to develop positive attitude in the eating pattern.

4. Nursing Diagnosis

Altered family thought processes related to clients' eating habits and alteration in body weight and shape of the child.

Goal

To develop clear understanding in imple-mentation of therapeutic nutritional plans and adopts change in eating practices; attains positive attitude in providing support to the client.

Interventions

- Guidance and counselling services to the family
- Teach adoptive/coping strategies to be implemented by the family members, accepts the suggestions and follows it for clients' welfare
- Provide empathetic support and guideline to improve the clients' condition.

OBESITY

Introduction

Obesity is considered as a symbol of wealth and social status in some European cultures. It serve more a visible signifier of 'lust for life'. It is also seen as a 'symbol' within a system of 'prestige'. Obesity is described in ICD-10, E_{66}; ICD-9, 278. It is a condition in which the natural energy reserve stored in the fatty tissue. It is a clinical condition viewed as a serious public health problem. Obesity is an epidemic in the United States and in other developed countries. Obesity means accumulation of excess fat in the body, and it is considered as a chronic disease. More than half of American adults are overweight, nearly 1/3rd children (1–5 years) are obese.

The food we eat everyday contribute to our wellbeing and provide us with the nutrients we need for healthy bodies and the calories we need for energy. If a person eats too much, the extra food turns into fat and is stored in the bodies and if one overeat regularly, they gain weight and if they continue to gain weight, they may become obese, obesity is often humorized in cartoons.

Obesity derived from the Latin word, Obesus, which means, 'stout, fat or plump' 'esus' is the past participle of edere (to eat), with 'ob' added to it. In 1651, the term was first used in English. Two kinds body fat-excess body fat distributed around the waist (apple shaped figure-intra-abdominal fat) carried more risk than fat distributed on the hips and thighs ('pear'-shaped figure, fat under the skin).

Prevalence

The health survey for England predict that more than 12 million adults and 1 million children will be obese by 2010, if no action is taken. In USA, obesity is a leading public health problem. It has highest rates of obesity in the developed world. From 1980-2002, obesity has doubled in adults and overweight has tripled in children and adolescents (2-19 years–17% were overweight and 20 years or above were obesed). The environment produces risk factors for decreased physical activity and for increased calorie consumption. It may be due to lack of activity, lower relative cost of food stuffs, increased marketing, changing work force pattern, ample number of restaurants.

Risk Factors

- Coronary heart disease
- Type 2 diabetes
- Sleep apnoea
- Secondary to diseases, e.g. hormonal problems like hypothyroidism, Cushing's syndrome; depression, polycystic ovarian diseases
- Smoking
- Hypertension
- Advanced age
- Family history
- Poverty–lack of education-tendency to rely on cheaper fast foods
- Over eating
- Sedentary habits (inactivity)
- Medications–steroids, hormonal drugs, anti-depressants.

Causes

- Obesity tends to run in family
- Genetic disorders like Prader-willi syndrome
- Overeating–when food energy exceeds energy expenditure, the excess is converted to fat cells through out the body
- Environmental factors–life style, eating habits, activity level take the energy and store it, when they can no longer expand, they increase in number.

- Sex–men have more muscle fibers than women; men burns more calories than women, even at rest; so women are more prone for obese
- Age–people tend to loose more muscle fibers and gain fat as the age advances; it lowers calories requirements
- Neurobiological mechanism–the adipokines are mediators produces by adipose tissue, their action is thought to modify many obesity related diseases; leptin and ghrelin are considered to be complementary in their modulating short term appetitive control (to eat, when the stomach is empty and to stop the stomach is stretched; leptin is produced by adipose tissue to signal fat storage reserves in the body and mediates long term appetite controls (i.e. to eat more when fat storages are low and less when fat storages are high)
- Neuroscientific approach–hypothalamus send signals related to metabolic state and energy storage and to shift the energy balance in either positive or negative direction, primarily by acting on appetite and energy expenditure. The lateral hypothalamus (hunger centre) and ventro medial hypothalamus is the satiety centre
- The imbalance between calorie consumption and expenditure vary by individual to individual
- Decreased or optional physical activity, increased caloric consumption
- Certain drugs. For example, antipsychotic medications, hormones
- A high glycemic diet (meals that gives high postprandial blood sugar)
- Weight cycling (caused by repeated attempts to loose weight by dieting)
- Stressful mentality–depression, hopelessness, anger, boredom, these feelings influence the eating habits, causing to overeat
- Pregnancy–women tend to increase weight an average of 4–6 pounds more after a pregnancy, it can compound with each pregnancy. It may contribute more weight.

Mechanical Complications Due to Obesity

- Cardiovascular diseases–congestive heart failure, enlarged heart, arrhythmias, dizziness, corpulmonale, varicose veins, pulmonary embolism
- Endocrine disorders–polycystic ovarian syndrome, menstrual disorders, infertility
- Gastro-intestinal diseases–gastro-esophageal reflux diseases, fatty liver diseases, cholelithiasis, hernia, colorectal cancer
- Renal and genitourinary diseases–erectile dysfunction, urinary incontinence, chronic renal failure, hypogonadism (male), breast cancer, uterine cancer, still birth
- Integument (skin and appendages)–stretch marks, acanthosis Nigricans, lymph oedema, cellulitis, carbuncles, impetigo
- Musculo skeletal diseases–hyper uricemia (predisposes gout), immobility, osteoarthritis, low back pain
- Neurologic diseases–stroke, paraesthesia, headache, carpel tunnel syndrome, dementia
- Respiratory diseases–Dyspnoea, obstructive sleep apnoea, hypoventilation syndrome, bronchial asthma.

Clinical Diagnosis

- Measuring body mass index (BMI)
- Waist circumference
- Presence of risk factors
- Co-morbidities
  In epidemiological studies only BMI is used as an indicator to define obesity.

Exams and Tests

- *Weight to height tables*: It gives general ranges of healthy weights and overweight for adult height. They are useful in identifying the risk of health problems related to weight. But they do not distinguish fat from muscle, water or bone.

- *Body fat percentage*: Percentage of body weight, i.e. fat is a alternative good marker of obesity; men with more than 25 per cent fat, women with more than 30 per cent fat are considered as obese. Simpler method for measuring body fat are: Skin-fold thickness test–a pinch of skin is precisely measured to determine the thickness of the subcutaneous fat layer, other methods are: bioelectrical impedance analysis (done at specialist clinics), computed tomography (CT scan), magnetic resonance imaging (MRI), and dual energy x-ray absorptiometry (DXA).
- *Body Mass Index (BMI)*: Simple and widely used method for estimating body fat. It is developed by the Belgian statistician and anthropometrist, Adolphe Quetelet, BMI is used to assess weight relative to height (kg/m^2) or lbs/inc^2); the greater the BMI, the higher the risk of developing health problems.

Steps to calculate: Weight (pounds) X 705 (Weight in pounds is MULTIPLIED by 705) and DIVIDED by Height in inches and the SUM is AGAIN DIVIDED by Height (inches).

Categories of individual based on weight and BMI are:

Under weight - BMI is less than 18.5

Normal weight - BMI is between 18.5-24.9

Over weight - BMI is between 25.0-29.9

Obese - BMI is between 30.0-39.9

Severely or morbidly obese - BMI of 40.0 or higher

Morbid obese–BMI of 35.0 or 40.0 in the presence of atleast one other significant co morbidity:

- Waist measurement/waist circumference: people with 'apple' shapes, who tend to put on weight around their waist, have a higher risk of obesity–related health problems. It includes women with a waist measurement of greater than 35" and men with a waist measurement of 40". Visceral fat or central obesity or apple type obesity have a much stronger correlation,

particularly with cardiovascular diseases than the BMI alone.

The absolute waist measurement circumference (> 102 cm in men and > 88 cm in women) or waist-hip ratio (> 0.9 for men and > 0.85 for women) are both used as measures of central obesity.

Treatment

- Eat less, 500 calories/day; low carbohydrate, non-energy restricted diets or low fat energy restricted foods are of helpful
- Consumption of vegetables and fruits, atleast 5 servings/day
- Consumptions of grains, atleast 6 servings/day
- Exercise will increase metabolism, individual who exercise for atleast 30 minutes/day for 5 days/week. Regular exercise helps in increasing heart and lung functions, lowers triglyceride levels, increases the HDL levels
- Modify the life style to loose weight. For example, Eat less, do more physical exercise
- Promote breast feeding among postnatal mothers to shed extra pounds
- *Medications*: Orlistat (xenical, reduces intestinal fat absorption by inhibiting pancreatic lipase and sibutramine)
- In the presence of DM, glucophage can assist in weight loss. The thiazolidinediones (Pioglitazone) can cause slight weight gain, but decreases the 'pathologic' form of abdominal fat, hence it will be used to combat obesity, laparoscopic procedure is used in which gastric band where a silicone ring is placed around the fundus of stomach to help restrict the amount of food eaten in a sitting. It is completely reversible technique, removing the implant returns the stomach to its pre surgical form
- Clients also requires to make life long changes to their diet, if they want to maintain the weight in the long term
- Behaviour modification techniques have to be used to change the attitude towards food and

exercise, to cultivate new habits that enhances loosing weight.

Prevention

- Avoid high caloric fast foods or snacks
- Modify the life style, eat more vegetables, fruits, less of fried foods
- Increase level of activities by physical exercise.

ANOREXIA NERVOSA

Anorexia Nervosa is common among teens; 10 percent of adolescent girls have anorexia, boys and men also can develop, but less often than girls and women; 1 per cent of older adolescents, young adults and women have anorexia. However, it can begin well before even puberty or well after that, even starting in midlife or beyond. The key elements are:

- People are intent on becoming too thin, may starve themselves or exercise excessively to prevent weight gain or to continue loosing weight
- It is a way to try and to cope-up with emotional problems, perfectionism and a desire for control
- Failure to gain weight in the absence of physical or psychiatric disturbance.

Definition

'It is an eating disorder, where people involuntarily refuse to eat'.

Risk Factors

- Excess dieting
- Unintentional weight loss after an illness or accident
- Weight gain–some one who gains weight may be dismayed with their new shape and may get criticized or ridiculed, in response, they may wind up dieting excessively
- Puberty: trouble coping with the changes in their body, go through during puberty, increased peer pressure, sensitivity to their comments

- Transition periods in life: going to the new school or new place or new job or broken up in relationships or death of a loved one or chronic illness; emotional distressing situations
- Athletics involved in sports and games; actresses, models working in artistic activities like dancing, are at high risk
- Professionals (men and women) may believe they will improve their upward mobility by loosing weight and then take it to an extreme
- Coaches, parents may contribute by suggesting young athletic to loose weight
- Media: Television and some other magazines frequently publishes beauties and their structure, people who are exposed to these images fascinated and they believe thinness will equates to success and popularity.

Causes

1. Genetics

   Some people may be genetically vulnerable to develop anorexia. Genetics contribute by creating a tendency toward perfectionism, sensitivity and perseverance, etc. traits associated with anorexia. In twins anorexia nervosa were observed more.

2. Neurobiological factors

   Serotonin, norepinephrine, dopamine neurotransmitters will inhibit feeding pattern, results into anorexia nervosa. Cholecystokinin peptide inhibits eating behaviour excessive stimulation of CCK activity may decrease appetite in anorexia nervosa cases.

3. Psychological factors

   People with low self worth, low self esteem, avoiding psychological maturation, extreme drive for perfectionism may go for poor feeding pattern; psychodynamic conflicts, rapid growth in physique massive fear of becoming fat or sensitive about being perceived as fat, to control emotions, to maintain strict control over food intake, denying hunger, asking excuses to avoid eating, emotional/physical sexual abuse.

4. Sociocultural factors
- Modern culture, western culture often reinforces a desire for thinness
- Peer pressure, heightened sensitivity to criticism or even casual comments about weight or body shape may fuel the desire to be thin
- Habituated to eat junk food
- To avoid familial conflict caused by marital problems, diffused, inappropriate relationship among family members, rigid or strict rules/standards regarding food pattern
- Chaotic family environment, attitude of family members towards body images
- Tremendous need to control their surroundings and emotions
- Unique reaction to a variety of external and internal conflicts. For example, stress, anxiety, unhappiness, feeling like life is out of control, etc.

Clinical Manifestations

- Involves extreme weight loss–atleast 15 per cent below the individual's normal body weight; refusal to maintain a body weight which is consistent with their built, age and height
- Looks emaciated, anasarea
- Eventhough person is under weight, having intense fear of gaining weight or becoming fat
- Denying the seriousness of having a low body weight or having a distorted image of one's appearance or shape
- History of amenorrhoea for the last three months; men often may become impotent
- Thin appearance, thin hair, falling of hair or break in hair
- Fatigue, brittle nails, dizziness or fainting
- Constipation
- Dry skin
- Cold intolerance
- Irregular heart rhythm, low blood pressure, low blood count
- Dehydration, muscle wasting (cachexia)
- Osteoporosis
- Refusal to eat, doing exercises

- Flat mood or lack of emotions, feels difficulty in concentration
- Typically starve themselves, eventhough they suffer terribly from hunger pains.

TYPES

- Under weight
- Emaciated
- Restricting
- Binge-eating/purging.

a. Emaciation

Body requires a certain amount of energy to keep basic life systems functioning. Body needs additional energy to accomplish the activities like growth and repair.

The synonyms for emaciation are: 'bonyness, gauntness, maceration, thinness, extreme/excessive leanness or thinness, scragginess.'

Definition

Emaciation is extreme thinness/leanness with one-third or more of the body's weight being lost either gradually or suddenly.

Causes

- Imbalance in the system, as a result of starvation of disease
- Anorexia and bulimia
- Lupus
- Polymyalgia reheumatica
- Infections
- Febrile diseases
  There are three types of people who are extremely thin:
1. Those who eat well and stay thin–some children born thin inheriting their parent's physical built. If the child has a good appetite, active, they may remain lean and healthy inspite of being overfed. Whatever the child consumes gets converted into energy because of their overactiveness.

2. Those who cannot digest whatever they eat and inspite of a good living, because of illness (vit deficiencies, progressive illness, chronic disorders). These anaemic children keep on loosing weight steadily. The low resistance of the body invites diseases leading to emaciation. The drugs and energy drinks, special foods will not be helpful to gain weight.

3. Those who are under nourished and over worked, poor eating habits or eating food that lack nutrition combined with hard work, beyond the enduring capacity of the body results in thinness.

When thin persons lack good health or suffer from diseases which make them to loose the weight, they experience exhaustion.

Signs and Symptoms

- Weakness in the limbs
- Lack of appetite
- Poor digestion
- Easily tiring
- Desire to lie down or sleep
- Insomnia
- Head ache
- Giddiness
- Physical or mental fatigue
- Lack of interest in any activity
- Walking and ascending stairs induces violent palpitations of the heart
- Bony prominence
- Shoulder blades are prominent.

Prevention

- Adequate nutrition
- Physical exercise
- Activity choice.

b. Under Weight

A child is said to be under weight, if his/her BMI for age and gender is less than the 5th percentile.

$$BMI = \frac{Weight}{Height} \ (kg/m^2)$$

Causes

- Not consuming enough food
- An underlying illness
- Emotional disturbances. For example, anxiety, depression
- Food allergy
- Excessive fear of being over weight
- Eating disorder
- Family problem, adverse situations.

Signs and Symptoms

- Feels weak or tired
- Trouble in focusing attention and concentration
- Stunted growth
- Delay in the onset of puberty
- Experiences food insecurity
- At risk of becoming hunger
- No interest in eating
- Discomfort after meals.

Treatment

- Advise the care taker to give high caloric diet
- Continue to promote physical activity
- Advise the child to take rest for atleast 15 minutes before meals
- Advise the child to avoid candy, soft drinks, high fat food from fast food restaurant (canned food, dried fruits, cheese, ice cream, pudding, cream soups)
- Menu planning, include all nutrients, limiting snacks is required
- Give plenty of vegetables, fruits
- Maintain regular eating habits, hygienic measures
- Provide congenial, healthy environment at home.

c. Restricting

People will loose weight by severely restricting the amount of food they eat and also try to loose the weight by exercising excessively.

d. Purging/Binge Eating

People try to control their weight by purging get rid of food or calories by vomiting after eating, misusing laxatives, diuretics or enemas, some may binge or eat excessive amounts of food and then purge, others may purge even after eating a small quantity.

SCREENING AND DIAGNOSIS

Physical Examination

- Measurement of height and weight.

  Body weight will be maintained atleast 15 percent below that expected (due to loss or never achieved) or

  Quitelet's body mass index estimation for 16 years and above

$$QBMI = \frac{Weight\ (kg)}{Height\ (m)^2}$$

- Check vital signs–heart rate, blood pressure, temperature, respiration
- Check the skin for dryness or other problems
- Listen to heart and lung sounds
- Abdominal examination
- Assist for laboratory investigations
  - Complete blood picture (CBP)
  - Serum electrolytes and proteins
  - Hormonal assay (to exclude hormonal disorders)
  - Urinalysis
  - X-rays (to exclude skeletal disorders)
  - ECG (to exclude heart irregularities)
- Psychological evaluation.

  Clinical psychologist or other health care professionals will conduct mental status examination, appearance, memory, verbal response, orientation, speech pattern, reliability, judgement, insight, etc. developmental aspects, habits, behavioural pattern-cognitive, conative and affective domains, developmental aspects, mental status examination, etc. either by using structured questionnaires or psychological self assessment tool.

Thorough history collection regarding menstrual irregularities, puberty events, specific psychopathology to exclude abnormalities to monitor clinical pathology.

- Family history

  To identify family and environmental stressors, genetic vulnerability, psychopathology, relationship of family members with the client, family environment, situational support, cultural values, boundaries, perceptions of food, body weight expectations, medical illnesses

- Socio-developmental history

  Collect history related to abuse like alcoholism, smoking, drugs, etc. suicidal tendency, symptom of craving for weight reduction, cause and effect relationship between stressors; functioning levels and the occurrence of eating disorder; concurrent evaluation of existing medical conditions; assess current and past core symptoms, collect information regarding past psychiatric illness and treatment, type of medications consumed.

TREATMENT

- Team approach (Medical providers, mental health professionals, dietitians) will be used to treat eating disorders
- Medical care: Anorexia nervosa causes many complications, hence frequent monitoring of vital signs, hydration levels, electrolyte levels and other physical conditions are needed; and symptomatic treatment is planned
  - Treat dehydration, electrolyte imbalance, hypotension, psychiatric problems, sometimes hospitalization may be required in severe anorexia nervosa cases or its complications

– At day care centres, in specialized clinics intensive treatment will be carried out for longer periods of time.

Psychotherapy

Individual Psychotherapy

To deal with the behaviour and thoughts that contribute to anorexia through cognitive behaviour therapy, to promote healthy life style pattern. Guidance will be provided to stick to treatment, so follow meal plans, to develop good realistic thinking, enhance self esteem, self confidence and a sense of control, individual psychotherapy is focussed.

Family Therapy

To resolve family conflicts and to provide moral support from the concerned members to the client, to promote healthy interaction pattern among family members and to avoid restrictive and rigid behaviour family therapy will be given.

Group Therapy

Informal support groups will be of helpful, but precaution has to be taken, some times the support groups can result in competitions to be the thinnest person. It fosters self esteem and gains deep insight into the feelings and behaviour. It promotes concern, constructive support and feed back from peers.

Behaviour Therapy

To identify triggering situations and to develop a plan of action, to deal with them by showing positive role models, developing healthy eating habits, corrects behavioural pattern, alters symptoms.

Nutritional Therapy

Dietitian provides guidance on healthy diet and supplementation pattern, etc. plans specific meal plans, based on calorie requirements and focusing on goals to be attained. In severe anorexia cases, some times it may require nasogastric tube feeding to meet the nutritional needs.

Interpersonal Therapy

To resolve interpersonal difficulties and conflicts; stress and strain, to maintain good interpersonal relationships interpersonal therapy will be used.

Complication

Anorexia nervosa is most severe, it can be fatal. Life threatening complications–anaemia, heart disorders like mitral valve prolapse, abnormal heart rhythms, heart failure, etc. bone loss, risk of fractures later in life, lung problems-emphysema, constipation, nausea, vomiting, electrolyte imbalances, kidney problems.

Severe malnourishment, every organ in the body can sustain damage of brain, heart and kidneys. Psychiatric disorders like depression, anxiety, personality disorders, obsessive compulsive disorders and drug abuse, etc.

The co-occurrence of these complications with anorexia can make the disease more difficult to treat.

Differences between Anorexia nervosa and Bulimia nervosa has been described in Table (Page 503).

BULIMIA NERVOSA

The word, 'Bulimia' derived from the Latin word 'Bulimia' and from the Greek word, 'Boulimia' which means ravenous hunger, compounded from 'Bous', 'Limos' means 'hunger of anox'.

People with bulimia are preoccupied with their weight and shape, often judging themselves severely and harshly for perceived flaws, they often live in a secret world of shame, self disgust and whose behaviour is embarrassing and socially unacceptable. It commonly begins in late adolescence or early adulthood, it is a serious potentially life-threatening condition.

Definition

'An eating disorder, characterised by episodes of recurrent binge, chaotic eating of large quantities of food within short time, followed by intentional purging in the form of inducing vomiting, inappropriate use of laxatives, enemas, diuretics or other medication or by doing excessive physical exercise'.

Risk Factors

- Dieting–people with bulimia may excessively eat, that dieting can trigger a binge episode, leading to purging and then more dieting and consequently it turns to a vicious cycle
- Puberty–some adolescents have trouble coping with the puberty changes in their bodies
- Increased peer pressure, heightened sensitivity to criticisms or even casual comments about weight or body shape
- Transition periods in life; like going to new place, taken new job and responsibility, etc. all these changes will bring emotional distress, to overcome it some may go over eating
- Secondary to endocrinal disorders
- Some special fields like athletics, gymnastics, certain games require good personality to play, to build-up their body shape.

Causes

- *Psychological causes*: Stressful situations, self depreciation, insecurity, substitution of food for affection or sex
- Deep psychological issues and profound feelings of lack of control, low self worth, trouble controlling impulsive behaviours, managing their moods or expressing anger 'emotional upheavals; depression'
- Environmental factors–the disorder is more prevalent in Caucasian groups, but is becoming a rising problem in the African-American and Hispanic communities
- Biological-genetically vulnerable to develop bulimia in twins, young women with a biological sister or mother with an eating disorder are at higher risk. The families of people with bulimia may tend to have more open conflicts along with more criticism and unpredictability

- *Neurochemical factors*: Serotonin, a Neurochemical receptor may influence eating behaviours as it regulates food intake. CNS serotonin concentrated in hypothalamus is involved in the regulation of satiety. Altered function at the presynaptic or postsynaptic neuron sites or nutritional intake may be responsible. Reduced CCK secretion, a neuropeptide, is observed in bulimia cases, alteration in neuropeptide secretion may lead to excessive stimulation of feeding behaviour as reflected by binge eating episode
- *Sociocultural factor*: Modern western culture often cultivates and reinforces a desire for thinness, worth is often equated with being fat, peer pressure may fuel this desire with being thin or fat.

Incidence

- Ten to twenty-five years of age; common in persons with heavy work loads
- Traumatic experiences in their life, e.g. child abuse or sexual abuse
- Common in higher socioeconomic groups, people with high intelligence; working for higher goals, work for perfectionism
- Can occur at all ages and in both sexes
- In Western industrialized countries 1–3 per cent of women experience bulimia during their life. The rate of bulimia in men is about 1/10 of that in women.

Bulimic Cycle

It vary from person to person
- Some might binge and purge several times a day
- Some bulimics may be able to vomit without gagging themselves after eating
- Bulimics may go through a severe binge/purge cycle, i.e. very devastating to the body
- They may hide or hoard food and over eat when stressed or worried or upset

- The bulimic may feel a loss of control during a binge and consume very large quantities of food
- Some may eat socially but may be bulimic in private
- Bulimics may appear to be underweight, normal weight or even over weight
- Every bulimic is completely different in 'how much' they purge. Some binge, some do not, often times when the urge 'hits' they will go to great lengths to purge as if an uncontrollable urge or force is making them to do so
- The chemicals released during purge may lead to extreme dehydration and electrolyte imbalances.

CLINICAL MANIFESTATIONS

- Clients will engage in episodes of binge eating followed by attempts to prevent weight gain
- Binge is, eating a larger amount of food than most people would eat under similar situations
- Once the binge episode ends, the purging begins may be vomiting or inducing vomiting or excessive exercise or fasting or taking diuretics, laxatives, enema.

a. Physical Manifestations

- Abnormal bowel functioning
- Damaged teeth and gums
- Swollen salivary glands in the cheeks
- Sores in the throat and mouth
- Bloating
- Dehydration
- Fatigue
- Dry skin
- Irregular heart beat
- Sores, scars or calluses on the knuckles or hands amenorrhoea in females
- Tends to have normal weight or overweight.

b. Emotional and Behavioural Manifestations

- Constant dieting
- Recurrent episodes of binge eating

- Feeling that they cannot control eating behaviour
- Eating until the point of discomfort or pain
- Eating much more food in a binge episode than in a normal meal or snack
- To prevent weight gain, activities like: self induced vomiting, using laxatives or diuretics, fasting or excessive exercise will be performed
- Unhealthy focus on body shape and weight
- Distorted, excessively negative body image
- Going to toilet after eating or during meals
- Hoarding food
- Depression or anxiety
- Guilty feelings, self condemnation.

Categories of Bulimia

- Purging–people regularly engage in self induced vomiting or misuse of laxatives, consumes tapeworms, or diuretics or ipecac; enemas to compensate for binges, as a means of rapidly extricating the contents from their body
- Non-purging–other methods will be used, to reduce the weight, e.g. over exercising or fasting; (6-8% of cases).

Consequences of Bulimia Nervosa

Malnutrition, electrolyte imbalance, hyponatraemia, esophageal reflux, peptic ulcers and pancreatitis, dry or brittle skin, oedema, muscle atrophy, orthostatic hypotension, anaemia, depression, infertility, insomnia.

Complications

- *Cardiovascular problems*: Electrolyte abnormalities or use of syrup of ipecac to induce vomiting can lead to cardiac muscle disorders and irregular heart rhythms. These can be life-threatening. Fainting and low blood pressure.
- *Tooth and gum problems*: Hydrochloric acid from stomach can wash over teeth and gums during vomiting. Repeated vomiting can cause a significant and permanent loss of dental

enamel. Teeth may become ragged and chipped and dental cavities may increase.

- *Throat and mouth problems*: Frequent or regular vomiting can cause sores in mouth or throat. Bleeding occurs, if one force to vomit.
- *Low potassium levels*: The purging process tends to dehydrate body and lower the level of potassium in blood. This can cause weakness and irregular heart rhythms.
- *Digestive problems*: Purging by vomiting or use of laxatives may irritate the walls of esophagus and rectum. In severe cases, esophagus can rupture, leading to life-threatening bleeding. Repeated purging may also cause constipation. Laxative abuse can lead to dependence.
- *Abuse of medications and drugs*: The variety of over-the-counter drugs one may use during urge cycle may cause a drug problem. Some substances used include laxatives, diuretics, appetite suppressants and ipecac, people with bulimia have higher rates of alcohol and substance abuse.

Diagnosis

- Physical examination: Auscultation of heart and lung sounds; anthropometric measurements–height, weight, body mass index
- Monitor vital signs
- Check the skin for dryness or other problems
- Assist for laboratory tests, e.g. x-ray, ECG, complete blood picture, urine analysis
- Psychological evaluation: Assess the mental status, eating habits, certain times standardized questionnaires may be used.

DSM Diagnostic Criteria

The following 5 criteria should be met for a patient to be diagnosed with bulimia nervosa, some people may not meet all of these criteria but still have an eating disorder and need professional help to over come or manage it

- Recurrent episodes of binge eating. An episode of binge eating is characterized by both of the following
  - Eating in a fixed period of time (within any 2-hour period) an amount of food that is definitely larger than most people would eat during a similar period of time and under similar circumstances
  - A sense of lack of control over eating during the episode (a feeling that one cannot stop eating or control what or how much one is eating)
- Recurrent inappropriate compensatory behaviour in order to prevent weight gain, such as self-induced vomiting, misuse of laxatives, diuretics or other medications, fasting, or excessive exercise
- The binge eating and inappropriate compensatory behaviours both occur, on average, at least once a week for three months
- Self-evaluation is unduly influenced by body shape and weight
- The disturbance does not occur exclusively during episodes of anorexia nervosa.

ICD-10, F$_{50.2}$

- There is a persistent preoccupation with eating and an irresistible craving for food, the patient yield to episodes of overeating in which the patient eats large amount of food in short time
- The client attempts to counteract the 'fattening' effects of eating by one or more of the following: self induced vomiting, purgative abuse, alternating periods or starvation, use of drugs such as appetite suppressants, thyroid preparations or diuretics. When bulimia occurs for a diabetic client, they may neglect their insulin therapy
- The psychopathology consists of a morbid dread of fatness and the patient sets himself a defined weight, well below the Premorbid weight that constitutes the optimum/healthy

weight in the opinion of physician. There is often, but not always, a history of earlier episode of anorexia nervosa, the interval between the 2 disorders ranging from a few months to several years. This earlier episode may have been fully expressed, or may have assumed a minor cryptic form with a moderate loss of weight or a transient phase of amenorrhoea.

Differences between anorexia nervosa and bulimia nervosa	
Anorexia nervosa	*Bulimia nervosa*
Underweight	As they cannot achieve the low weight, feels physically that they are at failure and this outlook infiltrates in all aspects of their life
BMI < 18.5 to 17.5 Refusal to maintain a normal weight by self starvation	Lacks control over eating Feels more shame and out of control with their behaviours, in severe cases they tend to be hospitalized
Does not engage in regular binging and purging sessions, though they may occur rarely, the patient binges and purges as well as fails to maintain a minimum weight	Uses compensatory behaviours aimed at preventing weight gain, e.g. self inducing vomiting with or without mechanical stimulation
Controls their intake, a symptom that calms their anxiety around food as they feel, they had control of it	Wide fluctuations in weight can be observed
They cannot see that they are underweight and is constantly working towards a goal that they will never meet	
Allows failure at achieving the 'perfect body' to define his/her self worth	

Both anorexics and bulimics have an over-powering sense of self that is determined by their weight and their perceptions of it. They both place their achievements and successes as the result of their body and are often depressed as they feel, they are consistently failing to achieve the perfect body. They never feel satisfied in their lives.

TREATMENT

Team approach is used which consists of medical providers, mental health professionals and dietitians. Early the intervention, effective the prognosis.

a. Residential Treatment Offers

- Long term support
- Counselling
- Symptom interruption
  Medical care–for early recovery of manifestations.

b. Psychotherapy

- Cognitive behaviour therapy
- Individual psychotherapy
- Family therapy
- Group therapy and informal support group therapy is not recommended, as there may be chance of sharing some tips on maintaining their condition.

c. Nutritional Therapy

- Nutritional guidance will be provided on healthy diet and healthy eating habits, specific menu has to be planned to achieve a healthy weight.

d. Drug Therapy

- Antidepressants. For example, Fluoxetine (Prozac) is of helpful; combination of therapies approach is used to deal bulimic cases; hospitalization may be necessary for intensive treatment over long periods of time.

e. Coping Skills

- Healthy life style has to be adopted
- Enhance positive health status

- Follow the menu as per nutritional guidance, maintains adequate supplementation
- Incorporates fun in life
- Resisting the urge to diet or skip meals
- Maintaining normal weight
- Identify the triggering situations and try to overcome or handling it carefully by developing plan of action to deal with them
- Following positive role models
- Encourage them to stick to the treatment, not skipping therapy sessions.

Prognosis

- With early diagnosis and prompt treatment, most bulimic clients will recover; depending on life circumstances complications, life time stress the condition may go into crisis or even fatal, 10 per cent of mortality can occur.

Prevention

- Parents can cultivate and reinforce a healthy body image in their children by reassuring them that they are of normal or healthy size
- Never criticize or tease any child for his/her weight or large body frame
- Never keep a nick name to the child
- Encourage the children to develop adaptive/ healthy behaviour.

FAILURE TO THRIVE

It is common in infants and in young children.

Causes

- Disturbed parent-child relationships
- Less experience in child rearing practices
- Eating inedible foods
- Over anxious mother
- Wrong selection of food stuffs.

Manifestations: Serious failure to gain weight.

Management

- Family therapy to enhance parent-child relationships
- Diet therapy, adequate nutritional supplementation
- Small and frequent feeds; never pressurize the child for feeding purposes.

PICA

Formulating the habit of eating non-nutritive or non-edible substances such as mud, dirt, wall plaster, chalk, paint, clay, etc. is called as 'Pica'. Tasking or mouthing of strange objects is normal in infancy and children upto the age of 2 years. Persistence of this habit beyond the age of 2 years may be a behavioural manifestation. Pica is commonly observed in low socio-economic group and in malnourished, mentally sub-normal children. It is also seen among pregnant women.

Causes

- Parental neglect
- Poor supervision by the parents or elders in the family
- Lack of affection
- Strained interpersonal relationship among family members
- Stressful situation or painful environment (hospitalization, entering to school)
- History of neonatal insults.

Clinical Manifestations

- Child complaints of pain abdomen
- Pallor, anaemic
- Slow in motor and mental development
- Exhibit neurologic defects
- Deviant behaviour
- Hysteric clients eat ash, salt, vinegar
- Epileptic clients feel strong taste before attack
- Schizophrenic client will have peculiar taste at certain times

- Separation, anxiety
- Maturational lag
- Prone for lead poisoning.

Management

- Nutritional and emotional needs of children have to be met
- Regularize the meal pattern, serve the food in pleasant manner
- Supplement with iron to treat iron deficiency anaemia
- Counselling of child and parents is essential to overcome deviant behaviour
- Drug therapy: Benzodiazepines
- Behaviour modification techniques
- Client education
- Milieu therapy.

Assess the neurological defects, if needed consult the neuro-physician.

BEHAVIOURAL PROBLEMS AMONG CHILDREN

In an individual's life, from birth to end of life at every stage of growth and development, there are some problems that are part of passing from one stage of development to another. For example, child who changes his life from helplessness to gradual independence may have certain adjustment problems, which has to be solved, where the child has to adjust to the new roles otherwise it will emotionally affects the entire family by slowing down their activities with disturbed emotional environment.

Definition

'Behavioural problems are the reactions and clinical manifestations which are resulting due to emotional disturbances or environmental maladjustments'.

The emotional environment of young child consists of entire relationship of the child with their parents and family members. Behavioural problems are less common, where the child is loved, accepted and who is living in favourable environmental conditions. Child's basic emotional needs like love, affection, good understanding, care, concern, a sense of belongingness and security, etc. has to be satisfied to ensure optimal development whereby child will attain emotional maturity and able to relate his life meaningfully with the society. Parents have to train up their children to cultivate socially acceptable behaviour. In times of stress, child should be cared properly, touch the distressed child, hug the child in comforting and relaxing manner.

Parents have to inculcate child's emotional stableness where the child always will be cheerful, friendly and cooperative in nature. Make the child to establish satisfactory relationship with others specifically the family members. If the children are often criticized and rejected will not cared properly and often parents does not show keen interest among their children, child will develop the feeling of insecurity and inferiority which will be reflected either one or other form of behaviour problem. Parents along with their children should enjoy conducive loving environment to prevent the occurrence of behavioural problems.

Causes

- Hereditary potentials
  Certain emotions characteristics like aggressiveness, temperament of the parents will transmit to their children by vertical transmission
- Deviations in the psychological development
- Unfavourable home conditions and lack of parental love, support and concern
- Poor health
- Inadequate nutrition
- Parental deprivation
- Lack of appreciation, incentives for accomplishing the activities by the parents
- Past or present emotional environment of the child and his family
- Sibling rivalry
- Pressure of highly competitive and stressful environment

- Unfavourable environmental factors or stressors
- Decreased educational and career opportunities
- Pressure of peer group
- Social tensions
- Maladjustment of children with siblings or parents
- Too much or too rigid discipline or over-protection of parents may prevent the child to develop the sense of independence and sense of autonomy, the child resists parental interference in his life
- Too much expectations of parents without seeing the abilities or intellectual levels of children related to scholastic achievements thus conflicts between the child's achievement and parent's desires increases the stress
- Parents may seek unrealistic attainment from the child
- The child will be given too many gifts as indication of love
- Lack of warmth in parental attitude
- Some parents wants to take pride in the achievements of their children and thereby they will impose their own value system, aspiration and philosophy on the child
- Over domination of child's personality, which may built-up stresses in the child's interaction with parent
- Unhealthy criticism and unfavourable comparison–children are sensitive to open negative criticism and unfavourable comparison with other children or their siblings which results in maladjustment
- Broken family
  Disharmony between parents, separation or divorce will have impact on child's development
- Reaction to the new situations
- Poor health
  Inadequate nutrition
  Lack of incentives
  Hormonal deficiency disorder (cretinism).

Assessment

The diagnosis of the behavioural problems in the child requires assessment and evaluation of child, his parents, family and its interactions, environment.

a. History Related to

- Antenatal period, birth, newborn and neonatal period
- Feeding pattern
- Developmental pattern
- Immunization status
- Past illness
- Present illness
- Interactions and relationships within the family
- Scholastic environment
- Attitude of parents or caregivers towards the children
- Parental child relationship
- Screening
- Physical examination of the child
- Psychological testing
- Testing of vision and hearing
- Assessment of family situation and environmental factors.

Principles of Dealing with Social and Emotional Problems

Management of behavioural problems is based on theory of behaviour modification. Education of the parents and continued help may be necessary in prevention and control of behavioural problems.

Specific Interventions

- Discipline the child
  Parents have to formulate certain rules and regulations which have to be followed by the children to develop socially acceptable behaviour, to maintain good discipline and to protect the children from dangers thereby builds good character.

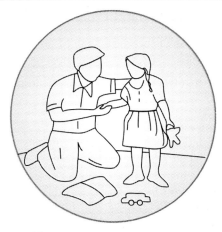

Fig. 15.1: Guiding children: Role of teachers and parents

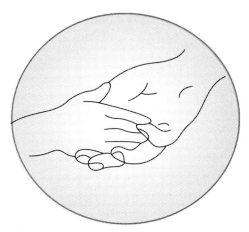

Fig. 15.2 : Coping with socio-emotional problems

- Behaviour modification

In behavior modification technique both positive and negative reinforcement methods will be used, based on type problem. During this process, child's emotional environment (internal and external) has to be assessed. The elders have to formulate and emphasize the importance of expected behaviour of the child. By using positive reinforcement in the form of a reward, praise or token where the child will follow repetitively the socially accepted behaviour in an interesting and enthusiastic

manner and learns cultured behaviour. By encouraging children to behave in specified ways will reduce the tendency of the child to misbehave.

Discourage the misbehaviour or misconduct of the child by punishment or timeout or disincentive or verbal disapproval whereby the child will not repeat the same type of misbehaviour.

Behavioural problems are common during childhood. Some of these difficulties will subside naturally as children grow. They learn to adopt to the situations and get over the hurdles in due course. Most of the children show difficulties in coping with these problems at some stage of development or the other.

Parental Guidance and Counselling

Parents have to

- Maintain relaxed state and emotional stability when they are taking care of emotionally instable children. They have to give self instructions like 'let me be calm', 'let me see what the child needs', 'let me take the charge of the situation', etc. are helpful
- Assure the child with empathetic reception that the child is important to entire family and he can make independent decisions
- Treat and respect late childhood children as individuals in their own right neither as babies nor as adults
- Select judiciously; either restraint or punishment
- Adults need to take time and trouble to provide opportunity for natural outlets of children in group activities. For example, picnic enjoyment, involving the children in community activities
- Provide outlets from self expression
- Assign responsibility in a group activity which will help them in a long way to grow smoothly
- Express faith in children and confidence in their growing independence is essential
- Promote the child in active participation in implementing group activities

- Involve the child in planning and organizing group activities and in decision-making of family affairs and consistently without betraying annoyance and emotional instability
- Children who does not cause trouble also needs adult attention
- Undue comparisons and making generalizations related to children should be avoided
- Encourage the child to participate in peer activities
- Have an idea of growing needs and changing characteristics and provide opportunities for its expression.

Parents, elders and teachers have to carry out the follow-up activities after intervening any of both, positive or negative reinforcement. Techniques to modify the psychopathology and to rectify the misconduct of the children, parents sometimes have to consistently sometimes have to ignore the wrong deed committed by the child and they should not pay attention, finally child will stop the misbehaviour as everybody ignored it. If it is persistence then only parents have to take some steps for its correction. For example, the child does the mistake or develops misbehaviour; parents have to explain the act and its effect in a calm and quiet manner. They should not shout or discourage or going on commenting destructively or doing unhealthy comparisons or going on probing the same issue for several times, etc. activities have to be avoided as it may affect emotional pattern of the child and prone for deviant behaviour. Instead, if the parents are silent and ignoring that situation, by not showing any attention or interest will calm-up the emotional impact on the child and the child will feel at ease, tries to modify the behaviour and develops good characteristics. Behaviour therapist has to guide the parents to understand the child and his emotions; and train up parents to assist in the activities related to behaviour modification techniques.

Specific Behavioural Problems

Colic

It usually starts within first week after birth, reaches peak by 4–6 weeks, improves after 3–4 months.

Causes

- Commonly seen in over active infants
- Over stimulation by parents
- May be manifestation of hunger in some infants
- Adoption of improper feeding techniques
- Allergy to cow's milk or lactose intolerance
- Low progesterone level
- Congenital hyper tonicity of intestines
- Physiological immaturity of infant.

Treatment

- Mother should be counseled about the transient nature of illness
- Baby has to be fed in upright position, after feeding, burping of the baby has to be carried out to promote the exhalation of air which engulfed by the infant during feeding
- For symptomatic relief of colic, based on the cause, doctors may prescribe phenobarbitone/chloral hydrate/analgesics/antispasmodics
- Undue attention by the parent have to be avoided.

Breath Holding Spells

It occurs between 6 months of age to 5 years.

Causes

- Manifestation of anger/frustration/fear
- May be seen in the clients with mild injury.

Clinical Manifestations

- Usually the child will cry after emotional outburst, e.g. anger, fear, frustration; after about of crying air in the lungs are exhaled, narrowed vocal cord closes, breath is held in expiration for a few seconds and the child will be cyanosed

- Rigidity
- Opisthotonous
- There after child recovers but becomes less active
- In some cases, the child becomes unconscious and apneic following an unexpected painful stimulus.

Treatment

- Measures to be taken to avoid precipitating factors (emotional imbalancing situations)
- Kindness and understanding the child's emotional distress by the parents is necessary and develop positive climate; reassure the child
- Over anxiety of the parents has to be avoided.

Sleep Problems

Newborn usually sleep for 4–5 hours uninterruptedly. By 2–4 months of age majority of infants acquire to sleep throughout the night. Parents are interested that their baby has to go to bed without any resistance and sleep throughout the night. Guidelines to be followed by the caregivers to cultivate the regular habit of sleeping and to prevent sleeping problems in their children are:

Newborn upto 3 Months

- Place the newborn in the crib, when they are drowsy
- Gentle rocking and cuddling will help the most, hold the baby for all fussy crying during the first 3 months
- Carry the baby for atleast 3 hours to reduce fussy crying
- Avoid sleeping for more than 3 consecutive hours during day, attempt to be made to awake the baby gently and entertain them
- More frequent daytime feeds lead to frequent awakening at night by crying, may be tired, bored, lonely so hold the baby comfortably at the time of need. Do not keep on feeding the baby, as a pacifier at times of crying

- Make the daytime feeding intervals to atleast 2 hours. Avoid 'grazing' (the child expects whenever he cries he will be getting feeding, whenever caregiver holds him)
- Make midnight feed brief
- Cultivate longer periods of play time in day so that child will sleep longer periods at night
- Change the diapers only when it is soiled, while changing use the light as little as possible and do it quietly.

Four Months Old Baby

- Give last feed at parent's bed time
- If the child cries during night, comfort them with a back rub and with some soothing words instead of feeding
- Don't allow the baby to hold the feeding-bottle and go to bed
- Make middle of night contacts brief
- Normally child will have 4–5 partial awakenings each night. They need to learn the procedure to go back to sleep on their own. If the child cries, gently pat them, don't turn on the light, play with them or take the child out of the crib; comfort the child with soothing words.

Six Months Old Baby

- Provide a soft toy to the child to hold in the crib; as the babies are worried and become anxious about separation from their parents, a stuffed animal doll or soft blanket can be given for comfort and security when he wakes up during the night
- Respond to 'separation-fears' by holding and reassuring the child for lessening night time fears
- For mild night time fears, check the child promptly and reassure them by keeping the interaction as brief as possible. Keep the light off, don't take the baby out of the crib; provide what ever needed for comfort and sit next to the crib with the hands rests on baby's chest.

One Year Old Child

- Formulate bedtime rituals. For example, telling stories
- Comfort the child by keeping the child's security objects nearby
- If the child is having temper tantrum at bed time and leaves the bedroom, tell them to return to bedroom and avoid any further conversation. If the parents are entertaining or responding to their protest, they will learn not to prolong bedtime tantrums
- Reassure the child during nightmare of fears, never ignore child's fears or punish for that. If the nightmares are frequent, assess the causative factors or stressors
- The amount of sleep required will vary from child to child
- Infants will have less than 2 hours naps; children stops morning naps between 18–24 months of age and give up their afternoon naps between 3–6 years of age.

Bedtime Resistance in Toddler Period

Toddlers above 2 years of age certain times refuses to got to bed or to stay in bedroom, they prolong their wakeup time by ongoing questioning, interacting, unreasonable requests, protests, crying or other temper tantrums; in the morning these type of children wakes up late.

Causes

- Children who are in need of attention seeking
- Sharing parent's bed or wants to speak to the parents more, feels more attachment with their parents
- Too much crying when put to bed as the child may not feel sleepy or distractions within the environment with TV/guests or wants to play with other children, who are playing nearby
- Resistance to nap
- Trying to come out of the crib before parents are ready to take the child out of the crib

- Colic or gas formation, wakening up before the usual wakening time.

Management

- Start the night with a pleasant bedtime ritual have to be followed, e.g. taking bath before going to bed, brushing teeth, reading stories, telling prayers or songs and other interactions with other children.

  To have familiarity and comfort repeat the same pattern of ritual daily, try to keep the same sequence each night. Ask the childs' preference, give a kiss and hug before sleep.

  Provide calm and quiet environment and avoid distractions to the child, make the child to sleep comfortably. When the child is drowsy, place them in the crib.
- Formulate rules to go out of bedroom without sleeping or having naps in between
- Establish regular bedtime and stick to it; don't force the child to sleep
- Ignore the verbal requests like ongoing demands or questions of child from the bedroom
- Close the bedroom door for screaming or for coming out
- Lock the bedroom door if the child repeatedly comes out
- Praise the child for good sleeping behaviour
- Advice for medical check up, if the child is subjected to colic pain or gas disturbances.

Sleeping Problem in Preschool Period

In early preschool period, more difficulty was observed for putting the child to bed; they will resist to go to bed.

Interventions

- Keep the child in bed at an appropriate time
- Ignore cry or other attention seeking behaviour
- Allow the child to read stories or have favourite play in night light

- At bedtime caregivers should not interact and they have to be out of bedroom stating that, 'No, it's bedtime'
- Caregivers reinforces the child, it is bedtime and only choice to go to sleep
- Reward the child who sleeps throughout the night with praise and positive reinforcement.

Night Mares

In all ages (after 6 months of age) occasionally, bad dreams may disturb the child's sleep pattern and prevents peaceful sleep.

'Nightmares are scary dreams that awaken a child'.

Nightmares will disturb the children especially, e.g. infants will cry and scream until someone comes carry them; preschoolers if they have nightmares they cry and run to parents' room; older children tries to understand what a nightmare is by themselves and tries to go back to sleep without waking their parents.

Causes

- Bad or dreadful dreams as they help the mind process by complicated events or information
- Fairy tales
- Content of nightmares usually relates to developmental challenges
- Separation from their parents among toddlers and preschoolers
- Darkness
- Excessive napping during the day
- Listening to devil stories
- Fear about death or real dangers
- Alone feeling
- Violent TV shows or dreadful movies
- Boredom and insufficient interactions with adults.

Interventions

- Listen to the tale of the dream or nightmare
- Parents have to answer to child's questions and discussions

- Returning the child to bed promptly
- Provide night-light
- Avoid or refuse to let the child into the caregiver's bed
- Until the child settles down, be with the child or in front of the bedroom door, open the bedroom door if the child is having fear of darkness
- Reward the child with praise and positive reinforcement who sleeps throughout the night without any disturbance
- Keep the bedtime hour a quiet time when the parents and the child feel greater interdependency
- Promote self assertiveness among older children
- Explain to the child that they might have had bad dreams; reassure the child during the bad dreams, help them to imagine a good ending to the bad dream; ask the child to draw pictures or write stories of bad dreams which will have happier ending
- Have several conversations with the child about the dream and take measures to keep the child's fear away
- Discourage the child (before 13 years of age) to see horror movies or violent scenes at bedtime which may develop fears or nightmares
- Consult clinical psychologist if the nightmares become worse or constant or if fear in interfering with daytime activities or persistence of several fears.

Night Terrors

Night terrors will be observed in 2 per cent of children with one to eight years of age. The episode lasts for 10–30 minutes, but the child will not remember the episode in the morning. It usually occurs within 2 hours of bedtime, the problem disappears by 12 years of age or sooner.

Causes

- An inherited disorder, where the child tends to have dreams during deep sleep from which it is difficult to awaken

- Over tiredness triggers night terrors
- Family stress.

Manifestations

- Child is frightened but cannot be awakened or comforted
- Agitated child may sit up or run helplessly
- Screaming or talking wildly or fall down or even break a window
- Eyes are wide opening and staring
- Unaware of surroundings which includes persons, place, etc.
- May mistake objects or persons in the room for dangers.

Interventions

- Help the child to get away from agitated sleep to normal sleep.
- Make soothing comments repetitively, e.g. you are alright, you are at home, you can take rest now, etc.
- Don't shout or shake the child which may prolong the attack.
- Protect the child against injuries, gently direct them to go back to bed.
- Parents should not overreact to the episode, understand the child provide protective measures.
- Prompted awakening exercise has to be implemented consecutively for seven days or more, e.g. observe how many minutes elapse from falling asleep to the onset of the night terror, then awaken the child 15 minutes before the expected time, keep the child fully awake and out of bed for five minutes.
- Consult pediatrician or clinical psychologist if the child is having day time fears, episode lasts longer than 30 minutes; any drooling or jerking or stiffening occurs.

Sleep Walking (Somnambulism)

Fifteen per cent of normal children (4–15 years of age) will have inherited tendency to wander during deep sleep. It occurs within 2 hours of bed time. This episode may last 5–20 minutes. This type of behaviour will usually stop by adolescence.

Causes

- Fatigue
- Lack of sleep
- Exhaustion.

Manifestations

- Child walks while asleep with blank open eyes
- Child will not be able to coordinate when awakes
- Child will perform the activities like dressing/ undressing; opening and closing doors, switching the lights on and off
- During the episode the child cannot be awakened, inspite of any effort.

Interventions

- Take the child to bathroom, assist for toileting and gently make them to get back to bed
- Don't put efforts to awaken the child, however, before they return to normal sleep
- Protect the child from accidents
- Avoid exhaustion
- Eliminate the child distressing sleep pattern
- Observe the episode pattern for several nights for the onset, duration, activities done by the child during sleep
- Make the child to be fully awaken 15 minutes before the expected time
- Carry out these prompted awakening for 7 consecutive nights.

Early Morning Riser

Among toddlers, some children who have rested well in the night will wake up early in the morning and excited, and wants to share this enjoyment with everyone at home in early morning hours as they no longer tired and awake early with no purpose.

Causes

- Child may be put to bed too early in the night before or had too many naps or had naps that were too long
- Some children may have reduced sleep requirement.

Interventions

- Reduce naps during the day, shorten the nap to 1½ hour
- Plenty of exercise has to be planned for the child as it promotes sleep during night time
- Delay bed time until 9 pm or 10 pm
- Formulate rule for the child, e.g. child has to play quietly in their bedroom until parents wake up, explain the child in a polite way that parents and others in the family also needs their sleep
- Keep some toys in a crib, the child will play with them and sleep off and after awakening also they will be playing with toys without disturbing the parents
- Praise the child or give a reward or special treat for not waking other people in the early morning
- Consult a physician if the child does not improve after trying this approach for 4 weeks and if the child has other behavioural problems also along with this complaint.

CONDUCT DISORDERS

Conduct of a child is "the behaviour of the total individual as expressed in psychological as well as physical activity; behaviour conforms to the standards established by the person's social group". Conduct disorders are marked by repetitive, persistent, aggressive conduct in which basic rights are violated.

It encompasses a range of dysfunctional behaviours that emerge over the course of childhood. Commonly seen in older children and adolescents. Conduct disorders have more deleterious consequences for individual, family and society at large.

For example, Hostile and defiant behaviour toward authority like disobedience, temper tantrums, argumentativeness, school refusal, rule violations; lying, fighting, bullying others

- Aggression towards others
- Destruction of property, theft, deceit
- Disruptive behaviours lead to impairment in everyday functioning
- Physical violence against persons or property like vandalism, rape, breaking, fire setting, assault behaviour; purse snatching, mugging, aggression and violence
- Conduct problems like peer rejection, school problems, conflictual interactions with parents, shyness, withdrawal
- Comorbid among adolescents–depression is strongly associated with suicide, substance abuse.

Types

- Aggressive type
- Group type, undifferentiated type.

Aetiology or Risk Factors

- Child temperament: Negative mood
  - Lower levels of approach towards newer stimuli
  - Less adaptability to change.

Psychosocial Factors

- Children often neglected or abused
- Brought up in chaotic situations, e.g. angry, disruptive, demanding, unable to progress or develop tolerance for frustration no role model for ego ideal and conscience; little or no motivation to follow societal norms.
- Neuro psychological deficits and difficulties, e.g. deficit in diverse functions related to language like verbal fluency, verbal (learning, IQ); memory, motor coordination, disintegration of auditory and visual clues, deficit in executive functions of the brain, i.e. abstract reasoning, concept formation, planning, attention and its control.

Parental Factors

- Prenatal and perinatal complications–maternal infection, prematurity, low birth weight, minor birth injury, impaired respirations at birth
- Parental psychopathology and stress
- Poor parental practices–Coercive parent–child communications, faulty child rearing practices, parental psychopathology, child abuse, inconsistent discipline, harsh or corporal punishment; over controlling parenting; Poor supervision, establishment of few or no rules;
- *Family factors*: Broken family, negligence, sociopath, negative attitude, substance abuse, less parental acceptance, less warmth, affection, attachment and emotional support, large family size; sibling with anti-social behaviour; high risk families–low socio–economy, low educational attainment, high stress living conditions
- *Marital discard*: Marital detachment, unhappy or strained marital relationship, interpersonal conflicts and aggression of parents
- *Social problems*: Poverty, overcrowding, unemployment, poor housing
- *Scholastic factors*: Little emphasis on academic work, little teacher guidance, infrequent usage of positive reinforcement by the teacher for child's accomplishments, e.g. less appreciation for school work; little emphasis on individual responsibility of the students; poor working conditions; unavailability of teacher; low teacher expectations.
- *Socio–cultural factors*: Socio–economically deprived children
- *Organic factors*: Brain damage
- *Neuro biological factors*: Decreased production of noradrenaline.

Clinical Features

The behaviours must be repetitive, persistent and associated with impaired functioning.

Childhood Onset Conduct Disorder

Aggressive, disturbed peer relationships, school drop outs, lower attainments.

Adolescent Onset Conduct Disorder

Antisocial personality disorder, vandalism, illegal behaviours.

Adolescent Onset Continuity in Adulthood

Aggressive type engage in fighting; antisocial personality, isolated symptoms (anxiety, somatic complaints), criminal behaviour; arrest records; shorter history of employment, lower status in jobs, more frequent change of jobs, lower wages, depends more frequently for financial status; higher rates of divorce, remarriage, separation; less contacts with friends and relatives little participation in social aggregations; higher rate of hospitalization and death.

Major Diagnostic Symptoms

Obviously exhibiting antisocial behaviour
- Bullying or threatening others
- Fighting
- Causing harm physically to others or to animals by using weapons;
- Stealing while confronting a victim (e.g. Mugging, purse snatching, extortion, armed robbery)
- Rape or forcing someone into sexual activity
- Fire setting
- Destroying property of others, e.g. damaging some body's house, building or car
- Frequently 'lying' or 'connecting' others
- Staying out late at night despite parental prohibitions
- Running away from home
- Being truant from school
- Physical aggression

- Exhibiting hostility and cruel behaviour with peer group
- Hostile
- Verbal abuse
- Impudent
- Defiant
- Negativistic towards adults, low self esteem
- Frequent truancy, destructiveness, using physical violence
- Socially withdrawn, isolated
- Substance abuse like tobacco, liquor or drugs
- Unusual sexual behaviour
- Lacks concern, feeling, wishing and welfare of others
- Easily frustrated
- School refusal, failure, disobedient, exhibits reckless behaviour.

Clinical Course

Conduct disorders can emerge in childhood or in adolescence. Adolescence onset is more common and is equally distributed among both sexes. Childhood onset conduct disorders are more severe form and leads to antenatal behaviour and other psychiatric disorders.

Assessment

Assess
- Parental practice
  Parent–child interactions
- Parental psychopathology
  Child's peer relationships
- If school or learning problems are suspected, perform educational assessment
  Functional analysis of behaviour patterns base line follow-up ratings
- Self report analysis: Inventories or check lists for child over 10 years of age can provide a valid report of their conduct
  Reports of significant others (parents, relatives, teachers)

Parents are in a unique position to provide accounts of a child's functioning and changes over a time. Their reports correlate significantly with clinical judgement.
- Child behaviour checklist, specific scales
- Direct observations
- Institutional and societal records will be used to measure anti-social behaviour as they represent a significant indicator of the impact of the problem on society
- Management: Multimodal Approach.

TREATMENT

Pharmacotherapy

Aims:
- To alleviate aggression
  To reduce reactivity, moderate levels of emotional arousal
  Psycho stimulants, e.g. Methylphenidate Amphetamine
- Mood stabilizers, e.g. Lithium Carbamazepine, Valproic acid
- Anti psychotics, e.g. chlorpromazine Haloperidol, Clozapine
- Adrenergic agents, e.g. Clonidine Propranolol, Metaprolal.

Evidence Based Psychosocial Treatments

This treatment has to be utilized considering child's age, severity, range of problems, family needs and commitment
- Parental guidance is needed
- Psychotherapies
- Parent management training
  - Parents are trained to interact with the child in ways to promote pro social behaviour and child's adaptive behaviour
- Develops interactions between parents and the child to promote positive parent and child behaviour

- To decrease disruptive behaviour
- Cognitive problem
  - solving skills training to resolve inter-personal problems
- Approaches in interpersonal situations to promote alternative consequences of actions.
- Multi systemic therapy: focus on child behaviour within the context of various systems (e.g. family, peer group and schools); help will be given to alter the child behaviour; to promote communication, to reduce negative interaction and to improve the parental functioning
- General relationship therapy
  Home making services, special school
- Residential placement
  Behaviour modification technique
      Child will be treated either in home or in foster homes or in the hospital.

Prevention

- Identify high risk families and supportive services have to be provided
      Provide counselling related to maternal care includes antenatal care, postnatal care
- Provide support in the home to reduce stress
      To prepare the parents for child rearing demands and practices
- Counselling services have to be provided to develop cognitive skills of the child and to enroll the child in school and make him to participate actively in scholastic programmes, selection of peer groups, develops positive skills and success experiences in the school and at home
- Encourage the family members to develop bonding relationships.

CHILDHOOD DISRUPTIVE BEHAVIOUR/ ANTISOCIAL DISORDER

Commonly seen in older children and adolescents. Conduct is the 'behaviour of the total individual as expressed in psychological as well as physical activity', behaviour that conforms to the standards established by the person's social group.

Conduct disorders are marked by 'repetitive, persistent, aggressive conduct in which basic rights are violated', e.g. Physical violence against persons or property

- Vandalism
- Rape
- Breaking Burning private/public property Mugging
- Assault
- Purse snatching.

Aetiology

1. Parental Factors
   - Attitude of parenting
     Faulty child rearing practices
   - Development of maladaptive behaviour
     Chaotic home condition
   - Broken family
     Parental psychopathology
   - Child abuse
     Negligence
   - Sociopath
     Alcoholism
   - Substance abuse
2. Socio-cultural factors
   - Socio-economically deprived children
     Socially unacceptable means and behaviours
3. Psychological factors
   - Neglected or abused children
     Children brought up in chaotic situation easily become angry
   - Disruptive
     Demanding
   - Unable to progress or develop tolerance from frustration
   - No role model for ego-ideal and conscience
   - Children are left with little motivation to follow societal norms
4. Neurobiological factors
   - Decrease non-adrenaline

5. Other factors
   - The temperament of the child in the later age
   Brain damage.

Clinical Features

- Bullying
  Physical aggression
- Cruel behaviour towards peer
- Lacks sustained normal peer relationship
  Hostile
- Verbally abusive
  Impudent
- Deviant
  Negativistic towards adults
- Low self-esteem
  Persistent lying
- Frequent truancy
  Vandalism
- Destructiveness
  Stealing
- Physical violence
  Obvious antisocial behaviour
- Socially withdrawn
- Isolated
  Regular use of tobacco, liquor, unusual sexual behaviour
- Lack feeling, wishes and welfare of others
  Easily frustrated
- Group type people could form age-appropriate peer relations or friendship
- School failure
  Disobedient
- Reckless behaviour.

Course and Prognosis

- Commonly starts in the early school age, but usually get corrected before adolescence
  Treatment
- Multimodal
  Individual psychotherapy
- Family therapy
  Special schooling

- Pharmacotherapy
  Home-making services
- Residential placement
  Behaviour modification therapy.

Conversional Syndrome

Whenever the child feels stress in going to school due to varied factors such as fear of new school, insults and beating from the teacher or bullying by classmates, etc. the child may exhibit certain manifestations like convulsions, paralysis of the limbs, fear, anxious, which are originating because of psychological stressors. Whenever the child faces such problem and is unable to find the solution the body responds to stress; when the parents tries for the salvation of the problem, the manifestations disappears. Guidance activities to be carried out:

- Allow the child to talk about her problems
  Identify the cause and attempts to be made to remove the cause
- Advise the parents to develop calm and quiet environment within the family and its surroundings
- Parents should not pay excessive attention for undue complaints by the child
- Teach better strategies for salvation of problem.

Passive Rebellion

Child will have stubbornness, sullenness, pouting, refuses to answer to questions. It usually occurs when the baby is punished to the open rebellion behaviour by the parents or elders.

Going back to the childish behavioural patterns:
If child's desires are not fulfilled, they will go back to certain behaviours like:

- The child after attaining bladder and bowel control again starts wetting or enuresis; wants to be fed by parents, thumb-sucking, etc.

Remedial Measures

- Taught the child how to use their skills and decision-making power

- Train them to meet their demands independently on their own
- Parents should not take this normal phase of negativism too personally; this phase is critical to the development of independence and identity
- Try to look at it with a sense of humour and amazement
- Try to explain the situation to the child, if he is able to understand and punish the child for what he does, not for what he says 'no', ignore it, if the parents are arguing with the child it may prolong the behaviour
- Increase the child's sense of freedom and control by giving plenty of choices as the child gains a feeling that he is a decision-maker and he will become more cooperative
- Avoid threatening the child, if the child has to follow compulsorily for his welfare, make him to understand and follow it. For example, following road safety rules to prevent accidents
- If the child has to change the activities, give advance information to the child, so that they can prepare the mind to change the activities, e.g. the child will be enjoying the play activities, as lunch time approaches give the child 5 minute advance notice
- Don't insist excessive rules to be followed; if rules are less, the child may agree about following them
- Help the child to have more positive interactions than negative ones each day
- Avoid responding to the child's request with 'no'. For example, The child may ask a glass-doll to play with, say sorry and give the reason so that the child will try to understand.

Spoiling

Child with self-centeredness, who wants everything and not wiling to give anything in return. Parents should not give too much attention by pampering them and giving whatever they asks, as it may spoil them. Usually first-born, last-born and one-child are having more chances of spoiling. However, any baby can be spoiled. Parents should show attention what the child requires to enhance normal growth and development of their children.

Remedies to prevent spoiling
- Answer child's cries once in a while, let them wait when something more important comes up
- Parents have to find things, that the child can enjoy it by doing themselves
- Encourage the child to observe and listen to other people, when they are performing the activities and give them chance to talk with others
- Assign simple tasks for children to help each other, when they are able to do so. If they accomplish the tasks, elders have to praise them for performing well.

Jealousy

Usually jealousy among children is observed, when one more baby arrives in the family, the elder child will feel that the newborn is give more attention and they feel jealousy. Children with jealousy always will exhibit angry. They will feel that their place in someone's affection has been taken by another person, i.e. intruder, hence these children will try to show their anger by fighting with intruder by kicking, hitting, biting or he will try to hurt the feelings of intruders. As the child is afraid of loosing love, so he will expose his feelings by crying.

To prevent jealousy behaviour among toddlers, the parents should meet the toddler's need, show their attention and love, allow them to stay around when the new baby's physical needs are being taken care of and encourage them in taking care of their own siblings. It will lessen the toddler's anger.

Selfishness

Development of a sense of ownership is necessary before they can learn to be generous with others. Slowly they learn the joy of giving and of sharing with others. Children should be allowed to decide whether to give or refuse their toys to another child.

Adults can help child, learn to share with others. Group play encourages the habit of sharing.

Hurting Others

If the hurting is accidental, the incident should be overlooked. But if the children persistently try to hurt others adult help is needed to prevent serious injury to another child. Adults should not allow their children to hurt others. Hurting may be with the mental state. Children should know that some one who loves them deeply will control them and so prevent the unpleasant consequences of their behaviour. They need to feel secure within limits beyond which they are not allowed to go. The adult takes the actions in situations in which children are likely to hurt others, other children are directed in some activity they all enjoy in happy play. Encourage the child to participate in group play to enhance the security.

Destructiveness

Destructive children are usually unhappy, unable to control their feelings of jealousy, helplessness, aggression or anger. They may feel unloved, disliked by peers or bored by inadequate play things. The parents should avoid scolding or punishment. They should help direct the children energy into appropriate activities.

Developing Self-esteem

The sense of initiative, children enlarge their concept of self by relating it to the world. Through playing the roles of adults, children assign qualities to their self-concept. Consistency and sincere encouragement by parents, family members, teachers and peer opinions regarding adequacies and acquisition of motor, language and self-care skills.

Physiologic-Biologic needs

Control of bodily functions

By the end of preschool period, children are adequately independent in toilet skills. Accident may still happen during periods of stress illness, or if children are involved in play activities.

Anxiety Disorders

In normal growth and development, anxiety has an adaptive function, to alert an individual. Anxiety becomes pathologic, when it interferes with normal development by preventing the children from mastering major developmental tasks like academics, social integration and self perception. Anxiety is an anticipatory response to perceived threat, either internal or external.

Aetiology and Risk Factors

- Children are born with biologically or constitutionally predetermined temperaments, children with 'inhibited temperaments' are at risk for development of social phobia
- *Environmental factors,* e.g. Neurobiologic insults, exposure to trauma; when needs were not met, peer teasing, parental discord
- Extreme behavioural inhibitions in toddler period results in social anxiety in adolescents and adults
- The stress of school entry due to separation of primary care giver
- *Familial background or environment,* e.g. If parents had anxiety, children also imitate the same behaviour
- Children with serious illness
- Disruptive change in the school or home environment
- Death or illness of a loved one
- Social phobia in first degree biological relatives, e.g. specific phobias aggregate within families, e.g. fear of blood or injury
- Neuro transmitters interactions disturbances, e.g. GABA (r–amino butyric acid) Nor epineplirine (NE), serotonin (S) Neuropeptide–Y (NPY) and Cholecystokinin (CCK)
- Stress related to separation either temporary or permanent

- Disturbance in the functioning of limbic system, prefrontal cortex or Brain stem, e.g. Phobic anticipatory anxiety are associated with the cingulated portion of the limbic system; Phobic avoidance is associated with the prefrontal cortex, panic reaction is associated with the brain stem.

Clinical Features

- Fear
  - A response to actual threat
- Distressing 'fight or flight' reaction
- Plethora of other physiologic responses that may affect multiple systems including cardiac, pulmonary, GIT and Neurologic.
  Cognitive symptoms, e.g. Feelings of loosing control or loosing one's mind, unwelcome or intrusive thoughts, Inattention, Insomnia
- *Perceptual disturbances,* e.g. Depersonalization or vague visual images.

Types

Separation anxiety disorder (SAD)
Developmentally inappropriate anxiety when faced with separation or anticipated separation from home or loved ones, (including pets) will be killed, lost or kidnapped.

- Afraid to go to sleep by themselves and often sleep with their parents, refused to let them sleep in their bed, these children may sleep on the floor outside the bed room parents, may need to sit with them until they fall asleep
- Unusual experiences, e.g. seeing monsters or feeling that they are being watched
- Sleep disturbances, nightmares related to catastrophic events that destroy the family, e.g. fire, earthquakes
- Fearful of being alone in a room; always wanting their parent in eye sight at all times, may even follows the parent into the bathroom
- Somatic complaints are common in morning, study time or school days dizziness, nausea, vomiting

- School refusal, school phobia because of fear and separation
- When they feel separation, they may be aggressive or tempertantrums are common.

Significant Impairment in Functioning

- Developmentally inappropriate, worries about loss or harm be falling loved ones.

Generalized anxiety disorder (GAD)
GAD Children are characterized by worry about all i.e. school, family, friends, games, safety of their loved ones, possibility of occurrence of natural disasters like earth quakes, nuclear wars etc.

- Complaints many somatic concerns, e.g. headache, abdominal pain, tiredness, muscle pains, etc.
- Cognitive symptoms for example, decreased attention or concentration, irritability
- Worry interferes usual daily functioning for example, difficulty in completing assignments, avoidance of school activities, reluctance to participate in sports and games
- Often questioning about perceived threats, dangers, unanticipated difficulties they may face and they are not easily reassured
- Do not feel confident to cope with all dangers, they think that they could occur
- Always looking for dangers, potential threats and the unexpected
- Do not like surprises; limit participation with their peers
  Commonly 'wide–eyed' or vigilantly scanning their environment
- Social and academic derailment occurs; avoidance by peer group; too distracted by their worries
- Limits participation in usual teen activities, limit peer relationships, may decline to go on family vacations or family gatherings as they feel ill, worried about getting sick or hurt
- Prone to brooding, which tends to distance them from their family and friends; dropping out from

school, as they feel ill or unsafe in school environment or not able to keep up with peers socially

- Depression, adapts substance abuse, excessive worry, i.e. difficult to control, associated with restlessness or the feeling of being on edge, fatigue, difficulty in concentration, mind going blank, irritability, muscle tension, sleep disturbances
- In adults, the symptoms often affect their work performance and marital relationship.

Phobia Disorders

Heterogeneous, excessive, unreasonable fear either involved a single object or a situation, exposure to the phobia stimuli provokes an immediate response and social phobia.

Specific Phobia

Fear and avoidance occurs in response to exposure to a specific object or situation; development of intense and immediate anxiety

Children may appear panic with physiologic arousal when they are frightened by the object or situation or become agitated.

Interferes with social relationships and they may refuse to visit other homes or friends also.

Social Phobia

A marked and persistent fear of one or more social situations, i.e. fear of being placed in social situations

- DSM–IV, TR; Intense anxiety is situated when placed in social settings.

Children with social phobia tend to withdraw from group activities and stay in periphery; they dislike situations in which other scrutinizes them. Often, they cling to familiar adults

- Feeling of separation from a loved one, 'shy' in public

- They do not answer the questions in the class rooms, often they will be mute; school refusal, school failure, truancy begins
- Avoid participating in social gatherings
- Eating may become aversive when he has to eat infront of others
- Same may become paranoid as they avoid talking to others or reluctant to talk over by phone
- Avoids all meaningful social relationships, forego in developing friendships or attachment with peer groups
- A marked and persistent fear of performing one or more social functions, they feel humiliating and embarrassing
- They may cry, have tantrums when exposed to unfamiliar situations
- Unreasonable fear or distress experiencing in group situations.

Panic Disorder

Children with panic disorder become withdrawn; They make many excuses about why they cannot go out; they become distressed, withdrawn or refuse to mingle with others; getting impairment in most domains of life; persistent worry; fear of losing control; a significant change in behaviour; irritable, tantrums.

Panic Attacks

Discrete episodes of intense anxiety that begin without warning and generally peak within 10 minutes:

- Panic attacks are characterized by autonomic arousal, e.g. chest pain, palpitations, numbness, tingling, diaphoresis, child with hot flashes, nausea, vomiting, trembling, dizziness, shortness of breath, feeling of choking, abdominal distress, dizziness
- Cognitive symptoms
  - feelings of being unreal or detached from oneself, fear of dying or going crazy;

unprovoked tantrums, manipulative or controlling, e.g. throwing and destroying objects

- It may occur at least 4 times per week followed by 1 month apprehension about additional attacks
- Irrational, irritable and having tantrums without warning.

Assessment

- Mental status examination
- Rating scales and checklists.

Treatment

1. Cognitive Behavioural Therapy

- Multi-modal, e.g. cognitive behavioural therapy, family therapy, pharmacotherapy and exposure and response prevention (EPR)
- Involve school staff, family members, primary care clinicians and therapists in all the treatments.
  Aim: To modify the child's maladaptive behaviour into adoptive behaviour.

Procedure

- Identifying automatic 'thinking errors' that perpetuate the anxiety, i.e. a wide range of internal thought constructs that organize how children perceive, code and experience their world and then fuel their emotions, e.g. over generalization (e.g. all monkeys are going to bite me); catastrophic thinking (e.g. I know this world going to end, earth quakes occurs)
- Restructure their thinking and develop a plan to cope with anxiety arousal by stressful situations.
- Home work assignment, practicing coping skills
- Treatment gains also tend to be maintained 3 years follow-up
- An attitude of 'readiness to change' has to be there for children when they come for treatment.

2. Exposure and Response Prevention (ERP)

- ERP focusses on identifying a hierarchy of fearful stimuli; helpful for specific phobia
- Teaching the child relaxation techniques and desensitizing the child to fearful stimuli via graded exposure
- ERP process is repeated until treatment goals are obtained
- Children were given home work assignments and allowed to practice coping skills while being exposed to anxiety provoking situation
- Parents are involved in a supportive role as consultants and learned to use coping skills and learn how to support the child in implementation of adaptive responses
- Encourage the parents to form support groups/networks with other parents as group strategies found to be very effective. The family involvement augments the benefits of individual therapy.

Barrett and short developed the 'FRIENDS' Programme

F– Feeling worried? Educate the children to recognize anxiety

R– Relax and feel good. Relaxation skills are taught and practiced

I– Identify the children's inner thoughts

E– Explore plans; problem solving skills are taught and practiced

N– Need rewards; evaluate children's performances and reward themselves for little perfection

D– Don't forget to practice; children are learnt to practice skills, what they learned

S– Stay calm; as they know how to cope-up with worries.

3. Family Therapy

- To change family maladaptive patterns to adaptive patterns

- To improve competence and functioning pattern
- To increase family bonding and coping strategies.

4. *Pharmacotherapy*

Anti depressants–1st line
Benzodiazepines–2nd line
Antipsychotics–3rd line
Anticonvulsants
B–blockers.

JUVENILE DELINQUENCY

Definitions

'A juvenile delinquent is a person between the ages of 15–17, who indulges in anti-social activity'.

'Juvenile delinquent, who breaks the law, is a vagrant, persists in disobeying orders, whose behaviour endangers his own moral life as well as the moral life of other'.

'Juvenile delinquent involves wrong doing by a child or a young person, who is under age specified by the law of the place concerned'.

—Dr Sethna

'A delinquent is a person under age, who is guilty of anti-social act and whose misconduct is an infraction of law'.

Causes of Juvenile Delinquency

1. Social causes
   Defects of the family: In broken families, where family ties and mutual intimate relationships have been destroyed.
   Parent-child relationship: When the child is deprived of love and is scolded constantly on every occasion, child develops feeling of revolt and hatred, so that he runs away from the house and falls into a life of criminals. It induces a feeling of insecurity and develops mental complexes. If the parents have negative attitude, hurt the child's feelings and lead to insecurity children's tendency towards crime is aggravated.

Character and conduct of parents at home: The child's personality is considerably influenced by the character and conduct of their parents. Child has been able to mould their behaviour according to socially accepted values and conceptions. If parents are indulged in such behaviour like telling lies, hypocritical behaviour, sexual immorality and thieving will have effect over the child's development.

Influence of siblings or criminal relatives: Child's personality is susceptible to the influence of his siblings' personality apart from the personality and mutual relationship of the parents. If the siblings in the family manifest criminal tendencies and immoral behaviour the youngsters are invariably influenced by it.

2. Defects in the school
   - Next to the family, the child's personality is influenced by the school
   - Theft and sex crimes
   - Low intelligence level
   - Roaming outside the school (vagrancy)
   - Criticism by parents and teachers
   - Gaining membership of a gang and criminals
   - Punishment by teachers
   - Weakness in some subject
   - Level of education is too high
   - Lack of companionship or influence of bad companion.

3. Influence of cinemas or movies
   Mass-media activities.

4. Physical abnormalities
   Like handicapped children have to overcome their insecurity develops deliquescent behaviour.

5. War and post war condition
   While the father is in war zone and mother is in some occupation due to this the children's education is considerably affected. In war time, wherever there is bombing, the adolescents took the greatest part in looting and smashing the houses.

6. Social disorganization
   Disorganization of society leads to increase in criminal activity. Modern industrial societies where lack of synthesis and equality, creates tension. This tension inspires young men and women to perform delinquent activities.

7. Displacement
   Displacement of thoughts, ideas, attitudes, in a negative manner influence child's conduct and demoralize the child's values.

8. Psychological causes
   • Intellectual weakness
   • Mental diseases
   • Psychopathic personality.
   Total absence of love, affection and control. The individual is unsocialized, irritable, cruel, obstinate, suspicious, self-centered, lonely, full of feelings of revenge, backward and hyper-sexual or uncontrolled sexual behaviour. In extreme cases, the person lacks the ability to sympathize completely devoid of repentance over their own cruel doings and the pain or suffering of others.

9. Personality Defects
   The method of an individual's adaptation to environment. Criminal children resort to illegal modes of such adaptation.

• Degree of freedom
• Irresponsibility
• Revolt
• Homicidal tendency
• Suspicious
• Lack of control
• Sadism
• Emotional and social maladjustment
• Extrovert behaviour
• Immaturity in sentiment
• Lack of emotional balance, unbalanced through lack of love and affection
• Disobedient and unsocial
• Inferiority complex.

10. Economic Causes
• Poverty
• Poor working condition
• Unemployment
• Child labour
• Unfulfilled desires.

Control of Juvenile Delinquency

a. *Probation*

Juvenile delinquents are kept under the supervision of a probation officer, whose job is to look after the delinquent, to help him in getting established in normal life and to see that the delinquent observes the rules of bail-bond. Thus, the delinquent not only gets a chance to reform himself, but also gets advice and concrete help.

b. *Reformatory Institutions*

To reform inmate delinquents, the institutions provide an all round personality development by sufficient means of separating the inmates by providing adequate facilities to meet the basic needs such as proper sanitary arrangements, water supply, food, clothing and bedding for the inmates and vocational or industrial training. When delinquent becomes sick medical aid will be provided.

c. *Certified Schools (Fit Persons Institution)*

These are established for the treatment of juvenile delinquent. The schools are of two types:
• Junior school < 12–13 years of age. (Primary education)
• Intermediate school 13–15 years of age. (Technical education)
• Senior school between 15–17 years of age. (Industrial training)
   The children are generally confined there upto a certain age limit and for about 2–3 years, but the school authorities can make an early discharge.

After their release, they are kept under the charge of a welfare officer or probation officer.

d. *Auxiliary Homes*

These are attached to certified schools, here the delinquents are kept for sometime and studied by a social worker and then they are sent to the certified schools according to the nature and aptitude of a young offender.

e. *Foster Homes*

These are specially for delinquent children of under 10 years of age, who cannot be sent to approved or certified schools unless the court is satisfied that they cannot be dealt with otherwise. These are generally run by voluntary agencies, aided by government.

f. *Uncared Children Institutions*

The children in the pre-delinquent or near delinquent stage, who are mostly found in a state of destitution or neglect, are cared for. All over the country they are situated, managed by private philanthropists.

g. *Reformatory School*

These are meant for the education and vocational training of delinquent children with much regard to the type of crime committed. The delinquents are removed from bad environments and placed in the reformatory school for sometime after which they can adapt some vocation learnt in the school. Young offenders, under 15 years of age are imprisoned for 3–7 years.

h. *Borstal Institutions*

It is a system of detaining juvenile delinquents, first correctional purpose of reformatory is at borstal. Special treatment is provided for adolescent offenders between the ages of 15–21 years.

Two Types of Borstal Institutions

Open institutions: Open environment with no surrounding wall.

Closed institutions: Converted prison building where maximum security provided.

Industrial training, where arduous physical training and education will be given according to the age, record and character of the inmate so as to deter them from committing crime again. The training is different for boys and girls. For example, Mixed farming, building and engineering laundry, cooking and housework. 2–3 years is the term of borstal but the date of release is decided by the borstal authorities according to conduct and progress of the inmate. The person is attached to borstal associate or probation officer, whose duties are to see that he is fitted in the trade for which he has been trained.

i. *Psychological Techniques*

*   Play therapy
    The delinquent children are given opportunities to participate in play, which give expression to the repressed motives and help in the development of creative energy.
*   Finger painting
    The child is given plain papers and some colours. Child is allowed to paint in his own way. The purpose is not painting, but expression of repressed motives in the child, which leaves them sensible and healthy.
*   Psychodrama
    The child is allowed to participate in different roles in group drama and thereby manifest their repressed motives. The Psychologists reform delinquents by creating healthy atmosphere in the family and by providing adequate healthy recreation. Coordinated and concentrated efforts of teachers, guardians, and government are required to organize psychodramas by delinquent children.

j. *Government Measures*

- Formal education
- Vocational training in a number of trades is imported to the inmates. Certified, reformatory and borstal schools enable them to settle down in trades learnt in school.
- Follow-up services are given. Training in citizenship of democratic living. The juvenile delinquents are encouraged to take part in extra-curricular activities, e.g. Sports, debate, dramas, music and scouting.
- Rehabilitation–guidance and training. Family community based programmes have to be organized to improve environment and to reduce the peer group influences.
- Behaviour therapy
  Motivate the child by reinforcing good habits, which modify maladaptive behaviour.
- Family therapy.
- To establish intimate relationship safeguards child's freedom by engaging them in useful activities.

Prevention of Juvenile Delinquency

- Team work of private and public agencies.
  These agencies assist parents and guardians in locating difficult children in danger of maladjustment and in recognizing early symptoms of unhappiness, conflict and insecurity.
- Training of members and staff of all organizations.
  Counsels to recognize the juvenile delinquents and to overcome the difficulties.
- Establishment of child guidance clinics
  Diagnostic facilities are established in the schools to treat seriously disturbed and maladjusted children.
- Education of the family
  Health professionals educate the family members about preventive measures and rehabilitation of the clients with juvenile delinquency.

- Establishment of recreational agencies
  Provision for sport activities, cultural activities, organizational activities.
- Assistance to under privileged children
  Character building agencies like schools, churches should be encouraged to serve under privileged children.
- Propaganda
  Through mass media like newspaper, magazines, radio, TV, motion pictures, to encourage the parents for good child rearing practices.

Unsocial Behaviour

Shyness of the child appears between 4–6 months of age. Its peak is observed around one year, gradually reduces with each passing month. The babies with shyness should be given an opportunity to see, to touch and to hear new things and exposes to new people slowly to remove fear. Allow the child to explore new and different things under parent's supervision. Give the objects/toys to children which are safer to handle. For example, If the baby is approaching for glass items, change the baby movement in safer side (away from glass items).

Encourage the child to share their toys with other children in play, which will promote cooperative and parallel play among children; prevents the child from fighting and grabbing their toys. If the child is cooperatively sharing their toys with other children, parents have to show their appreciation and encourage the children for sharing, concern and affection.

Head Banging

When the toddler is under stress, he may bang his head against the bed or rocking in bed in rhythmic movements as it gives pleasure and diversion for the child. To prevent injuries to the child, parents have to take proper precautions like protective clothing over the bed and try to explain to the child to avoid that habit formation.

Temper Tantrums

Temper tantrums usually seen among toddlers and preschoolers. If they are persistent and severe, it may become pathological; otherwise it can be relieved. These behavioural syndromes are violent and short lived in nature. It results from frustration or when the child's desires are blocked; when the child's independence was asserted and discipline wad objected. During temper tantrum the child may lie down on the floor, kick their feet, scream out at the maximum living capacity, tear off their clothes and holds the head.

Management

- Behaviour therapy and play therapy are indicative in treating the child with temper tantrum.
- Encourage the child to express his anger and other emotions in a socially acceptable manner
- Measures to be taken to relieve child's emotional tensions whenever it is possible
- Parents have to be close with the child during temper tantrum, acknowledge orally to the child and efforts have to be implemented in inculcating self control in the child
- During temper tantrum, parents have to observe the child carefully to prevent the child from self injury or from injuring others
- Remove the stressor, place the child in calm and quiet environment, divert the child's mind and attention by providing toys
- Child should be given time and space to recover
- Adult must be firm and consistent in train-up the child's personality development.

Obsessive-Compulsive Disorder

Obsessive-Compulsive disorder appears in late childhood; child will often follow rituals like repeatedly doing the activity and again checking it. Obsessional thoughts more often concerned with contamination, illness related to parents or others.

Management

- *Behavioural therapy.* For example, response prevention strategy, i.e. train-up the child to become aware of the cues that trigger the obsessional idea or compulsive ritual and then using distraction techniques to interrupt the obsessional idea or to make the performance of ritual impossible
- Drug therapy, e.g. Clomipramine
- Family therapy
- Psychological counselling.

Dissociative Disorders

Common in adolescence. Partial or complete loss of the normal integration between past and present, immediate sensation, control of body movement.

Manifestations

- Paralysis
- Gait variation
- Inability to see or hear.

Management

- Behaviour therapy
- Psychotherapy
- Deep breathing and other exercises.

Mood Disorders

Common in children and adolescents.

Manifestations

- Depression
- Irritable mood
- Lack of interest
- Failure to make expected weight gain
- Insomnia or hypersomnia
- Psychomotor agitation or retardation
- Fatigue
- Decreased ability to think, concentrate
- Recurrent thoughts of death.

Management

- Cognitive therapy
- Psychotherapy–psycho-education, counselling
- Behaviour therapy–modelling, role playing, problem solving approach
- Social skill training
- Drug therapy–antidepressants or antimanics based on symptoms
- Family therapy.

Depression

Early onset depression often persists, recurs and continues into adulthood. Depression in childhood may also predict more severe illness in adult life. Depression in young people is often accompanied by psychological manifestations or other anxiety disorders. It also occurs in conjunction with illness like diabetes mellitus.

Risk Factors

- Family history
- Teen cigarette smoking
- Stress
- Loss of parent or loved one
- Attentional, conduct or learning disorder
- Chronic illness
- Abuse or neglect
- Orphans.

Incidence

- In childhood, boys and girls appear to be at equal risk for developing depression
- Adolescent girls however, may be more at risk than boys.

Clinical Manifestations

- Irritable mood
- Loss of interest in activities
- Significant change in appetite or body weight
- Difficulty in sleeping
- Over-sleeping

- Psychomotor agitation or retardation
- Lack of energy
- Feelings of worthlessness or inappropriate guilty
- Difficulty in concentration
- Recurrent thoughts of death or suicide
- Vague, non-specific physical complaints, e.g. headache, muscle ache, pain abdomen
- Easily tiredness
- Frequent absence from schooling or poor performance in school
- Talk or effort to runaway from home
- Outburst of shouting, complaining, unexplained irritability
- Crying a lot, cry easily at smallest pretext or not to talk to anyone, not showing interest in anything
- Being bored
- Lack of playing with friends
- Alcohol or substance abuse
- Social isolation
- Poor communication
- Fear of death
- Extreme sensitivity to rejection or failure
- Increased irritability, anger, hostility
- Reckless behaviour
- Difficulty with relationships
- Moody and cranky.

Somatoform Disorders

Causes: Over protection, rigidity, avoidance of conflicts, emotional struggle.

Manifestations: Body aches, fatigue, malaise, other areas focussing pain, anorexia, weight loss or increase in weight.

Treatment

- Reduction of stressful situations
- Psychotherapy
- Drug therapy, e.g. anxiolytics, antidepressants based on symptoms.

Negativism/Being Stubborn/ Ornery/Contrary

Children with negativism usually does the opposite of what others want, they will resist to the demands made by the others or who are in authority. It begins around 6 months of age onwards, it tends to get stronger by passing each month, reaching its peak around 2–3 years. It starts when children discover that they have the power to respond negatively to many questions including pleasant ones. In general they are stubborn rather than cooperative. They get happiness in extremely frustrating the parents. The baby cries, screams, kicks, bites and slashes. If anyone is within reach, the child will bit, hit or throw objects at the person.

Nail Biting

Commonly observed among preschool age and school age children. It is an attempt when the child wants to humiliate and annoyed by his parents. Usually, anxiety causes the child to bite the nail, cuticle or skin margins of the nail bed and surrounding nail tissue. As it is painful, the child wants to punish by himself in order to cope-up with hostile feelings towards parents.

Treatment

Parents and teachers have to encourage the child to express true/open feelings.

Parents have to increase self-confidence among children recognition, encouragement and praise the child for their achievements.

For example, Provide manicure set and praise them for well maintained hands and nails.

Masturbation

In preschool age children, it is observed that boys and girls feel pleasurable sensation by touching and manipulating genitals. For example, Rubbing of thighs against each other; rhythmic swaying movement. In adolescent boys, this behaviour is observed and they are curious to explore the sexual impulses as it may cause sexual excitement, erection of penis; it develops sense of mastery over sexual impulses and capacities which helps the adolescent to prepare for heterosexual relationships; and this act releases the anxiety and tension among the teens. If the parents focusses a great deal of attention on masturbation activity of their children, the child will develop parent-child conflict.

Management

- Allay/reduce the parents' anxiety as it is generally harmless and normal
- Child's curiosity has to be channelized in other directions
- Educate the child that masturbation is a private affair and can be done in privacy
- Motivate the child to develop self-control
- Parents must show love, affection, attention and concern to their children, encourage and divert the child's mind in exploring knowledge and they should teach about sex education, sex hygiene
- Channelize the child's curiosity in other useful directions by diverting the mind with other constructive and purposeful activities.

School Refusal

Some children are emotionally dependent on their mother and they will have difficulty in adjusting to the school set-up.

Clinical Features

- Fearful
- Anxious
- In the beginning, crying a lot for going to school is a natural phenomenon, in course of time the child will be used to go to school. But if it persists for a long period, teacher has to handle the situation very carefully.

For example, During initial days of the school, mother is allowed to stay with the child in the class room and make the child to get acquainted with classroom and the other children. Slowly the mother has to reduce the stay with the child and after few days/weeks she has to accompany the child upto the gate.

Problems in Toilet Training

Enuresis

The neuromuscular maturation of bladder occurs among toddlers usually around three years, i.e. myelination of nerves completely occurs to the urinary bladder and anal sphincters and when they can walk, the child is considered to be physically ready for toilet training. Parents have to remember that children can be toilet trained, only when they are completely ready (physical, psychological and intellectual) and are able to control urination and defecation.

Definition

'Repeated or frequent involuntary emptying of bladder or bed wetting results after bladder control occurs'.

Enuresis may occur either in day time or nocturnal period.

Incidence

- It is commonly observed in children over 5–6 years of age
- It is also noticed that boys will suffer more than girls
- Fifteen per cent of children between the ages of 5–10 years are known to be enuretic
- One per cent of children may continue to wet the bed upto 15 years of age.

Types

- Primary enuresis
  The child will never attain bladder control.
- Secondary enuresis
  If the child has once attained bladder control and then subjected to enuresis. It may be nocturnal or diurnal.

- Functional enuresis
  Generally, it occurs after the age of 5 years, may be due to improper toilet training, delayed bladder development, stressful situation, hospitalization and entering to the school.

Causes

- Faulty or defects in toilet training techniques may be adopted by the parents. For example, lack/too early/too severe/over training
- An organic problem, e.g. neurologic defect, incomplete neuromuscular maturation of bladder, mental sub-normality, urinary tract infections, epilepsy, neurological disorder, deformities
- Irritable bladder that cannot hold large quantity of urine
- Over activity of sympathetic nervous system
- Environmental factors, e.g. dark wall, where the child has to walk to reach to bathroom
- Reluctance to get out of a warm bed
- Emotional conflicts, e.g. hostile-dependent parent-child relationships; excessive attempts by the parents in toilet training, emotional disturbances, parent-child maladjustment, disturbed family, marital discard, broken family, separated parents, divorce, death or illness of a parent, school phobia, anxiety, birth of sibling, regression, attention seeking, depression, anger, punishment, rejection by care takers, parents making criticism in front of others
- Subconscious desire of the child to gain care and attention from their parents
- Subconscious resentment against the parents
- Feeling of shame and guilt, fear and nightmares
- Social pressure felt in the new environment
- Familial tendency
- Usually the child may sleep very deeply at night, it may be difficult to arouse them; signals from distended bladder indicating the need to empty the bladder do not reach the conscious level of the mind during sleep results in involuntary emptying of the bladder
- Sleep disorder.

Assessment

- Enquire whether the child is having enuresis problems either in day or at night
- Thorough physical examination and investigations like urinalysis, urine culture and sensitivity have to be carried out to exclude physical deviations.

Management

Parental counselling, behavioural modification techniques and individual psychotherapy.

- As enuresis is generally harmless and self limiting, reassure the child and parents
- All attempts should be reinforced to minimize the emotional impact of enuresis on the child
- Advise the parents not to nag/criticize/embracement or reprimand the child for wetting the bed as it results in low self-esteem in child
- Measures to increase the self-confidence to control the elimination in the child have to be implemented
- Discourage humiliation and punishment of the child
- Refrain the child from taking beverage like tea, coffee after 5 pm. Less fluid should be given after dinner
- Inculcate the habit of emptying the bladder before going to bed, again after 3 hours of sleep, persuade the child to walk unaided to the toilet to empty the bladder
- Motivate the child to control the bladder
- Attempts should be made to attain a positive attitude towards free from enuresis, i.e. always interested to be dry both in day time and night. Train the child to retain the urine for a longer time or to accommodate larger volume of urine in the bladder for a longer time
- Bladder stretching involves the child to hold the urine for increasing length of time
- Conditioning therapy by using the alarms is the safest effective technique to control enuresis, i.e. one type of device goes off as soon as the child begins wetting and other goes off when the bed becomes wet. Restricting fluid before bed time.

Pharmacotherapy

- In very resistant cases after 6 years of age, tricyclic antidepressant, e.g. imipramine 25–50 mg orally at hour of sleep for 2 months may be given or amitriptyline 25 mg at Hs, tincture of belladonna 5–10 drops TID
- Desmopressin, synthetic anti-diuretic hormone given as nasal spray at night for about 4 months may be helpful.

ENCOPRESIS

The child continues to have uncontrolled stool passages beyond the time where bowel control is expected, i.e. about 3–4 years of age. Certain times, school children have bowel movements in unacceptable situations (passing stools in the under garments) such children becomes tense and anxious that their peers may come to know about this problem.

Definition

Encopresis is the 'repeated voluntary or involuntary passing of faeces in inappropriate places after the age at which bowel control is usual, in the absence of known organic cause'.

Causes

- Emotional disturbances
- Too rigid toilet training
- School stress
- Peers may make this situation as embarrassing and humiliating results in with holding defecation rectal and anal sensations may cease
- Constipation
- Parental over concern
- Congenital anorectal anomalies
- Fissures
- Over aggressiveness

- Fear related to toilet
- Attention deficit
- Prolonged gastroenteritis
- Psycho-social stress
- Poor parent-child relationship.

Types

- Primary encopresis.

Present at Birth

- Secondary encopresis
- Starts after a period of continence, faeces may be passed in clothing or deposited inappropriate places, e.g. on the floor of the living room. Children who soil their clothing may deny what has happened and try to hide the dirty clothing. Some children smear faeces on walls or elsewhere.

Clinical Manifestations

- If the child withholds defecation, abdomen becomes distended with faeces and gas
- Diarrhoea results due to irritation of the intestinal tract
- Tensed up.

Diagnosis

- Obtain developmental history of bowel training
- Collect information about current pattern of toilet use, e.g. where the child passes stools, how long, etc.
- Ascertain about family situation.

Management

- Establish regular bowel habits, e.g. ask the child to sit on toilet seat for atleast 10 minutes twice a day
- If the child is able to understand, explain the physiology of bowel elimination and importance of regular evacuation

- Liquid paraffin, a mild laxative may be used for 4–6 weeks
- Provide roughage diet with adequate fluids
- Reestablish a pattern of bowel elimination
- Psychiatric assistance may be required to treat persistent unresolved psychological problems.

Thumb Sucking

Sucking is a normal reflex which has a soothing and calming effect for the child and pleasurable sensation is derived by the child from self stimulation and common instinctual behaviour pattern. Most of the children who habituated thumb sucking will give-up this habit when they are 2 years old or the maximum by the time of schooling. After the age of 7–8 years if the child continues the habit it indicates sign of stress.

Causes

- Emotional insecurity
- Boredom feeling to the child
- Isolation
- Lack of stimulation.

Management

- Parents should avoid excessive anxiety
- Encourage the child to relieve fear, anxiety and other stressors
- Direct the mind with other suitable activities
- Reward technique has to be used, e.g. appreciation, praising the child for constructive behaviour
- If the child cooperates, cover the thumb with either bitter edible substance or with high grade plastic.

Teeth Grinding/Bruxism

It is an involuntary act usually occurs during sleep among school age children. Certain stressors predispose continued bruxism more among school children.

Stressors

- Periodontal disease
- Facial pain
- Possible loss of teeth.

Intervention

- Correction of the alignment of teeth surfaces
- Use of a dental appliance
- Exercise–instruct the child to clench the teeth tightly for 5 seconds and then relax, repeat several times each day for 2 weeks
- Counsel the child regarding the specified stressors.

Personality Disorders

A person's bodily characteristic traits, coping styles and ways of interacting in the social environment emerge during childhood and normally crystallize into established patterns by the end of adolescence or early childhood. The patterns constitute the individual's personality; the unique pattern of traits and behaviours that characterize the individual. For some individuals, personality formation has led to some traits that are so inflexible and maladaptive that they are unable to perform adequately atleast some of the varied roles expected of them by their societies. These people might be diagnosed as having personality disorders. Personality disorders are grouped into 3 clusters on the basis of similarities among the disorders.

Cluster 1: Includes paranoid, schizoid. People with these disorders often seen odd or eccentric with unusual behaviour ranging from distrust and suspiciousness to social detachment.

Cluster 2: Includes histrionic, narcissistic, antisocial and borderline personality disorders. Individuals with these disorders have in common a tendency to be dramatic, emotional and erratic. Their impulsive behaviour, often involving antisocial activities is more forceful and more likely to bring them into contact with mental health or legal authorities than the character disorders in the first cluster.

Cluster 3: Includes avoidant, dependent and obsessive-compulsive personality disorders. Anxiety and fearfulness are often part of these disorders, making it difficult in some cases to distinguish them from anxiety-based disorders. People with these disorders, because of their anxieties are more likely to seek help.

Treatment

Electro-convulsive therapy, psychotherapy, supportive services, guidance and counselling.

Aggression and Tension

One time or the other, children will express anger; aggression or tension. It is the parent's responsibility to observe the reason for the outburst and control the child. Their anger is easily aroused but channelized toward solution of the problem, stop the physical attack and protect the child from harmful activities. Allow older children to express their feelings and make reasonable rules and limitations which the child can follow. These emotional outbursts are common in preadolescents and adolescents.

Causes

- Stressful situation
- After hospitalization
- During illness
- When alone.

Clinical Manifestations

- Nail biting
- Stuttering
- Chewing pencils
- Developing facial twitches.

Remedy

- Control the child and protect from injury
- Lay down the rules, explain the child to follow them

- Find situation in which they shine, praise for successful accomplishment of activities
- Avoid too much noise, violent movies, TV which will arouse tension
- Avoid stressors, provide conflict free conducive environment for the child to learn about his own family and society first, then they tries to control emotions and have control over their environment
- Make the child to learn coping methods, i.e. usage of defense, mechanisms to cope-up during stressful environment or situation.

If all above said measures fails, consult the Psychiatrist for counselling to solve the problem.

Childhood Schizophrenia

Causes

- Disturbed mother-child relationship
- Extreme frightening or threatening experience.

Symptoms

- Inability to respond emotionally
- Frustration-tolerance level is low
- Autistic thinking
- The child is unable to relate to others
- Decreased motor activity
- Child may adapt a bizarre posture, extreme restless, sudden kicking, screaming
- Refusal to talk or to eat
- Loss of interest in play or continuously playing with one toy only
- Irregular sleep pattern
- Head banging.

Treatment

- Psychotherapy
- Play therapy
- Family therapy
- Behaviour therapy
- Use of day hospitals.

Emotional Outbursts

These are unchecked expressions of child's emotions. Emotions like happiness, anger, jealousy and fear. Negative emotions outburst are annoying and troublesome. Too much of anything is not good, either positive or negative moods. With curiosity, the child wants to explore the things by themselves. For example, Removing parts and tries to assemble it again; breaking things, spilling them on furniture causing extra work to the elders.

Remedies

- Babies are not mature enough to express and control their emotions or curiosity, they act out patterns of response that are natural to them
- Parents have to provide relaxed and pleasant environment in the home so that inculcation of destructive behaviour among the children will be prevented
- Elders should not use harsh ways in punishing the child to control the childs' emotions, e.g. by beating, slapping, harsh words, forcibly putting the child in the crib or in the rooms where the doors and windows are closed, thinking that they are keeping the baby away from bothering environment, but it will worsen the emotional pattern of the child
- Choose the method to attack the problem, which will suit the developmental level of the baby
- As babies have shorter attention span, shift the baby's attention to something else, such that child can forget their emotional bursts.

Violent Behaviour

Aggressive/violent behaviour is common among preschoolers, during aggression, the child may loose grip on vocabulary. To express his frustration, always the child will demonstrate by hitting or pinching or biting or showing aggressive tendency defiant or destructive or annoyed behaviour like quarreling, restlessness, etc.

Causes

- Lack of impulse control, e.g. child may be knowing pinching will hurt, but he may not be able to stop it from doing so
- Frustration, e.g. he will understand, he can not control his environment, so he responds in a better way what he knows, e.g. biting, pinching, snatching a toy from his friend or sibling
- Urge for being independent and he want to proove, he is important and need to be recognized
- Unable to visualize the consequences of hitting or biting, he will not have control of himself
- Inadequate attention, negligence by care givers and siblings
- Children will express their feelings, desires or needs with action rather than with words.

Measures to Handle violent behaviour

- Try to respond quickly, when the child is getting an aggressive mood
- Remove the child from the situation for the brief period
- Utilize negative reinforcement behaviour modification techniques like time out, make him to understand, he will be the sufferer by missing out fun and other desirable things
- Handle the child in gentle manner, avoid physical punishments like hurting him by beating or other strainful situations or activities
- If the child exhibits acceptable or desirable behaviour, give him a reward or appreciate the child, which encourages him to perform it efficiently
- Keep a note how many times the child does well, give a prize or incentive, whatever he feels to have, let the child enjoy it
- Provide opportunity to the child, to minimize his frustration or anger through appropriate outlets, e.g. making the child to learn specific skills constructively, e.g. dancing, swimming, play, etc. to regain physical or muscular strength

- Anticipate child's interest and encourage him to perform the activities effectively
- Help the child to work through the emotions that tend to lead aggression and control his behaviour in future
- Counsel the child, if he is able to understand, provide rational emotive training to control aggressive behaviour.

Child Guidance Clinic

In 1909, in Chicago first child guidance clinic was started and then the number of clinics has increased. It deals with all children upto adolescents, who are not fully adjusted to their environment.

Aim: To prevent children from the possibility of becoming neurotics and psychotics in later life.

Team

- Paediatrician–takes care of physical health of the child
- Clinical psychologist–observe the psychological status of the child
- Psychiatrist–diagnoses and treat mental illness
- Educational psychologist to restore positive feelings of security in the child
- Psychiatric social worker by lessening parental tensions, reconstruction
- Public health nurse assists in assessment and meet the needs of children
- Speech therapist will help the child to develop good seech pattern
- Occupational therapist assists in developing vocational skills
- Neurologist assess the neurological status and treat the illness, if identified.

Therapeutic Modalities Used in Childhood Psychiatric Disorders

Therapeutic Play

Based on age, developmental abilities, potentialities and needs of children the 'therapeutic play activities' will be selected.

Values

- To overcome resistance, fantasy and developmental fears
- To abreact the emotional experiences
- To develop mastery and competence over the skills
- To acquire creative thinking
- To catharsizes or ventilate the emotional feelings
- To relieve tension, worries, it acts as an emotional outlet
- To enhance the social relationship and social network

Children Games

To develop skills and imagination, to improve child's motor abilities, concentration, frustration tolerance, coping pattern: to resolve internal conflicts and to provide pleasurable experience, to divert child's mind from tension and worries, games will be introduced for children. For example, Musical Chairs, Hide and seek, Finding out the coin, etc. the choice of preference of games or selection of appropriate game is based on child's developmental pattern, age, coping behaviour and anxiety levels or other emotional pattern.

Expressive Therapy

Child's creative process will be stimulated and whereby he can express openly or freely their views. It is a way of ventilating the child's mind and by relieving internal tensions or inner conflicts, diverts the mind in a relaxed manner. It enhances group interaction and participation.

Materials like puppets, audio visual aids, etc. will be given to the child to express their views freely without any hesitations or inhibitions, e.g. drawing pictures, diagrams, painting, writing, singing, dancing, movement, etc. will be encouraged. Instruction will be given to describe and interact their experiences with others, promotes imagination process. Nurse has to identify the child's views by observing child's behaviour and through the activities performed, the factors associated with child and able to diagnose child's pathology and plans for remedial measures.

Enacting/Role Play

Provides an opportunity for the child to practice or enact certain role, where he can learn to interact with others and able to participate in structured activities.

Story Telling

To relieve distress, to teach new coping skills, morals, ethics, appropriate problem solving technique, a valuable intervention, 'story telling', will be used. The child will imaginate the story life into his own life situation. Encourage the child to understand the morals and develop some stories (autogenic story telling). Morals can be applied into the real life.

Bibliotherapy

Based on the age, developmental ability, nature, interests or likings, attention span of the child, appropriate reading material has to be selected carefully. The child will always correlate and compare the material or stories to his life situations, child will be able to identify and express the feelings, child's imaginative process will be enhanced. If the material possesses pictures, illustrations, child will enjoy it more. Nurses have to interpret child's reaction towards the reading material, e.g. the enjoyment, interests and learning capacities of children.

Cognitive Behaviour Therapy

To modify cognitive distortion, to promote reasoning and self control, to develop appropriate healthy coping behaviour and competence, to learn problem solving skills and techniques, to improve cognitive skills which has to be utilized in specific situations, this technique will be used.

Therapeutic Milieu

To provide continuity of care, multiple interventions will be used in a psychiatric milieu based on developmental needs of the children. Safe, caring environment and planned activities are essential in providing safer milieu, either in inpatient department or in day treatment programmes. Family participation, staff cooperation are essential in successful implementation of milieu.

Restraint Method

Restrictive interventions are recommended. Nurses have to carefully select and use these methods in inpatient care.

NURSING MANAGEMENT OF THE CHILD WITH PSYCHIATRIC DISORDERS

Nursing Assessment

- Establish and maintain therapeutic nurse-patient relationship. Win their confidentiality by providing friendly atmosphere and cooperation.
- Collect the history from client (if the child is able to narrate), parents, the teachers and significant personalities (if they know the situation in detail), encourage them to talk spontaneously the factual information, assess their feelings and attitudes while they are narrating.
- Observe the child, while he is expressing his views, as younger children are less efficient in usage of words to express their views or ideas.
- Find out the reason for referral, what they are expecting from the referral system.
- Description of present event/problem: onset, course, consequences on family, interaction, aspects of family life involved based on child's health.
- Recent behaviour and emotional status.
- Enquire about general health-pattern and habits related to likes, dislikes, interests, disinterests,

intelligence levels, educational achievements, schooling, child's behaviour with peer group, scholastic environment, scholastic abilities, scholastic difficulties, school report, disciplinary measures implemented.

- Pattern of social relationship and network with family, peers, others, reaction to the new situation.
- Moods or emotions- either positive or negative and its extension, attention, concentration, understanding, coordination.
- Motor activities-tics, mannerisms, ritualistic behaviour, activity performance
- *Family history*: Family size, family type, interaction and relationship of family members, participation of the child in family activities, difficulties experienced by family H/o any psychiatric disorders in the family, disciplinary measures were used to control child's behaviour.
- Religious activities, interest and participation.
- Particulars of child in detail, e.g. age, education, gender, address, nativity, etc.
- Maternal factors–type of pregnancy (wanted or unwanted), any complications, delivery (home or institutional), type of delivery (normal/abnormal/difficult).
- Birth weight of the child, fulfillment of neonatal needs, H/o any difficulties in neonatal period, toddler period, any H/o temper tantrums.
- Temperamental pattern–with new people, new situations or environment, new relationships, sensitivity to the environmental stimuli.
- Physical examination: head to foot examination, posture.
- Anthropometric Measurements: height, weight, mid upper arm circumference, chest circumference, head circumference, skin fold thickness.
- Mental status examination: general behaviour, mood pattern, activity levels, attention, concentration, speech pattern, intellectual abilities.
- Neurological assessment, sensory and motor aspects–muscle tone, muscular rigidity.
- Type and nature of personality.

1. Nursing Diagnosis

Alteration in growth and development.

Goal

Enhances Mile Stones.

Interventions

- Establishes and maintains therapeutic nurse-patient relationship.
- Assess the growth and development pattern of the child, identify the deficiencies related to it.
- Educate the mile stones of children to the parents, provide needed assistance and guidance, regular health check-up, growth monitoring, checking anthropometric measurements, adequate supplementation of nutrients, treatment of minor ailments, protective measures against accidents and injuries, etc.
- Teach the child appropriate tasks as per age, if child accomplishes it, appreciate it and positively reinforce the task.

2. Nursing Diagnosis

Potential for anxiety, fear and other emotional disturbances.

Goal

Maintains emotional balance and integrity.

Interventions

- Observe the child's emotions and mood pattern
- Provide calm and quiet environment, less stimulating environment, if the child has disturbed moods
- Encourage the child in play and other activities
- Allow the parents to stay with the child, to provide moral support and comfort to the child
- Assess the mental status of the child
- Divert the mind of the child in creative activities, promote the child's interests (if it is desirable and acceptable)

- Process recording has to be carried out about child's activities and report to the appropriate authority
- Maintain consistent schedule for activities
- Orient the child to health professional and to the environment policies and procedures
- Engage the child in diversional activities to overcome emotional disturbances.

3. Nursing Diagnosis

Lowered self-esteem, altered social interaction process.

Goal

Enhances self-esteem.

Interventions

- Encourage the child to develop direct, trusting relationship with parents and peer group
- Develop creative independent roles, teach the child creative skills, adequate coping strategies to attain frustration tolerance and cope-up the situations
- Works as a liaison or connective link between various groups like, parent groups, professionals and other community agencies
- Monitors child's behaviour, which requires consultancy services
- Coordinates various activities, follows therapeutic instructions given by concerned specialist in the field, reports if any hurdles, traumatic experiences
- Utilizes problem solving approaches and varied interventions to attain specific goals
- Enhances optimum development of the child.
- Nurses will assume various roles like teacher, counselor, parent, care taker, guardian, etc. meets the developmental needs of children
- Guide the child to utilize adequate coping strategies to cope-up with the developmental crisis
- Appreciate the child for his accomplishments

- Motivate the child to do the activities independently and participate in therapeutic play activities as early as possible
- Help the child to identify stressors and cope-up with them
- Provide safe environment in home and in school
- Enhance healthy interaction between the child and parents and peer group.

4. Nursing Diagnosis

Altered family process related to child ill health.

Goal

Reestablishes good familial environment.

Interventions

- Involve the family members or supportive system in the treatment process
- Clear the doubts of care takers and assist them in solving interpersonal problems
- Identify the stressor and teach the family members the coping strategies to resolve the crisis
- Motivate for healthy interaction among family members
- Enhance good child rearing practices.

5. Nursing Diagnosis

Alteration in sleep pattern related to emotional disturbances.

Goal

Promotes sleep pattern.

Interventions

- Avoid or remove anxiety prone situations
- Motivate the child to practice deep relaxation exercises and techniques
- Encourage the child to develop bed time rituals, e.g. taking warm water bath at bed time, listening to melodious music, or reading moral based stories.

6. Nursing Diagnosis

Prone for injury and violence.

Goal

Prevent the child to become violent or aggression and protect the child from injuries.

Interventions

- Handle the child's conflicts in a smooth and gentle manner
- Never hurt inner feelings of the child
- Don't encourage aggressive prone situations
- Explain the child the reasons for limitations or restrictions related to their activities
- Appropriate behaviour modification techniques have to be used based on the environmental situations and nature of the problem, e.g. time out, self control, shaping, modelling, positive or negative reinforcement techniques, etc.
- Provide constructive feed back related to child's activities
- Avoid hazardous materials near to the child to prevent injuries and to protect the child from harmful environment.

Preventive Care

To prevent childhood psychiatric disorders the services like: family counselling, parental guidance, antenatal care, institutional deliveries, establishment of adequate parent-child relationship, effective implementation of interventions.

Family health care services and school health services, etc. has to be organized.

Family oriented programmes includes implementation of ICDS activities, i.e. care of the child in Anganavadi centres, day care centres, planned parenthood activities, home care or residential care, etc. has to be provided.

Societal programmes focusing on mental health planning, implementation of Mental Health Policy, Health Maintenance, Educational Guidance and supportive services, etc. have to be implemented.

Primary prevention services includes Genctic Counselling, Essential obstetrical care, provision of safe environment, fulfillment of emotional needs, immunization, health education, counselling, regular health check-ups, Monitoring of child growth and development, provision of good familial environment, Family planning, Management of crisis situations, Protection of high risk groups, etc.

Secondary Prevention services includes Early identification of childhood behavioural problems through Appropriate Screening, Regular Health Check-ups, Organizing Training Programmes for parents, school teachers in early detection of Behavioural Problems and implementation of appropriate Remedial Measures, Provision of Community based services through domiciliary care, etc.

Tertiary Prevention Services comprises of Disability Limitation, Provision of Supportive Services, rendering Specialized Institutional care, Professional Guidance, Counselling, Rehabilitation services, Restoration of families for better functioning for promotion of healthy behaviour, promotion of Child Advocacy to meet the specific needs of focus groups, e.g. abuse (physical/psycho-logical/sexual), delinquency, victims of calamities and crisis, etc.

Review Questions

1. Explain the Nursing Management of a patient with Juvenile Delinquency. (7.5M, GULBU, 1994, 99).
2. Character disorder. (2M, GULBU, 1994).
3. Delinquency. (5M, GULBU, 1999; 5M, MGRU, 2001; 2M, RGUHS, 2001).
4. Juvenile Delinquency. (5M, MGRU, 2000; 5M, RGUHS, 2000, 06, 2M, 07).
5. What are the factors contributing to the development of Juvenile Delinquency? (2M, RGUHS, 2001).
6. Role of a Nurse in Mental Retardation. (15M, NTRU, 1992).

7. What are the causes of Mental Sub-Normality? How can you help public to prevent Mental Sub-Normality? (15M, GULBU, 1997).
8. Classification of Childhood Psychiatric disorders. (5M, 10M, RGUHS, 2001).
9. Behavioural disorders in children. (2M, 1999, 5M, 2004, 06, RGUHS; 5M, 1996, 2000, MGRU).
10. Enuresis. (2M, 2001, 02, 5M, 2004, RGUHS; 2M, GULBU, 1997).
11. Care of enuretic child. (5M, RGUHS, 2004).
12. Clinical features of School Refusal. (2M, RGUHS, 2004).
13. Autism. (2M, RGUHS, 2003, 05, 06; 4M, NIMS, 1995).
14. Hyper kinetic disorder. (5M, Oct, 07, RGUHS, 2003).
15. Childhood disorder. (10M, RGUHS, 2003).
16. Classification of Mental Retardation. (5M, RGUHS, 2003, 06; 3M, 7M, MGRU, 2003).
17. Conduct disorder. (5M, RGUHS, 1999, 2002; 5M, PCBSc, 2005; 5M, MGRU, 2000, 02).
18. Refusal of food. (5M, RGUHS, 2000, 02).
19. Classify Mental Retardation and write its significance. (5M, RGUHS, 2001).
20. Care of children with Conduct disorder. (5M, RGUHS, 2001).
21. Habitation of Mentally Retarded child. (5M, RGUHS, 2001, 07).
22. Outline the causes of Mutism. (5M, RGUHS, 2001).
23. What are the factors associated with Enuresis? (2M, RGUHS, 2001).
24. Infantile autism. (5M, RGUHS, 2000).
25. Four causes of Mental retardation. (2M, RGUHS, 2000).
26. Mental Retardation. (5M, RGUHS, 1997, 98, 99, 2000, 2006; 5M, GULBU, 1994).
27. Mental Sub-normality. (5M, MGRU, 1991).
    A. Enumerate the important causes of Mental Retardation.
    B. Explain the role of the Nurse in the Rehabilitation of a Mentally Retarded child. (5M, MGRU, 1991).
28. Define Mental Retardation. Explain the nurse's role in taking care of the children with various levels of mental retardation. (1+11 M, MGRU).
    A. Mental retardation.
    B. Describe the psychopathology and causes of Mental Retardation.
    C. Discuss the assessment, classification and Nursing Management of the mentally retarded persons. (2+5+8 M, MGRU, 5M, GULBU, 1994).
29. Rehabilitation of the mentally Handicap. (5M, RGUHS, 1999).
30. Profound Mental Retardation. (10M, RGUHS, 2005).

31. Anorexia Nervosa. (5M, RGUHS, 2006, Oct, 2007).
32. Aetiology of Mental Retardation. (5M, 2000, 04, 06).
33. Specific learning problems among school age children. (5M, 2005).
34. Child Guidance Clinic. (5M, RGUHS, 2006).
35. Prevention of Mental Retardation. (4M, NIMS, 1995).
36. Define Mental Retardation. Write Causes and Nursing Management by using Nursing process. (1+2+6, NIMS, 2004).
37. Role of a Nurse in the prevention of Mental Retardation. (5M, RGUHS, 2006).
38. Nursing Management of Autistic child. (5M, RGUHS, 2000).
39. Childhood Schizophrenia. (5M, RGUHS, 2007).
40. Ritualistic Behaviour. (5M, RGUHS, 2003).
41. Attention Deficit Hyperactive disorder. (5M, RGUHS, 2002, 03).
42. Nursing Management of a child with Hyperkinetic disorder. (5M, RGUHS, 2006).
43. Mutism. (5M, RGUHS, 2001).
44. TIC disorder. (5M, RGUHS, 2002, Oct, 07).
45. Nursing Management of Childhood Psychiatric disorders. (10 M, RGUHS, 2006).
46. Neurotic disorders of childhood. (5M, RGUHS, 2003).
47. Childhood Psychiatric disorders. (10M, KSDNEB, 2007).
48. Eating disorder. (5M, RGUHS, Oct, 07).
49. Altruism. (2M, RGUHS, Oct, 07).
50. Kleptomania. (2M, RGUHS, 07).

16 Organic Brain/Mental Disorder

'The syndrome attributed to cerebral or brain disease or disorder'.

It may be acute or chronic, behavioural or psychological disorders associated with transient or permanent brain dysfunction. Organic Mental Disorders are described in ICD-10 F_{00}-F_{05} chapters.

DEFINITION

'A pattern of organic psychological and behaviour symptoms associated with permanent or transient brain dysfunction but without reference to etiology'. —*DSM-III*

Causes

- Cerebral diseases
- Brain injury/head injury or trauma
- Insult leading to cerebral dysfunction
- CNS systemic diseases or disorders
- Metabolic disorder complications
- Toxic conditions
- Encephalitis, systemic infection
- Brain tumour or cerebral arteriosclerosis
- Fever.

Manifestations

- Impairment in cognitive functions, e.g. thinking, memory, reasoning, orientation, judgement, intelligence, emotional adjustment
- Impaired processing of incoming information
- Depression
- Mild motor disability tremors
- Loss of dexterity
- Imbalance.

Classification of Organic Brain Disorders as per ICD-10

F_{00}- –F_{09} Organic, including symptomatic, mental disorders

F_{00} –Dementia in Alzheimer's disease

$F_{00.0}$ –Dementia in Alzheimer's disease with early onset

$F_{00.1}$ –Dementia in Alzheimer's disease with late onset

$F_{00.2}$ –Dementia in Alzheimer's disease, atypical or mixed type

$F_{00.9}$ –Dementia in Alzheimer's disease, unspecified

F_{01} —Vascular dementia

$F_{01.0}$ —Vascular dementia of acute onset

F_{01} —Multi infarct dementia

$F_{01.2}$ —Subcortical vascular dementia

$F_{01.3}$ —Mixed cortical and sub-cortical vascular dementia

$F_{01.8}$ —Other vascular dementia

$F_{01.9}$ —Vascular dementia, unspecified

F_{02} —Dementia in other diseases classified elsewhere

$F_{02.0}$ —Dementia in Pick's disease

$F_{02.1}$ —Dementia in Creutzfeldt-Jakob disease

$F_{02.2}$ —Dementia in Huntington's disease

$F_{02.3}$ —Dementia in Parkinson's disease

$F_{02.4}$ —Dementia in human immunodeficiency virus (HIV) diseases

$F_{02.8}$ —Dementia in other specified diseases classified elsewhere.

F_{03} —Unspecified dementia

A fifth character may be added to specify dementia in F_{02} - F_{03} as follows:

X0 Without additional symptoms

X1 Other symptoms, predominantly delusional

X2 Other symptoms, predominantly hallucinatory

X3 Other symptoms, predominantly depressive

X4 Other mixed symptoms

F_{04} —Organic amnesic syndrome, not induced by alcohol and other psychoactive substances

F_{05} —Delirium, not induced by alcohol and other psychoactive substances

$F_{05.0}$ —Delirium, not superimposed on dementia, so described

$F_{05.1}$ —Delirium, superimposed on dementia

$F_{05.8}$ —Other delirium

$F_{05.9}$ —Delirium, unspecified

F_{06} —Other mental disorders due to brain damage and dysfunction and to physical disease

$F_{06.0}$ —Organic hallucinosis

$F_{06.1}$ —Organic catatonic disorder

$F_{06.2}$ —Organic delusional (schizophrenia-like) disorder

$F_{06.3}$ —Organic mood (affective) disorder

—30 Organic manic disorder

—30 Organic bipolar affective disorder

—30 Organic depressive disorder

—30 Organic mixed disorder

$F_{06.4}$ —Organic anxiety disorder

$F_{06.5}$ —Organic dissociative disorder

$F_{06.6}$ —Organic emotionally labile (asthenic) disorder

$F_{06.7}$ —Mild cognitive disorder

$F_{06.8}$ —Other specified mental disorder due to brain damage and dysfunction and to physical disease

$F_{06.9}$ —Unspecified mental disorder due to brain damage and dysfunction and to physical disease

F_{07} —Personality and behavioral disorders due to brain disease, damage and dysfunction

$F_{07.0}$ —Organic personality disorder

$F_{07.1}$ —Post-encephalitic syndrome

$F_{07.2}$ —Post-concussional syndrome

$F_{07.8}$ —Other organic personality and behavioural disorders due to brain disease, damage and dysfunction

$F_{07.9}$ —Unspecified organic or symptomatic mental disorder.

DEMENTIA (CHRONIC BRAIN SYNDROME)

Introduction

Dementia is not a disease by itself, but rather a group of symptoms that are caused by various disease conditions. If it is severe, it will interfere with a person's daily functioning. It has been described in ICD-10 (F_{00} - F_{07}) ICD-9 (290-294). It is a late life disease, as it tends to develop mostly in elderly people. The word, 'dementia' derived from 2 Latin words 'de' means 'apart' or 'away' and 'mens' or 'mentis' (genitive) means 'mind'. In Latin 'dementia' means 'irrationality'.

Definitions

'The progressive decline in cognitive functions (particularly affected areas like thinking, reasoning, memory, attention, language, and problem solving) due to damage or disease in the brain beyond, what might be expected from normal aging'.

—Wikipedia Encyclopedia

'A chronic progressive disease of the brain affecting higher cortical functions in multiple ways and resulting into disturbances or decline in intellectual functioning. For example, memory, thinking, orientation, comprehension, learning capacity, calculation, language and judgement but not affecting consciousness commonly associated with deterioration in emotional control and social behaviour. *—ICD-10*

Prevalence

In western countries and Australia (1.03% of total population) are commonly affected. The prevalence of dementia is rising as the global life expectancy is rising. 5–8 per cent of all people over the age of 65 have one or other form of dementia, and this number doubles every five years above that age. It is a disease which is strongly associated with age (1% of 60–65 years of age; 2% of 65–69 years of age; 6% of 75–79 years of age; 20% of 85–89 years of age; 45% of 95 years of age and older suffer with the disease).

Causes

Common Causes

- Degenerative disease like Alzheimer's disease
- *Vascular causes,* e.g. Multiple infarct dementia, Binswanger's stroke, hypertensive encephalopathy, arteriosclerosis
- *Toxic reactions,* e.g. alcohol induced persisting dementia or drug abuse induced
- *Fronto-temporal lobar degeneration,* e.g. Pick's disease (degenerative disorder)

- Fronto-temporal dementia
- Semantic dementia
- Progressive non-fluent aphasia
- General paresis
- Senile dementia.

Less Common Causes

Consequences of
- Creutzfeldt-Jakob disease
- Huntington's disease (degenerative disease)
- Parkinson's disease
- HIV infection (AIDS dementia complex)
- Head trauma-dementia, subdural, epidural hematoma, contusion
- Down syndrome may develop Alzheimer's type
- Infections that affect brain and spinal cord-meningitis, encephalitis
- Metal poisoning-heavy metals (lead, mercury, manganese, carbon monoxide)
- Anoxia, e.g. secondary to respiratory syndrome, anaemia.

Potentially Treatable Causes

- Endocrinal disorder, e.g. hypothyroidism, myxoedema, Addison's disease
- Vitamin deficiencies (B_1, B_{12}) and Vit-A deficiencies
- Illnesses other than in the brain, e.g. complications of kidney, liver, lung diseases
- Depression-depressive pseudodementia, hysteria, catatonia
- Normal pressure hydrocephalus
- Brain tumours
- Syphilis
- Hypoglycemia
- Neoplastic lesions-space occupying lesions, abscesses
- Post anaesthesia
- Chronic respiratory failure.

Types: Based on etiology of disease
- Reversible dementia
- Irreversible dementia.

Manifestations

- Affected persons may be disoriented in time, in place and in person
- Forgetfulness with effects at work; they may forget names or appointments as memory function is declined
- Difficulties with familiar activities, e.g. absent mindedness like keeping vessel on the stove and forgetting
- Language difficulties, e.g. difficulty in finding right words, inappropriate filling-up of words, which others cannot be able to understand it (aphasia)
- Problem with spatial and temporal orientation, e.g. forgets the day of the week or they may lost in unfamiliar surroundings
- Impaired capacity of judgement, i.e. people with dementia can not be able to judge the things by themselves like wearing inappropriate clothes based on seasonwise
- Problems related to abstract thinking, e.g. the clients cannot be able to do simple calculations
- Leaving things behind, e.g. clients will forget where they left their belongings like purse, umbrella
- Clients may have sudden mood swing, depressed
- Pronounced personality changes suddenly or over a longer period of time, e.g. a person who is friendly in nature, with dementia suddenly becomes aggressive without any reason, mentally fatigue
- Looses interest in their work and hobbies, manifests lack of interest or zeal in cultivation of new activities
- Possesses stereotyped behaviour
- Neurological syndrome: drowsiness, confusion, ataxia
- Catastrophic reactions, e.g. agitation
- Impairment in thinking and reasoning capacity, reduction in flow of ideas (Alzheimer's type)
- Not able to attend more than one stimuli at a time
- Unable to follow social norm
- Isolation, withdrawal
- Inappropriate, indecent behaviour, e.g. lack of interest in hygiene
- Lack of emotional control
- Development of functional reactions, e.g. anxiety, depression, paranoid delusions

Diagnosis

- Referral to a specialist like Geriatric psychiatrists, Neurologists, Neuropsychologists or Geropsychologist
- Based on the cause the investigative procedure will be selected
- Mini mental status examination
- Abbreviated mental test score
- CT scan and MRI scan–based on cause like alcoholic
- Neuropsychological testing
- Hormonal assay
- Assessment of activities of daily living.

Treatment

- Training of thinking and memory functions are carried out carefully
- Reality orientation training
- Improve brain function by using drugs, e.g. psychotropic drugs, antipsychotic drugs, antidepressants, antianxiety drugs
- Organization of environment
- Cognitive and behavioural interventions may be appropriate
- Educating and providing emotional support to the caregiver is of importance
- Validation therapy–when the client has degenerative, irreversible cognitive impairment, the clients' sense of being will be understood by the nursing fraternity, in order to enhance the quality of life, reduce the incidence of agitation and catastrophic reaction, the nursing staff tries to attempt to enter the clients' world and render care-oriented activities, to meet the clients' needs

- Remotivation therapy
  - To provide opportunity for the client to derive pleasure and sensory stimulation by experiencing the world to feel safe and comfortable
  - To interrupt self-absorption
  - To overcome isolation
- Briefly theme has to be explained
- Clients are motivated to reminisce in relation to group's objective or theme
- If the client attends meeting and contributes, nurse will appreciate for his unique contribution
- Makes the client to touch some objects (e.g. flowers) to attain sensory stimulation.

Prevention

- Lead an active life, both mentally and physically
- Proper screening and treatment of underlying diseases is essential
- Provision of situational support, mutual concern are of much importance.

SENILE DEMENTIA

It is a progressive, degenerative brain disease affecting memory, thinking, behaviour and personality. The clients' brain function will gradually deteriorates resulting in alteration in mental functioning, usually associated with old age.

Risk Factors

- Vascular problems, e.g. Longstanding HTN, atherosclerosis, stroke
- Head trauma
- Manganese toxicity
- High levels of homocysteine (heart diseases, depression)
- Infection–lyme disease
- Chronic illnesses
- Deposition of aluminum/lead/mercury other substances in the brain
- The destruction of nerve cells leads to decrease in neurotransmitters results in structural and chemical alteration in brain tissue, causing dementia.

Causes

- Alzheimer's disease (generalized atrophy)– most common form, causing deterioration in memory and thought process
- Multi infarct dementia–results from series of strokes
- Damage of brain tissue–encephalitis, meningitis
- Drug abuse or poisoning–high dose steroid abuse
- Medication side effects or drug interactions
- Chronic alcohol abuse
- Huntington's disease, a progressive degenerative disease that causes dance like movements and mental deterioration
- Multiple sclerosis
- HIV
- Parkinson's disease, a degenerative disorder of part of the nervous system
- Creutzfeldt-Jakob disease, a rapidly progressing disorder of the nervous system causing problems with walking, talking, and the senses
- Normal pressure hydrocephalus or increased CSF
- Chronic subdural hematoma
- Brain tumour
- Wilson diseases, a rare disease causing an accumulation of copper in the liver, brain, kidneys and corneas
- Neurosyphilis causes weakness and mental deterioration
- Progressive supranuclear palsy (Steele-Richardson-Olszewski syndrome) a rare disorder of late middle age that causes widespread neurological problems
- Endocrinal disorders- hypothyroidism, hyperthyroidism
- Nutrients deficiency–Vit B_1, B_{12}, Niacin.

Incidence

Ten per cent of all people over 60 years have significant memory problems, above 80 years of age 20 per cent of people suffer with Alzheimer's disease, having a close blood relative will increase the risk and early onset; it will run in families and involves autosomal dominant, inherited mutations that may be the cause of the disease. The role of genes is less direct and definitive, so far 3 early onset genes have been identified, they may likely form plaques and tangles, which may give rise pathology in brain. Female are more likely to develop, as women live longer than men.

Clinical Manifestations

Early Stage (2–4 years)

- Forgets recent events and faded distant memory as the disease progresses, progressive loss of memory and mental abilities
- Experiences difficulty in reasoning, calculation and accepting new things
- Noticeable personality changes
- Confused by overtime, place and direction
- Declining interest in environment
- Affects the activities of daily living
- Impaired judgement
- Hesitates in initiating actions
- Passive, lower performance at work.

Middle Stage (4–12 years)

- Less cognitive ability, e.g. ability to learn, judge, reason and memory loss
- Emotionally unstable, easily looses temper and becomes agitated
- Irritable, anxious, wandering
- Needs help from their family members for activities of daily living, neglects personal hygiene
- Feels difficulty in following instructions
- Confuses night and day, disturbs family's normal sleeping time
- Hesitates to respond to the questions
- Socially isolated.

Later Stage

- Looses all cognitive abilities, communication activities
- Confusion may be punctuated by moments of lucidity, with memory and reasoning impaired, person looses interest in activities, which were once enjoyable, habitual behaviours which make up 'personality' breakdown, increase in emotional and physical instability, unpredictable switches between apathy and aggression, social inhibitions and sometimes sexual inhibitions also go out of the window
- Entirely incapable of self care activities like eating, bathing etc.
- Neglects personal hygiene
- Unable to recognize family members
- Incontinence of urine and faeces
- Looses the ability to stand and walk
- Looses weight gradually as inadequate food consumption, walks unsteadily and becomes confined to bed
- Death results due to aspiration pneumonia (common cause).

Diagnosis

- Obtain history of the client either from the client or family members and other significant members
- Explore family history, genetic predisposition
- Observation of manifestation, e.g. impairment in memory, attention span, decision making ability, judgement
- Observe conversation problem, e.g. language difficulty; personality changes.

Treatment

- Identify the cause and try to eliminate or exclude the cause
- Gingko biloba (herbal)
- Low dose of lithium (Mineral)
- Vitamin supplementation, B-complex

- Explain the family members about the disease condition, to gain knowledge and to extend support and cooperation in meeting the needs
- Family members provides suitable care and assistance to the client, show extra loving and concern
- Care giver education is the important aspect in the treatment of disease
- Avail social services assistance, e.g. daycare centres for elderly
- Make alterations in home environment to prevent accidents
- Establish a daily routine for the client to reduce the feelings of confusion
- Identification card is worn by the client like a bracelet, in case if he gets lost.

ALZHEIMER'S DISEASE

Introduction

It causes 50–60 per cent of all dementias. It is a brain disorder that destroys memory and undermines personality. Brain cells disappear in the cerebral cortex, hippocampus (which is responsible for intellectual activities like memory and reasoning). This interferes with the intricate process of cell-to-cell communication. This disease was first described in 1907 by the physician Alois Alzheimer. Symptoms usually occur before the age of 60 years and progresses rapidly, the probability of developing Alzheimer's disease increases with advancing age. It occurs primarily middle or late in life.

Risk Factors

Interaction of several factors probably leads to the onset of disease
- Family history
- Lack of exercise
- Smoking
- Advanced age
- Alcoholism
- Hypertension
- Viral infections
- Head injury

- Stress
- Estrogen loss following menopause
- Environmental factor.

Causes

- Head injury
- Excessive exposure to metals like aluminium
- Nutritional deficiencies, e.g. Vitamin–A, B_{12}, E, carotenoids
- Genetic defects, e.g. apolipoprotein-E gene defect
- Immunodeficiency disorders
- Progressing destruction of nerve cells in the brain
- Reduction in neurotransmitters like acetylcholine, choline-acetyltransferase, serotonin, etc.

Incidence

- More in western countries, 25,000 new cases are diagnosed annually. The probability of occurring disease is higher for women and for people having a low educational standards.

Manifestation

- Illness begins slowly, usually manifests by itself initially as bouts of forgetfulness (occasional first, but later it becomes more frequent) or memory lapses
- As the disease progresses, the individual must depend on others for all their needs
- Individual experience a range of progressive symptoms, e.g. disorientation, dysphasia, aphasia, apraxia, sudden and unpredictable mood swings, hallucinations, delusions, wandering without purpose, incontinence, neglecting personal hygiene, confusion (acutely/suddenly and limited in time), limitation of concentration, planning and judgement, personality changes, speech and walking disorders, impairment in social relationships. Impaired ability to learn new things or cognitive recall previously learned information difficulties; failure to recognize or identify objects (agnosia)

disorganized thinking, depressive mood, labiality, impulsivity, aggression, lack of social skills and not able to carry out functions independently.

Stages of Alzheimer's Disease

Slow unfolding progressive disease which is accompanied overtime by changes in appearance of patient. The individual's course of disease is however variable.

Mild or early stage or first stage
- Impairments of mental abilities
- Mood swings, incoordination
- Restlessness and anxiety.

Moderate or mid stage or second stage
- Blunting of emotions and apathy
- Hemiparesis
- Akinesia
- Increased muscle tone.

Third or final or late or severe stage
- Physical problems are dominant
- Psychotic syndrome-perception disturbances, e.g. hallucinations and delusion
- Cognitive decline
- Incontinence
- Loss of personality.

Diagnosis

- Based on symptoms
- Exclude the other diseases which predisposes the disease.

Treatment

- Hospitalize the client
- Symptomatic treatment.

DELIRIUM (ACUTE ORGANIC BRAIN SYNDROME)

Definition

'It is a state of clouded consciousness in which attention cannot be sustained, the environment is wrongly perceived and disturbances of thinking are present'. —*ICD-10*

'An acute organic mental disorder characterized by impairment in attention, concentration and consciousness added by disturbances in thinking and perception'.

Incidence

- 20–40 per cent of geriatric clients in hospitalization
- In postoperative cases highest incidence was noticed.

Causes

- Head trauma
- Postoperative cases
- Heat stroke
- High fever in children
- Metabolic-thiamine deficiency, uremia, liver disorders, diabetic coma
- Toxic-metallic poisoning, e.g. lead, manganese, mercury, carbon monoxide
- Intoxication, withdrawal effects of alcoholic, sedative, hypnotic drugs
- Infections, e.g. pneumonia, meningitis, encephalitis
- Vascular-hypertensive encephalopathy, arterio-sclerosis, intracranial haemorrhage
- Neoplastic, e.g. space occupying lesions
- Anoxia, e.g. anaemia, cardiac failure/congestive heart failure
- Epilepsy and cerebral tumors
- Lupus erythematosus, respiratory insufficiency
- Sensory deprivation.

Manifestations

- Impaired consciousness-cloudiness consciousness ranging from drowsiness to coma
- Disorientation
- Mental confusion
- Disturbance in memory and comprehension of factual knowledge
- Impulsive, irrational and violent behaviour

- Transcient and reversible changes
- Lack of insight
- Moods are liable to change from apathy to sudden panic
- Disturbances in perception, e.g. hallucination, illusion, delusion
- Disturbances in cognition, e.g. impairment in thinking, distorted thinking
- Dream-like content in thinking
- Disturbances in sleep, nightmares
- Psychomotor disturbances
- Emotional disturbances.

Treatment

- Identify the cause and treat the cause
- Symptomatic treatment
- Administration of sedatives and tranquilizers to calm-up the mind.

SENILE PSYCHOSIS

Definition

'Progressive, abnormally accelerated deterioration of mental faculties and emotional stability in old age'.

'A psychotic condition characterized by difficulty in orienting to reality (visual, auditory hallucinations, odd or bizarre thoughts) that has no identifiable cause, other than ageing'.

Causes

- Stroke
- Alzheimer's disease.

Manifestation

- Significant paranoid like delusional beliefs, fear
- Memory lapses
- Some individuals act or respond as though, they are living during another period in time, e.g. they speak to a dead loved one
- Perception of reality is different
- Bizarre thoughts

- Perceptional difficulties, e.g. hallucinations (visual and auditory)
- Inconsistency in activities
- Sometimes they also exhibits completely normal/rational functioning.

Treatment

Aim: To maintain appropriate level of independence.

- Medical treatment varies greatly among individual, according to age, health status and symptoms
- Family support is needed
- Utilization of community resources, social support networks for supportive services
- Home care.

ORGANIC AMNESTIC SYNDROME

Aetiology

Underlying organic cause for example,

- Thiamine deficiency, the most common cause is chronic alcoholism or 'Wernicke-Korsakoff syndrome'. 'Wernicke's encephalopathy is the acute phase of delirium preceding the amnestic syndrome, while Korsakoff's syndrome is the chronic phase of amnestic syndrome
- Head trauma
- Bilateral temporal lobectomy
- Hypoxia
- Brain tumours
- Herpes simplex encephalitis
- Stroke.

Clinical Features

- Recent memory impairment
- Anterograde and retrograde amnesia
- No alteration in consciousness.

Management

- Treat the underlying cause.

PERSONALITY AND BEHAVIOURAL DISORDERS DUE TO BRAIN DISEASE, DAMAGE AND DYSFUNCTION

Aetiology

Underlying organic causes
- Complex partial seizures (temporal lobe seizures)
- Cerebral neoplasms
- Cerebrovascular disease
- Head injury.

Clinical Features

- Premorbid personality
- No alteration in consciousness
- Emotional lability
- Poor impulse control
- Apathy
- Hostility.

Management

- Treat the underlying cause
- Symptomatic treatment with drugs like lithium, Carbamazepine and other anti-psychotic drugs.

NURSING MANAGEMENT OF THE CLIENT WITH ORGANIC MENTAL/BRAIN DISORDERS

1. Nursing Diagnosis

Alteration in cognitive functioning due to brain damage resulting in impaired mental functions in thought process, attention, concentration and memory.

Goals

Promotes mental functions of the client. Enable the client to adjust and accommodate memory changes.

Interventions

- Educate the family, friends (significant personalities) and the client about the disease and its effect and prognosis

- Encourage the family to show concern, love, support, and to have patience when rendering services to the client
- Stimulate memory of the client by showing pictures, discussing about past experiences, listening to music, songs, recalling them as it preserves quality of life
- Motivate the client to perform the activities or tasks of his liking, and use memory aids with the help of written reminders, object clues, e.g. timer setting for each activity, placing the item in the specific places like keys, spectacles, money, ornaments
- Encourage the client to have daily routine like eating, bathing, dressing, using telephonic reminders, e.g. the activities which they have to perform compulsorily to have pleasure like wishing family members and friends for their significant events
- Pursue the client to prepare memory wallets like about one topic, preparing 10–12 important activities, by seeing each step, elaborating it
- Orient the client to reality, i.e. time, place, person, as they may be confused
- Usage of memory tapes
- Motivate the client to discuss any topic which ever interests them
- Provide calm, non-stimulating environment to prevent agitation of the client
- Divert the clients' mind in relaxing manner
- Encourage the client to avoid stressors and calm the mind by engaging in useful activities
- Appreciate, if the client exhibits good expression of his thoughts.

2. Nursing Diagnosis

Self care deficit due to impaired physical functioning. For example, bathing, eating, bowel and bladder, tremors and motor retardation. Alteration in bowel functioning due to side effects of drugs or activity disturbances.

Goal

The client develops a sense of well being and accepted by others; prevents infection.

Interventions

- Provide barrier free environment
- Help the client to meet his physical hygienic needs, dressing, utilize adaptive or assertive devices
- Encourage to do frequent changing of positions
- Provide back care to prevent occurrence of pressure sores
- Provide things necessary to the client, so that it is easy to carry out his activities easily
- Give directions to the client to perform activities on his own
- Never hurry the client to do the activities
- Provide adequate clothing to the client according to season
- Provide fibre-rich diet to regulate bowel functioning, encourage the client to cultivate regular bowel habit
- Appreciate the person, when he does the activity adequately.

3. Nursing Diagnosis

Impaired nutrition related to eating difficulties like chewing, swallowing.

Goal

Obtains adequate nutrition by maintaining adequate food and fluid intake.

Interventions

- Well balanced diet; high protein and vitamin rich supplements are provided to meet caloric requirements (soft, easily digestible food)
- Fiber rich/roughage diet, e.g. fruits, green leaf, vegetables, whole wheat are given to prevent constipation
- Never serve too hot/too cold food; never scold the client, if he is not eating adequately

- Provide small and frequent feeds
- Never restrict the client to have the meals in the scheduled place and eat hurry, allow him to eat in his own pace
- Encourage for good chewing and swallowing techniques.

4. Nursing Diagnosis

Altered sleeping pattern related to depression, aloofness.

Goal

Enhances sleeping pattern.

Interventions

- Do not encourage the client to sleep in day time, make him busy in some constructive activities
- Motivate the client to take lukewarm water bath at night to promote sleep
- Provide calm and quiet environment
- If needed, provide back massage to promote sleep and relaxation
- Establish a bed time routine by encouraging him to have conducive or interested activity to get good sleep like listening to soft music, reading books, watching natural scenery
- Never encourage the client to have coffee at bedtime as it stimulate them to be awake all the night
- Provide safe place to avoid injuries due to wandering and sleep disturbances
- Instruct the care takers to observe/vigilance on the client in between, as they may have wandering tendency
- Provide ID card to the client, such that even if he gets lost, someone can trace him by checking the ID card.

5. Nursing Diagnosis

Impaired communication related to language difficulties, speech problems, difficulty in facial muscle movement.

Goal

Enhances interaction by adopting good communication techniques and exercise.

Interventions

- Motivate the client to take deep breath before conversation
- Demonstrate a caring attitude and concern by showing respect and regard, and positive reinforcement when the client is trying to converse
- Be brief, simple and clear, approach the client in slow and gentle manner
- Use soft voice when conversing with the client
- Develop and maintain good interpersonal relationship, help the client to establish closer relationship with others
- Promote socially acceptable behaviour
- Try to avoid over correction; ignore the client for his unacceptable behaviour.

6. Nursing Diagnosis

Potential for injuries because of sensory deficit.

Goal

Prevent injuries.

Interventions

- Provide safe environment, e.g. closed electricity circuits, dry flooring
- Remove any sharp instruments from the client's room
- Maintain adequate ventilation and pleasing environment.

7. Nursing Diagnosis

Social isolation related to mood changes and depression.

Goal

Reduces social isolation by enhancing socialization.

Interventions

- Encourage the client to interact with others
- Motivate the friends and family members to interact with the client frequently
- Be active listener, show attention and concentration, when the client is expressing or conversing his feelings
- Give respect, call by name, convey warmth, concern
- Never argue with the client
- Provide comfortable environment.

8. Nursing Diagnosis

Alteration in perception related to hallucinations and depression.

Goal

Adjusts to the perceptual difficulties.

Interventions

- Make the client to be familiar with his surroundings
- Promote sensitivity
- Always one member has to be available, to help the client when the need arises
- Speak clearly to the client and reorient him to the things perfectly without loosing confidence
- Remove the objects which promote perceptual disturbances
- Administer the drugs as prescribed
- Minimize sensory provoking environment
- Encourage him to perform the activities of his choice
- Provide supervision over clients' tasks
- Limit inappropriate behaviour
- Encourage the family members to provide support.

9. Nursing Diagnosis

Inadequate coping related to impaired cognitive abilities.

Goal

Client and his family members adopts adequate coping strategies in handling situation and meeting clients needs.

Interventions

- Accept the client as he is, reassure him
- Encourage the client to perform family activities, insist the family members to assist the client in performing the activities in a better manner
- Motivate the family members to discuss their problems openly, allow the client during discussion
- Permit the client to perform his interested activities like spiritual prayers, recreational activities
- Promote the client to interact and socialize with their own groups
- Avoid triggering stimuli or stressors which promote aggressive reactions
- Keep consistent and simple routine, provide some enjoyable activities
- Engage the client in meaningful activities
- Protect the client from being humiliated
- Provide supportive resources, guidance and counselling
- Assist family to take proper decision related to clients' care.

10. Nursing Diagnosis

Knowledge deficit related to the disease condition.

Goal

Enhance the clients' knowledge.

Interventions

- Arrange guidance, counselling services, educative sessions to enhance the clients' and family members' knowledge related to disease condition in detail
- Explain them to identify stressor and eliminate it
- Promote adequate family support to the client
- Encourage the client to join in family support group, as it will smoothen the pressure of looking after the client by sharing of their experiences.

REVIEW QUESTIONS

1. Delirium. (5M, RGUHS, 2004).
2. Discuss causes, manifestations and nursing management of an individual with Delirium. (15M, MGRU, 2002).
3. Toxic effects of Brain. (5M, RGUHS, 2003).
4. Senile Dementia. (5M, RGUHS, 01, 02, 04, 06; 5M, MGRU, 1999).
5. Dementia and Delirium. (5M, MGRU, 2002, 5M, RGUHS, 00.01, 02, 05, 06).
6. Psychological problems of Old Age. (5M, MGRU, 2000).
7. Organic functional disorders. (5M, MGRU, 2002).
8. What do you mean by Organic Psychosis? Write the Nursing Interventions for a patient suffering with Senile Dementia. (2+5M, IGNOU, 1999).
9. Alzheimer's disease. (2M, RGUHS, 98, 5M, KSDNEB, 2007).
10. Classification of organic mental disorders. (5M, RGUHS, 01).
11. Amnestic syndrome. (2M, RGUHS, 06).

17 Psychophysiologic Disorders/Psychosomatic Disorders

INTRODUCTION

The word, 'Psychophysiologic disorders' indicates 'alteration in physiological functioning of the individual due to psychological factors', changes occurs both in 'Psychic-Mind' and 'Somatic-Bodily', manifesting physical symptoms or bodily complaints, suggesting diseases without demonstrable organic pathology. People can convert transference of unexpressed emotions into physical symptoms is called as, 'Somatization'.

These clients neither obtains medical treatment as no organic cause or do not perceive themselves as having psychiatric problem, thus they do not obtain psychiatric treatment.

Franz Alexander, 'The father of Psychosomatic Medicine' described the classical illnesses.

DEFINITIONS

'A syndrome of multiple somatic symptoms that cannot be explained medically and are associated with psychosocial distress and long term seeking of assistance from health care professionals'.
—*Mary C Townsend*

'Disorders in which psychic elements are significant in initiating alterations in chemical, physiological or structure of the individual resulting in physical symptoms'.
—*Sreevani R*

'A group of ailments in which emotional stress is a contributing factor to physical problems involving an organ system under involuntary control'.
—*Bimla Kapoor, 1994*

'Psychological factors can influence the course of the general medical condition, which can be inferred by a close temporal association between the factors and the development or exacerbation of or delayed recovery from the medical condition'.
—*American Psychiatric Association, 2000*

Examples of Somatoform disorder are: Conversion reaction, pain disorder, hypochondriasis, body dysmorphic disorder, dissociative disorders–amnesia, fugue, depersonalization, identity disorder, mood disordermania, MDP, thought disorders–psychosis–schizophrenia, cognitive impairment disorder.

Incidence

- Age: below 30 years Psychosomatic Disorder are common.
- *Sex:* Females are more prone.

Aetiological Factors

Three essential factors are required to initiate exacerbate and maintain the physical symptoms of Psychosomatic disorders:

- Biological predisposition: Family history or hereditary; possible biochemical alterations
- Vulnerable personality: Type 'C' personality–suppression of anxiety, frustration, exhibits calm and placid, depressed, despair, low self worth and self-esteem, self pity
- Extreme or significant psychosocial stress: Severe emotional stress, crisis, traumatic life events
- The interaction between psychological, social and biological factors
- Social environment: Poor IPR, deprived bondages, cultural or religious factors; disharmony between family members, altered family dynamics, low socio-economic, educational difficulties, absence of support systems, unfulfilled needs for nurturing and caring
- Personality traits: Tense, under pressure, dependent, attention seeking, timid, weak ego
- Unresolved dependency conflicts
- Incidence is more in women and first degree relatives of persons and in twins, suggestive of genetic influence
- Poor or inadequate coping strategies
- Maladaptive health behaviour: Variations in eating pattern, lack of exercise, unsafe practices
- Stress related physiological or behavioural factors: Interpersonal factors, weak ego development; unacceptable emotions, repressed anger
- Occupational difficulties
- Smoking
- Chronic usage of anti-inflammatory agents
- Imbalance of angiotensin and prostaglandins
- Increased sympathetic nervous system stimulation

- Exposure to allergens like foods, drugs and for bright light
- Excessive exercises
- Perceptual and cognitive abnormalities, developmental difficulties, sickness, past experience with serious or life threatening illness.

Types of Psychophysiologic Disorders

Cardiovascular disorders
- Coronary heart diseases
- Essential hypertension
- Migraine headache
- Angina pectoris
- Myocardial infarction.

Gastrointestinal disorders
- Peptic ulcer/stress ulcer
- Irritable bowel syndrome
- Ulcerative colitis
- Esophageal reflux
- Crohn's disease
- Obesity
- Anorexia nervosa
- Eating disorders.

Endocrinal disorders
- Diabetes mellitus
- Hyperthyroidism
- Pre-menopausal syndrome.

Musculoskeletal disorders
- Backache
- Rheumatoid arthritis.

Immune disorders
- Viral infections
- Systemic lupus erythematosus.

Respiratory disorders
- Bronchial asthma
- Hyperventilation.

Skin disorders
- Neurodermatitis
- Eczema
- Psoriasis
- Alopecia
- Trichotillomania (Hair pulling)

- Pruritus
- Urticaria
- Acne vulgaris

Genitourinary disorders
- Non-specific urethritis
- Chronic prostatitis
- Menstrual disorders
- Dysmenorrhoea
- Amenorrhoea
- Menopause

Miscellaneous
- Accident proneness
- Headache
- Sleep disorders
- Visual disturbances
- Cancer
- Conversion disorders
- Tinnitus
- Hypochondriasis
- CNS disorders
- Hysteria

Flow chart 17.1: Dynamics of psychophysiologic disorders

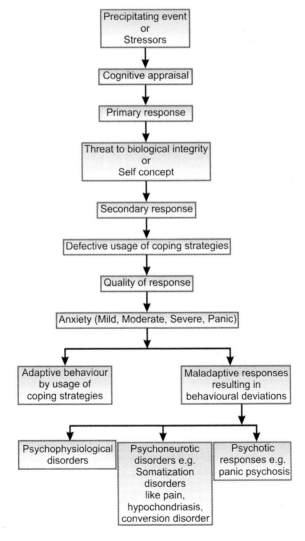

Clinical Manifestations

The symptoms varies based on cause associated to it, the symptoms or magnified health concerns are not under the clients' conscious control/voluntary control.

- Feelings of helplessness, guilty and insecurity
- Developmental regression
- Angry, hostility, aggressiveness
- Feelings of low self-esteem and worthlessness
- Bodyaches, headache, migraine, dysurea, dysmenorrhoea, dyspareunia
- Unpleasant activity
- Attention seeking behaviour
- Depression
- Unexplainable fears
- Social isolation
- Preoccupied with anxiety, fears, separation.

a. Psychoneurological Symptoms

- Signs and symptoms of conversion disorder, e.g. paralysis, aphonia, seizures, coordination disturbances, dysphagia, retention of urine, akinesia, deafness, blindness, double vision, hallucinations, pain sensation, amnesia, loss of consciousness other than fainting
- Sleep disturbances like insomnia, hypersomnia and parasomnias.

b. Sexual Symptoms

- Sexual indifference, ejaculatory dysfunctions, irregular menses, excessive bleeding, hyperemesis
- Significant impairment in social, occupational and other areas of functioning
- Withdrawal behaviour/socially isolated behaviour.

c. GIT Symptoms

- Nausea, bloating, vomiting, diarrhoea, dehydration, intolerance of certain foods.

The clients may exhibit primary gains: The direct external benefit that being sick. For example, relief from anxiety, stress or conflict or secondary gains–internal or personal benefits received from others. For example, attention from family members.

Dynamics of psychophysiologic disorders is described in Flow chart 17.1.

Treatment

- Exclude organic cause
- Psychotherapy
- Cognitive and behaviour therapy
  - Positive reinforcement
  - Role modelling
- Social therapy
- Drug therapy to relieve clinical manifestation
- Adaptive methods of stress management.
  - Progressive relaxation exercises, e.g. deep breathing
  - Meditation
  - Mental imagery or guided imagery
  - Assertiveness technique
- Provision of comfort measures, e.g. back rub, warm bath, cold/heat application
- Diversional therapy, e.g. music or dance.

Problem focussed coping strategies like problem solving techniques and role playing.

Nursing management of the client with psychosomatic disorder:

Assessment

Assess physical health status to exclude organic pathology, carry out

- Thorough physical examination
- Laboratory investigations
- Monitor vital signs
- Assess psychological and physiological functioning of the individual
- Assess psychological manifestations, e.g. self concept, thought process, mood and affect, judgement, insight
- Assess level of understanding about their disease process.

Nursing Diagnoses

Based on the disease process, the diagnoses will be varied

- Knowledge deficit related to physical and psychological illness
- Fear and anxiety related to past experiences with life threatening illnesses
- Low self-esteem related to unfulfilled childhood needs
- Alteration in physical and psychological dysfunctioning
- Disturbed body image related to anxiety
- Disturbed sleep pattern related to psychological disturbances.

Nursing Interventions

Help the client

- To recognize and accept the physical complaints eventhough no organic pathology
- To recognize the gains that the physical symptoms which are providing for the client, e.g. dependency, distraction, attention, deficit
- To withdraw attention to physical symptoms
- Refer the client if any additional symptoms occurs
- Advise the client to use possible alternating coping strategies
- Identify the ways to achieve recognition from others
- Ask the client to keep a record of physical symptoms and stressful situations
- Administer the drugs as per physicians orders
- Provide comfort measures
- Encourage the client to verbalize his psychological feelings, current life situations
- Teach the client to recognize different aspects of behaviour whether healthy behaviour or deviated behaviour
- Provide positive feedback for the acceptable behaviour of the client
- Counsel the clients, encourage them to participate in social activities
- Assist the client to recognize their own strengths/abilities, weakness, accomplishment, provide positive feedback by appreciation, small token to adopt socially acceptable behaviour
- Encourage the client to perform self-care activities
- Maintains non-judgemental attitude, when providing assistance to the client
- Encourage the client to perform independent activities when he is able to do, avoid dependency
- Allow sufficient time for the client to perform activity
- Encourage the client to express fears and anxieties related to stressful situations, validate the clients' feelings and counsel them
- Promote sleep by providing warm bath, soft music and relaxation exercises and provide a cup of warm milk
- Help the client to identify a resource person to provide situational support
- Educate the client to learn about their disease process with positive and coping strategies to be adopted at the time of stress or need; healthy behaviour, body-mind relationship; stress associated physical symptoms, relaxation techniques
- Establish daily health routine, e.g. adequate rest, exercise and nutrition
- Encourage the family to provide attention and concern, when the client is in 'sick role'
- When the client has fewer complaints, ask the family members to decrease special attention
- Motivate the client to identify the relationship between stress, physical symptoms and coping strategies
- Provide community based care–establish trusting relationship with the client; provide empathy and support, appropriate referrals, assistance from support groups, encourage the client to spend in pleasurable activities for attention and security, health promotion activities.

Evaluation

Somatoform disorders are recurrent and chronic hence slowly changes will occur. The positive coping techniques and counseling will help the clients' prognosis and improves functional abilities. Family support, situational guidance will assist the client for better prognosis. If the clients' condition does not improve, alternate coping strategies and health counselling, etc. may help them to overcome the problems.

DISSOCIATIVE DISORDERS

In DSM IV, the terms, 'Conversion and Dissociative disorders' were synonymously used. In ICD-10, F_4, it was indicated that both the terms are interchangeable and are described under 'dissociative disorders'. In these disorders, ability to exercise conscious and selective control is impaired to a degree, that can vary from day-to-day or even from hour-to-hour, i.e. onset or exacerbation of the symptoms. The disturbance may be sudden or gradual, transient or chronic. These are the mental illnesses that involve disruptions or breakdown of mental functions like memory, perception consciousness or awareness, identity, etc.

Definitions

'Dissociation reactions are the psychological manifestations which will occur when there is a partial or complete loss of the normal integration between past memories and awareness of identity, perception or consciousness due to underlying psychological conflicts'.

'Dissociation reaction' may take the form of amnesia, pseudo-dementia, fugue, stupor, trance, possession states, multiple personality disorder and pseudo-seizures (hysterical fits).

'Dissociation is one type of defense mechanism whereby the person will be protected from traumatic events by allowing the mind to forget or remove itself from painful situation or memory'.

Incidence

- Common in women and among first degree biological relatives of individual
- In adolescence or early adulthood, but any age it can occur.

Causes

- Psychological stress or conflicts or frustrations.
- Childhood trauma or sexual abuse is associated with adult dissociation symptomatology.
- Limbic system may be involved, traumatic memories are processed through limbic system and the hippocampus stores the information. Early trauma could remain detached from memory and stress could precipitate dissociation.
- Lack of attachment have effect on neurotransmitters like serotonin.
- Depersonalization cause block in neurotransmitter link.
- Drug abuse (like alcohol, barbiturates, benzodiazepines, hallucinogen).
- Traumatic life events–rape, incest, kidnapping, abuse, threats of death, physical violence, witness to violence.

Psychodynamics

- The disturbance is not under voluntary control but the symptoms occur in organs under voluntary control, e.g. symptoms will not develop intentionally
- Clients will benefit by both **Primary and Secondary gains**
- Primary gain is obtaining relief from anxiety by keeping an internal need or conflict out of awareness, e.g. an individual met with some problems suddenly, which he knows it, but he poses himself that he was not having any problem; temporarily gets relief from anxiety or frustration
- Secondary gain is support from the environment that a person obtains as a result of being sick,

e.g. Attention or support either financially or monitory benefit or regard and sympathy, e.g. an individual will get support (either financial or monitor) from parent or family members, when they become sick

- *La Belle difference* is clients' reaction like indifference to the symptoms and displaying no anxiety or lack of concern about the symptoms
- Clients will suffer with more number of problems in their private life
- Absence of medical and neurological abnormalities or organic deformities
- Amnesia or fugue related to a traumatic event
- Alteration in memory, consciousness, identity
- Interrupted family processes related to amnesia or other changing behaviour
- Symptoms of depersonalization
  - Feelings of unreality
  - Body image distortion
- Substance abuse
- Dysfunction in usual patterns of behaviour
  - Absence from work
  - Withdrawal behaviour
  - Alteration in functional aspects
- Feeling of absence of control over memory, behaviour, awareness
- Unable to explain the actions or behaviour in altered state.

Management

Aim

- Complete elimination of the symptoms by regular intake of medicines as per prescription
- Mild sedation or anxiolytics, e.g. Amobarbital
- Relaxation exercises
- Hypnosis
- Free association
- Teach stress reduction methods
- Abreaction therapy or pentothal review
- Psychotherapy (supportive, behaviour, hypnosis, etc.)
- Secondary gain has to be reduced to minimum.

Prognosis

Many cases will resolve spontaneously, when the client is removed from stressful situation.

NURSING MANAGEMENT

Aim

Ensure the client that he will recover completely.

Nursing Assessment

- Obtain history about past events in early life
- Any history of epilepsy, traumatic events, e.g. sexual or mental abuse, substance abuse
- Observe dressing pattern, interaction, working ability and primary and secondary gain pattern
- Complete assessment including physical examination, frequent observation and laboratory investigation (EEG, MRI, CT) to exclude organic pathology. Observe the mental and neurological status includes identity, memory, consciousness, life events, mood.

Interventions

- Try to understand the client, have tolerant, firm, kind and non-judgemental attitude
- Identify clients' psychological needs and attend
- Establish therapeutic nurse-client relationship
- Recognize the primary and secondary gains to the client
- Explore the clients' feelings, encourage the client to verbalize his stress, fears, anxiety and provide support in need of hour
- Assist the client to set the realistic goals
- Identify specific unresolved conflicts and the life situations that cannot be controlled and assist the client for possible solutions
- Withdraw attention of the clients' physical symptoms
- Provide safe, protective environment to the client
- Encourage the client to perform self care and therapeutic activities independently, provide

nondemanding and simple routine procedures to reduce anxiety
- Instruct the client that his disability should not be a limitation for participating in therapeutic activities
- Provide psychotherapeutic activities and encourage the client to use possible alternative coping strategies for problem solvation
- To promote ego integrity, support and adopting to the client to identify himself and give orientation to time and place
- Encourage the client to make decisions about his routine tasks and assist him for other decisions in his life
- Allow the client to progress at his own pace of recovery
- Accept the clients' negative feelings expressions
- Assist the client to reestablish relationships with significant personalities for situational support.

TYPES OF DISSOCIATIVE DISORDERS

a. Dissociative Amnesia

Impairment of integration of memories will occur, it is a form of psychogenic amnesia, common form of dissociative disorders.

Causes

- Genetic link
- Neurophysiological dysfunction–reactive inhibition of signals at synapses in sensorimotor pathways by negative feedback between the cerebral cortex and brain stem reticular formation
- Traumatic events after a severe psychosocial stress–when a person blocks out specific information
- Repression process–the painful events was stored in unconscious level
- Unexpected bereavements
- Stressful life situations or overwhelming stress
- Anxiety provoking internal urges

- Significant distress or impairment in social, occupational or other important areas of functioning.

Incidence

- Common in women than in men.

Clinical Manifestation

- Usually alert, a brief period of disorganization or clouding of consciousness
- Sudden inability to recall important personal information or loss of memory of recent events
- Depressive symptoms
- Memories still exist, but are deeply buried within the person's mind and cannot be recalled
- Memory gap spanning few minutes, few hours, few days, years
- Depersonalization
- Significant distress
- Trance state
- Regression.

Types of Amnesia

- Generalized amnesia
  Unable to recall information about their entire life time. It is diagnosed when a person's amnesia encompasses the present entire life.
- Localized amnesia
  Unable to remember all events of a circumscribed period (few hours to few days), the loss of memory is localized within a specific window of time, e.g. death of a loved person
- Selective amnesia.
  The ability to remember some events but not others for a short period, e.g. remembering the stressful events but not remembering the loss of people during that specific stressful situation
- Continuous amnesia
  Inability to recall events eventhough they are alert and aware. It occurs when the individual has no memory for the event beginning from a

certain point in the past continuing upto the present.

- Systematized amnesia
Individual cannot remember event that related to specific information or particular event.

Incidence

- Common among young adults
- People who are exposed to wars, accidents or natural disasters
- Women experience more than men.

Diagnosis

- Complete medical history
- Physical examination, X-rays and other lab tests like EEG, blood test for toxins and drugs
- Psychological examination
- Referral to psychiatric unit.

Treatment

Goal

- To relieve clinical manifestation
- To recall painful experiences or internal conflicts
- To control any problematic behaviour
- To facilitate the client to express or ventilate the painful memories
- To develop new coping and life skills
- To restore functioning pattern
- To improve social relationships
- To reduce anxiety associated with amnesia.

Types of Treatment

- Memory retrieval techniques–consent has to be obtained
- Psychotherapy–psychological processes will be sued for catharsis or ventilation to resolve the internal conflicts and to increase deeper insight into the problem and find the ways to resolve them. Hypnosis technique will be more helpful,

drug facilitated interviews (Amobarbital I.V) skill is very much essential to utilize the technique to reduce the anxiety

- Drug therapy–antidepressants or anxiolytics can be used based on manifestation
- Cognitive therapy–to change dysfunctional thinking pattern and behaviour
- Social therapy–is based on manifestation
- Family therapy and counselling–to provide situational support
- Diversional therapy, art therapy, music therapy–allows the patient to explore and express their thoughts in a creative manner
- Work therapy
- Relaxation techniques
- Prognosis–good, memory returns with time.

b. Dissociative Fugue

When the ability to integrate identity is affected or fragmented, results in 'dissociative fugue'. It increases in stressful situations. It is a psychogenic state, a sudden unexpected travel away from home or work place, a feeling of new identity, unable to recall the past. Self care is maintained, new identity may be maintained for few days, following recovery, they will not be able to recollect the events that took place during fugue and leads simple life; confusion about personal identity.

Causes

- Substance abuse
- Marital disharmony
- Financial upheavals
- Occupational distress
- Wars
- Depression
- Suicidal idea
- Personality disorders
- Epilepsy.

Prognosis

- Rapid and spontaneous.

Treatment

- Manipulation of environment; psychotherapy; hypnosis.

NURSING MANAGEMENT

Nursing Diagnosis

- Risk for violence related to fear of unknown circumstances
- Ineffective coping related to stressors.

Interventions

- Protect the client from harmful stressors thereby prevention of self harm
- Encourage the client to express his feelings related to anxiety
- Identify the resources, where client can be relieved from stress
- Gentle encouragement, persuasion, direct association is required.

c. Dissociative Identity Disorder or Multiple Personality Disorder

The aspects of the self may emerge as distinct personalities. Individual will loose the sense of who they are; women have a higher degree of prevalence, i.e. 5:1 to 9:1 (Women to Men ratio). If untreated, the disorder becomes a recurring one.

Definition

'A condition in which 2 or more distinct identities or personality states alternate in controlling the patients' consciousness and behaviour'.

In multiple personality disorder, the person is dominated by 2 or more personality of which only one is manifest at a time. One personality will not be aware of the other personality, suddenly one form to other form will change and the behaviour in each personality will be contrast of other, its own pattern of relating, perceiving and thinking about them and environment. Persons' behaviour will be controlled by these sub-personalities. It may be a culture specific syndrome found in western society.

Causes

- An innate ability to dissociate easily
- Repeated episodes of severe physical or sexual abuse in childhood
- Lack of supportive or comforting person to counteract abusive relatives
- Influence of other relatives with dissociative symptoms or disorders
- Physical or psychological traumatic experiences
- Absence of situational support
- Intolerable terror–producing event
- Absence of adaptive coping ability
- Intense anxiety
- Negative role models
- Unspecified long term societal changes
- Rigid religious beliefs
- Isolation from the community
- Lack of cooperation among the employees.

Manifestations

- Inadequate defenses to handle the intense anxiety
- Individual dissociates the event and the feelings associated with the event
- Clients with dissociative disorders experience their alters as distinctive individual assessing different names, histories and personality traits
- Dissociated processes are split off from the memory of the primary personality
- Dissociative part of personality takes an existence of its own, becoming a subpersonality
- The subpersonality learns to deal with emotional feelings which will overwhelm the primary personality
- When individual is facing with anxiety producing situation, one of the subpersonality takes over to protect the primary personality from disintegration and disorganization
- Usually the primary personality is religious and moralistic
- Subpersonality are aggressive, pleasure seeking, nonconforming or sexually promiscuous

- Sometimes the dominance will be changing, voice will have different sounds and intelligence level varies
- Cognitive distortions, amnesia or 'loose time' for periods when another personality is 'out'.
- Transition from one personality to another often occurs during time of stress.

Diagnosis

- Rule out physical conditions
- EEG–to exclude seizures
- Dissociative experiences scale and dissociative disorders interview schedule
- Structured clinical interview for DSM-IV dissociative disorders
- Hypnotic induction profile.

Treatment

Psychotherapy

- Initial phase for uncovering and mapping the patient's alters
- Treating the traumatic memories, fusing the alters
- Consolidating the patient's newly integrated personality
- Social skill training
- Family therapy–for personality reintegration
- Mixed therapy groups.

Drug Therapy

- Tranquilizers or antidepressants.

Hypnosis

- To recover repressed ideas and memories
- To control problematic behaviours.

  To 'fuse' the alters as part of the patient's personality integration process

  Adjunct or alternative treatments. For example, Hydrotherapy, therapeutic massage, yoga, art therapy, meditation.

Prognosis

Is excellent for children and better for adults.

NURSING MANAGEMENT

Nursing Diagnosis

- Prone for suicide related to unresolved grief
- Alteration in personal identity related to childhood traumatic experiences.

Interventions

- Assess the suicidal tendency of the client and sudden changes within the behaviour
- Assist the client to identify stressful precipitating factors
- Provide trusting relationship, support and reassurance to the client when he will discouraged more
- Administer the drugs as per doctor's orders
- The safety of the client is maintained
- Provide positive reinforcement for the client.

d. Depersonalization Disorder

Definition

'A persistent or recurrent alteration in the perception of the self to the extent that the sense of one's own reality is temporarily lost, while reality ability testing remains intact'.

Depersonalization is a dissociative symptom in which the patient feels that his/her body is unreal, is changing or is dissolving. Some dissociative disorders clients experience depersonalization as feeling to be outside of their body or as watching a movie of themselves.

Aetiology

- CNS diseases, e.g. Brain tumours, epilepsy
- Severe sensory deprivation
- Psychological conflicts
- Unpleasant emotions or emotional pain.

Manifestation

- The person experiencing depersonalization may feel mechanical, dreamy or detached from the body.
- Ego dystonic, e.g. perceiving the limbs to be larger or smaller than the normal
- The experience causes significant impairment in social or occupational functioning makes distress.

MANAGEMENT

- Teach relaxation technique and assertiveness techniques
- Administer drugs as per order
- Supportive services.

NURSING MANAGEMENT

Nursing Diagnosis

- Deprivation of sensory perception
- Anxiety related to ear of lack of control

Interventions

- Provide a sense of reality environment during stressful situation, e.g. calm and non-threatening environment
- Provide support and encouragement
- Assist the client to explore past experiences related to painful situation
- Arrange for role play, where the client will have the opportunity to observe the situation and faces the stressful situation in real life and to adapt coping strategies.

e. Dissociative Stupor

- Clients are motionless, mute
- Will not respond to stimulation
- Aware of surroundings.

Ganser's Syndrome

- Rarely occurs 4 cardinal symptoms

- Clouding of consciousness
- Hallucinations
- Psychogenic physical symptoms
- Answering approximately which are designed to test intellectual functions.

f. Dissociative Sensory Loss and Anaesthesia

- Sensory disturbances are common
- Hemi anaesthesia
- Blindness
- Deafness
- Glove and stocking anaesthesia (absence of sensation at wrist and ankle)
- Detailed examination will not reveal any abnormalities.

g. Dissociative Motor Disorders

- Motor disturbances
- Paralysis–monoplegia, paraplegia, quadriplegia
- Abnormal body movements–tremors, gait disturbances
- On examination normal tone and reflexes will be observed.

h. Trance and Possession Disorders (Common in India)

- Total awareness of person's surroundings
- Narrowed attention
- Repeated body movements, postures, utterances.

i. Dissociative Convulsions (Pseudoseizures/Hysterical fits)

'Hysteria' is a Greek word means 'the womb'. It is a clinical manifestation which may mimic epileptic seizures in which 'body' movements are common. It is a state of trance partial loss of consciousness mimicking so many other diseases; shows abnormality in functions under voluntary control, physician often feels great difficulty in determining the true nature of the case. Hysteria is more commonly observed in young women.

Manifestations

- The trunk and limbs are strongly convulsed
- Struggles violently
- Retracting and extending legs
- Twisting of body, may prone for injury
- Thrown backward, flushing of the face, turgid neck
- Closed eyelids, tremulous, distended nostrils, irregular breathing
- Jaws are often firmly shut; trembling, spasms
- Violent agitation slowly calm down
- Whole attack frequently terminates in an explosion of tears, sobs and convulsive laughter
- Uneasiness in the abdomen, eructation
- Recovers consciousness, but remains depressed for some time, in spirits and fatigued
- Pseudo disease come to a sudden favourable termination under some strong mental or moral emotions.

Differences between epileptic seizures and hysterical fits is represented in the Table 17.1.

Treatment

- Reconstructive educational psychotherapy
- Family therapy
- Diversional therapy
- Task oriented approach
- Sometimes–suggestions therapy with I.V pentothal sodium may be of helpful.

Aims

- Counsel the client in handling problematic situations
- Cool-up and divert the clients' mind and engage the client in useful or productive activities.

Measures

- Educate the client the 'healthy coping behaviour' and strategies to overcome 'psychological stressors'
- Teach the client 'the problem solving techniques', 'assertiveness techniques' 'coping mechanisms and its utilization' to overcome the stressful situations

Table 17.1: Differences between epileptic seizures and hysterical fits		
Sl. No Clinical features	Epileptic seizure	Hysterical fits
1. Aura (warning)	Common	Uncommon
2. Duration	Clonic phase and tonic phase 30-70 seconds	Quarter of an hour to many hours
3. Time of the day	Any time even in sleep also attacks may occur	Never occurs in sleep (as it is voluntarily affected)
4. Place of occurrence	Any place	In safer environment, commonly indoor
5. Attack pattern	Stereotyped	Purposive body movements
6. Amnesia	Complete	Partial
7. Neurological signs	Present	Absent
8. Postictal confusion	Present	Absent
9. Tongue bite	Present	Absent
10. Larynx	Is closed	May be affected, never closed
11. Incontinence of urine and faeces	Can occur	Very rare
12. Injury	May result	Very rare

- Advice the client to explore the 'psychological stressors' which are troubling more, teach suitable coping strategies; ask them to avoid physical or mental excitement
- Provide counselling to the family members and motivate them to provide support to the client in times of stress
- After the paroxysm is over, ask the client to have shower-bath and have active purge
- Place the client in fresh cool air
- Iron and vitamin supplements can be given to enhance strength to the client.

CONVERSION DISORDER OR CONVERSION REACTION

Conversion reactions are partial or complete loss of normal integration between immediate sensations and control of bodily movements or deficits involving voluntary motor or sensory functions due to underlying psychological conflicts and anxiety. 'La Belle difference' (lack of concern or distress) is a vital feature.

Physical symptoms caused by psychologic conflict, unconsciously converted to resemble neurologic disorder (pseudo-neurological).

Aetiology

- Traumatic events/unacceptable emotions
- Sexual abuse in childhood
- Disturbance in CNS arousal
- Lack of situational support.

Clinical Manifestations

- Motor deficits
  Tremors, mutism, hysterical convulsions, aphonia, lack of coordination or balance, weakness, dysphagia, akinesia, urinary retention, lack of clients' social, occupational or other area of functioning, paralysis
- Sensory deficits
  Anaesthesia, paraesthesia, hyperaesthesia, loss of one of the special senses like blindness,

double vision, deafness, sensation of a lump in the throat, lack of pain sensation, hallucinations, environmental misperceptions, hysteric symptoms.

Conversion symptoms promote secondary gain for the individual by enabling them to avoid difficult situations.

Diagnosis

- Conversion symptoms rarely conform fully to known anatomic and physiologic mechanisms
- Extensive physical examination and laboratory test fail to reveal a disorder that can fully account for the symptoms and its effects
- A trusting therapeutic nurse client relationship is essential
- Reassure the client, that the symptom do not indicate a serious underlying disorder; the client feels better when the symptoms fade.

Treatment

Psychotherapy
- Hypnotherapy–when the client is hypnotized, the aetiologic psychologic issues were explored
- Narcoanalysis
- Behaviour modification techniques
- Relaxation techniques.

Prognosis

- Client may have a single episode or sporadic ones
- Client generally improve within 2 weeks
- 20–25 per cent have recurrences within a year at the time of extreme stress
- In some cases, symptoms may become chronic.

NURSING MANAGEMENT

Nursing Assessment

- Observe the psychological stressors
- Assess the motor and sensory functioning

- Observe the motor and sensory deficit
- Visualize the situational support.

Interventions

- Nurse has to be non-judgemental
- Encourage the client to accept and participate in decision making process and in group activities
- Identify the strengths, abilities, accomplishments
- Provide positive feedback and reinforcement for corrective behaviour
- Encourage the client to withdraw their attention on physical symptoms
- Assertiveness technique and communication techniques has to be taught to the client
- Assist in self-care activities
- Encourage independency in behaviour
- Explain the effects of psychological factors on physical illness
- Provide guidance and counselling service to the client and his relatives
- Advise the family to provide situational support to the client.

REVIEW QUESTIONS

1. Hysteric Fits and Epileptic Fits. (2M, RGUHS, 00).
2. Amnesia. (5M, RGUHS, 05).
3. Seizure. (1M, Gulb, 98).
4. Multiple personality. (5M, RGUHS, 06, 02).
5. Conversion Disorders. (5M, RGUHS, 03, 06).
6. Conversion Reaction and Dissociative Reaction. (2M, RGUHS, 00).
7. Psycho Somatic Disorders. (5M, RGUHS, 01, 02, 06).
8. Psycho Somatic illness. (5M, RGUHS, 01).
9. Psycho physiological disorder. (5M, Oct, 07, RGUHS, 06).
10. What do you understand by the term Psycho Physiological disorders? Name the disorders commonly found in our clients. Discuss the line of Nursing Management of any one such patient. (2+4+9M, MGRU, 92).
11. Write the dynamics of Psycho Physiological relations. List the various types of Psycho Physiological disorders. Discuss the Nurse's role in caring such patients. (5+3+7, MGRU, 90).
12. Dissociative disorders. (5M, RGUHS, 2000, 06).
13. Differences between Epileptic Seizure and Hysterical fits. (5M, RGUHS, 2000).
14. Somatoform disorders. (5M, RGUHS, 2000).
15. Psychogenic pain. (2M, RGUHS, Oct, 2007).
16. Puerperial Psychosis. (2M, RGUHS, Oct, 07).

18

Sexual Disorders

INTRODUCTION

Sexuality is a complex process, coordinated by the neurologic, vascular and endocrine systems. Sexuality incorporates family, societal and religious beliefs and is altered with aging, health status and personal experiences. Sexual activity incorporates interpersonal relationships, each partner brings unique attitudes, needs and responses into the coupling. A breakdown in any of these areas may lead to sexual dysfunction and sexual deviation.

Based on cultural milieu, the categorization of sexual behaviour will vary, either normal or abnormal, sexual behaviour is considered in the context of total personality of an individual. Emotions will strongly influence the sexual behaviour. Due to cultural barrier and social stigma associated with sexual behaviour, the people will develop inhibitions, hesitations to discuss about and will not come forward to report exact complaint related to sexuality and unable to express openly. Sexual difficulties can begin early in life or it may develop after an individual has previously experienced enjoyable and satisfying sex. Problems may arise suddenly or gradually over a period of time.

DEFINITION

'Sexual disorders are characterized by sexual dysfunction or sexual malfunction and sexual deviation, i.e. difficulty during any stage of the sexual act (desire, arousal, orgasm and resolution) that prevents the individual or couple from enjoying satisfied sexual activity due to varied reasons'.

CLASSIFICATION

ICD-10

F_{52}–Sexual dysfunction (ICD-9 302.7)

F_{64}–Gender identity disorders

$F_{64.0}$–Trans-sexualism

$F_{64.1}$ –Dual role transvestism

$F_{64.2}$–Gender identity disorder of childhood

$F_{64.8}$–Other gender identity disorders

$F_{64.9}$–Gender identity disorder, unspecified

F_{65}–Disorders of sexual preference

$F_{65.0}$–Fetishism

$F_{65.1}$–Fetishistic transvestism

$F_{65.2}$–Exhibitionism

$F_{65.3}$–Voyeurism

$F_{65.4}$–Paedophilia

$F_{65.5}$–Sadomasochism

$F_{65.6}$–Multiple disorders of sexual preference

$F_{65.8}$–Other disorder of sexual preference

$F_{65.9}$–Disorder of sexual preference, unspecified

F_{66}–Psychological and behavioural disorder associated with sexual development and orientation

$F_{66.0}$–Sexual maturation disorder

$F_{66.1}$–Ego dystonic sexual orientation

$F_{66.2}$–Sexual relationship disorder

$F_{66.8}$–Other psychosexual development disorders

$F_{66.9}$–Unspecified–Psychosexual development disorder.

CLASSIFICATION OF SEXUAL DYSFUNCTIONAL DISORDERS

Sexual arousal disorders or decreased libido

- Sexual arousal disorders. For example, Frigidity or arousal in women, impotence/erectile dysfunction in men
- Orgasm disorders
- Sexual pain disorders, e.g. Dyspareunia (painful intercourse) and vaginismus (an involuntary vaginal muscle spasm that interferes with vaginal intercourse).

Incidence

Sexual dysfunctions are more common in the early adult years and in the geriatric population. Majority of the people seeking care for these conditions during their late twenties through thirties, it is more common in addicts, i.e. alcohol and drugs, diabetics, degenerative neurological disorders.

Causes of Sexual Difficulties

Emotional factors affecting sex

a. Interpersonal problems, e.g. Lack of trust and open problems or conflicts, extra marital affairs, sexual/libido, desire or practices different from partner, poor sexual communication.

b. Ongoing psychological problems, e.g. Difficulty in maintaining relationships or chronic disharmony with the current sexual partner, depression, sexual fear or guilt, past sexual trauma, etc.

Life stressors: Financial problems, family or job problems, illness or death.

c. Medical diseases. For example, Benign prostatic hypertrophy, degenerative neurological disorders, injuries to the back, nerve damage (Spinal cord injury).

Endocrinal disorders: For example, Thyroid, pituitary, adrenal gland problems, diabetes.

Illicit usage of drugs or medication. For example, Antipsychotic, antihistamines, alcohol, nicotine, narcotics, stimulants, antihypertensive.

Physical or Sexual Abuse or Verbal Abuse

Hormonal deficiencies. For example, Low testosterone, estrogen or androgens.

Gynaecologic maladies and cancer. For example, Vaginismus, atrophy, strictures, vaginitis, prolapse, breast cancer, recurrent cystitis.

Gynaecologic changes related to a woman's reproductive life present unique problems and potential obstacles to sexuality. For example, Puberty–concerns regarding sexual identity.

Pregnancy and postpartum period, lactation–associated with a decrease in sexual activity, desire, satisfaction.

Menopause–The hypoestrogenic state of menopause may cause significant physical changes and alterations in mood or a diminished sense of wellbeing, effects negatively on sexuality.

d. Intrapersonal conflicts. For example, Religious taboos, social restrictions, sexual identity conflicts, guilt.

e. Historical factors. For example, Past or current abuse (sexual, verbal, physical) rape, sexual inexperience.

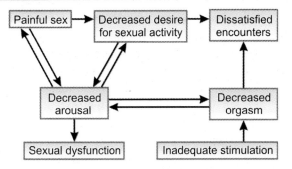

(Source: Philips NA. The clinical evaluation of dyspareunia. Int. J Impot res.1998:10 (Suppl-2) S117-20)

f. Life stressors: Financial problem, family problems, obstetric problems, illness of family members, death.
g. Birth defects.
h. Smoking results into erectie dysfunction, decreased sperm count.

The 4th edition of the DSM (Diagnostic and Statistical Manual of Mental disorders) list the following psychological sexual disorders:

- Hypoactive sexual disorder
- Sexual aversion disorder (avoidance of or lack of desire for sexual intercourse)
- Female sexual arousal disorder (failure of normal lubricating arousal response)
- Male erectile disorders
- Female orgasmic disorders
- Premature ejaculation
- Dyspareunia
- Vaginismus
- Secondary sexual dysfunction
- Paraphilias
- Gender identity disorder
- Post-traumatic stress disorder due to genital mutilation or childhood sexual abuse.

The cycle of sexual dysfunction was described in the above flow chart.

Diagnosis

- Obtain a detailed history of client
- Identify the causative or confounding medical or gynaecological conditions
- Elicit psychosocial information
- Physical examination, gynaecological examination
- Establishment of the client's sexual orientation is necessary for appropriate evaluation and management
- Be non-judgemental, ask direct questions
- Assist for laboratory examination and collection of reports, e.g. vaginal cultural swab, semen culture
- Routine screening tests.

TREATMENT

General Treatment

- Identify the aetiology and treat the cause to maintain satisfying sexual relationship
- Modification of life style
- Hormonal replacement therapy based on requirement of hormone, e.g. estrogen, testosterone, progesterone
- Integrated treatment approaches will be of helpful
  - Cognitive behavioural therapy
  - Couple's therapy
  - Traditional sex therapy
  - Client education and reassurance–about normal anatomy, sexual function, normal changes with aging; discuss sexual issues when a medical condition is diagnosed; encourage communication during sexual activity
  - Specialized counselling–individual or couple based on problem strategies to alleviate anxiety
  - Provide distraction techniques–pelvic muscle contraction and relaxation, Kegel's exercise with intercourse recommended the use of back ground music
  - Encourage noncoital behaviour– to promote comfort and communication between partners recommended sensual massage, sensate focus exercises, oral or noncoital stimulation, with or without orgasm

- Bio feedback, warm bath before intercourse, position changing
- Topical application of lubricants, e.g. Vit-E/mineral oils, lidocaine
- Non-steroidal anti-inflammatory drugs before intercourse.

Kegel's Exercises

Potential uses–Increased pubococcygeal tone, improved orgasmic intensity, correction of orgasmic intensity, correction of orgasmic urine leakage, distraction technique during intercourse, improved patient awareness of sexual response.

Teaching Kegel's Exercises

- Instructional examination with examiner's finger in vagina
- Initial patient home exercise with patient's finger in vagina
- Slow count to 10, with movement directed 'in and up'
- Hold for count of 3 slow release to count of 10 repeat 10–15 times daily
- Consider vaginal weights, biofeedback clinics.

Maintenance of Exercises

- Advise repetitions during routine activities schedule follow-up appointments to discuss progress.

NURSING MANAGEMENT OF SEXUAL DISORDERS

Nursing Assessment

Sexual History

- Establish therapeutic nurse-client relationship; first, ask general questions, approach the client gently in a friendly manner, after winning the confidence, start the discussion on sexual issues by open ended questions on menstruation, coitus, sexual changes with aging, menopause, any clarifications on sexual matters. For example, Masturbation, sexual frequency, safe sex positions, protective or precautionary measures; any other sexual issues related to partner, observation made regarding sexual responses after starting the treatment.

1. Nursing Diagnosis

Anxiety, fear and inhibitions related to expression of sexual feelings.

Goals

Expresses freely the problems related to sexual issues.

Interventions

- Establish and maintain therapeutic nurse patient relationship allow the client to express his views freely
- Attentively listen to the client's feelings and needs, show concern for the patient
- Never give false reassurance and false hopes
- Counsel the client, teach the appropriate measure to resolve the problems
- Needed referral can be made and encourage the client to seek medical help appropriately
- Teach relaxation techniques, movement and changing of position
- Provide alternative strategies to resolve the problem.

2. Nursing Diagnosis

Altered body image.

Goal

To enjoy worthful living.

Interventions

- Encourage the client to interact
- Nurse acts as active listener while the client interacts

- Motivate the client to discuss the physiological changes occurring in their body, quote significant examples with adequate meaning
- Review the clients' capabilities, strengths and limitations
- Be realistic with the client and set appropriate goals
- Make the client to understand their potentialities and utilize productively as it enhances utility values either in the family or to the society
- Understand the cultural values before providing counselling and guidance to the client.

3. Nursing Diagnosis

Impaired functional pattern evidenced by emotional distress.

Goal

Relieved from emotional distress.

Interventions

- Provide conducive support to the client, allow him to ventilate his problems openly in a comfortable manner
- Facilitate sharing and communicating the views, feelings
- Guide the individual to perform defined physical activities or exercises, healthy means of relieving stress and tension
- Encourage the client to meet his needs, provide some tips to fulfil it, e.g. adequate nutrition, rest and exercises.

4. Nursing Diagnosis

Distress related to inability to perform sexual acts satisfactorily.

Goal

To make the client free from internal conflicts related to sexual acts.

Interventions

- Assess the emotional status and problems of the client
- Encourage the client to perceive clearly about the treatment
- Clarify the doubts if appropriate; explain the importance of therapeutic strategies to achieve, cooperation in utilizing effective strategies
- Provide conducive or supportive environment to have emotional catharsis.

5. Nursing Diagnosis

Disturbed personality identity exhibited by maladaptive behaviour.

Goal

Adapts coping skills to develop adaptive behaviour.

Interventions

- Explain the consequences of maladaptive behaviour, make them to perform the 'right behaviour at their will'
- Make them to understand their responsibility
- Be non-judgemental
- Assist the client to explore alternative methods to overcome sexual dissatisfaction.

6. Nursing Diagnosis

Altered self-esteem evidenced by ineffective role performance.

Goal

Performs effectively their roles.

Interventions

- Teach the effective therapeutic means and its outcome in overcoming sexual problems
- Counsel the client, suggest varied methods to improve sexual performance
- Encourage him to share the views about sexuality openly

- Schedule the activities of client and motivate him to follow it adequately
- Explain the possible means of the solutions/ strategies.

7. Nursing Diagnosis

Impaired social interaction evidenced by improper communication.

Goal

Effectively interacts with others.

Interventions

- Maintains therapeutic relationship with the client
- Approach the client in a friendly manner
- Accept the client's feelings, encourage him to interact, first introduce to small groups, later extend to big groups
- Motivate to perform group activities
- Identify to cultural milieu of client and provide opportunities to accommodate within it so that they can live effectively and satisfactorily without any disturbances or cultural lag.

8. Nursing Diagnosis

Knowledge deficit related to treatment strategies.

Goals

Gains the knowledge and contributes effectively by active means.

Interventions

- Explain to the client adequately the treatment strategies, its effectiveness, contribution of client and their partners
- Provide alternative treatment choices
- Allow the client to select freely based on choice and suggest certain guidelines, if any help is required

- Teach the advantages, limitations, complications or delimitations of each strategy
- Explain the needed cooperation, appreciate if they are extending so
- Assist the client to accommodate satisfactorily and function effectively to the societal/cultural environment.

SEXUAL DYSFUNCTIONS (F_5)

Frigidity/Inhibited or Hypoactive Sexual Desire/ Sexual Aversion/Sexual Apathy.

Definition

'A low level of sexual desire and interest manifested by a failure or be responsive to a partner's initiation of sexual activity'.

Types

- Primary inhibited sexual desire–where the person never felt much sexual desire or interest
- Secondary inhibited sexual desire–where the person used to possess sexual desire, but no longer has interest
- Situational to the partner–where he/she has interest in other persons, but not towards the partner
- General–where he/she lacks sexual interest with anyone
- Extreme form–the person not only lacks sexual desire, but also finds sex repulsive, revolting and distasteful
- Discrepancy in sexual interest, levels between two partners, both of whom have interest levels within the normal range.

Causes

- Relationship problems, e.g. One partner does not feel emotionally intimate or close to their mate
- Emotional struggles and conflicts
- Communication difficulties
- Lack of time, lack of affection

- Restrictive upbringing concerning sex
- Negative attitudes towards sex
- Traumatic sexual experiences, e.g. incest, rape, sexual abuse
- Dietary variations
- Fatigue, insomnia
- Erection problems ,e.g. Impotence or erectile dysfunction
- Persons whose marriages are lacking in emotional intimacy.

Treatment

- Individualized to the factors that may be inhibiting sexual interest
- Relationship enhancement work through marital therapy
- Psychotherapy and counselling towards conflict resolution, enhancement of loving relationship, overcome strained relationship
- Communication training, showing empathetic understanding.

Steps to Resolve Differences

- Drug therapy, e.g. Bremelanotide–increases sexual desire
- Referral to the sex therapist.

Complications

- Barometer of emotional relationship
- Eventual feelings of resentment; emotional distance
- Conflicts and frictions.

Prevention

- Advise the client to maintain closer relationship among couple and utilize good communication techniques, skills
- Reserving time for intimacy with partner (both sexual or non-sexual), e.g. couple alone going for outing without any other family members, closeness feelings and enhance sexual desire.

ERECTILE DYSFUNCTION/IMPOTENCE

Erectile dysfunction affects the lives of many middle aged men, it can occur at any age. History of an occasional episode is normal; it may also a sign of physical or emotional problem. Described in ICD–10 (N.48.4) and ICD-9 (607.84).

Definitions

'The inability to obtain an adequate erection for satisfactory sexual activity'.

'A sexual dysfunction characterized by the inability to develop or maintain an erection of the penis'.

'Recurrent or persistent partial or complete failure to attain or maintain an erection until the completion of the sex act, which cause marked distress or interpersonal difficulty'.

—DSM-IV

Physiology of Erection

Penis contains two cylindrical sponge like structure that run along its length, parallel to the tube that carries semen and urine. When a man becomes sexually aroused, nerve impulses cause the blood flow seven times more than normal, this sudden influx of blood expands the sponge structure and produces an erection by straightening and stiffening the penis. Continued sexual arousal or excitation maintains higher blood flow, keeping the erection firm. After sexual excitement passes, the excess blood drains out of the sponge tissue and the penis returns to its non-concrete size and shape.

The hormonal component–adequate levels of testosterone and an intact pituitary gland are required for the development of healthy male erectile system. Release of non-adrenaline, non-cholinergic neurotransmitter acts directly on the smooth muscle to produce relaxation. Alpha-adrenergic receptors produce contraction.

Causes

- Physiological factors–marital discord, communication and expressiveness

- Physical cause–diabetic neuropathy, low blood supply to the penis, surgery for cancer prostate, fractures that injure the spinal cord, multiple sclerosis, hormonal disorders, alcoholism, drug abuse, smoking
- Drugs–thiazide diuretics, antihypertensive drugs, H_2 receptors antagonists
- Endocrinal disorders–hypogonadism, hypothyroidism, diabetes mellitus
- Psychiatric conditions–schizophrenia, Alzheimer's disease, stress, Madonna syndrome, Coolidge effect (couple no longer finding excitement), Widower's syndrome (occurs when a widowed male feels pressured to have intercourse before he has completed the grievance process for his wife)
- Nutritional disorder–obesity, protein caloric malnutrition.

Manifestations

- Regular or repeated inability to obtain or maintain an erection
- Erections may take longer to develop, may not be as rigid or may require more direct stimulation to be achieved
- Interfere with a man's self image as well as his or partner's sexual life.

Pattern

- Inability to have any erection at all from the beginning of a sexual experience
- First experiencing an adequate erection and then loosing tumescence when attempting penetration
- Having an erection, i.e. sufficiently firm for penetration but then loosing tumescence before or during thrusting
- Being able to experience an erection only during self masturbation or on awakening
- Lack of nocturnal erection

Diagnosis

- Duplex ultrasound to evaluate blood flow and calcification
- Penile nerves function test, nocturnal penile tumescence, penile biothesiometry, penile angiogram, magnetic resonance angiography, neurologic evaluation.

Treatment

- Identify the cause and eliminate the stressor/ cause
- Counselling to rule out psychological stressor and treat the cause, provide support for couple
- Drug therapy, e.g. sildenafil, tadalafil, vardenafil
- Based on cause, the treatments like needle injection therapy hormone replacement therapy, vascular surgery, etc.

PARAPHILIA/SEXUAL PERVERSION/ SEXUAL DEVIATION

Paraphilia is derived from two Greek words 'para' means 'besides' 'philia' means 'friendship'. Sexual perversions are conditions in which the sexual excitement or orgasm is associated with acts or imagery, to avoid problems associated with acts or imagery, to avoid problems associated with the stigmatization of labels, the neutral term, 'paraphilia' has been used.

Sexual deviation is any sexual behaviour, i.e. regarded significantly different from the standard establishment of sub-culture or set culture.

Definition

'A condition in which a person's sexual arousal and gratification depends on a fantasy theme of an unusual situation or object that becomes the principle focus of sexual behaviour'.

'Sexual impulse disorders are characterized by intensely arousing, recurrent sexual fantasies, urges and behaviours considered deviant with respect to cultural norms and that produce clinically significant distress or impairment in social, occupational or other important areas of psychosocial life functioning'

—*DSM-IV*

'Persistent, intense fantasies, urges, behaviours involving sexual arousal to non-human objects, pain or humiliation experienced by oneself or one's partner or children other non-consenting individuals'.

Paraphilia may interfere with the capacity for reciprocal affectionate sexual activity. It also involves sexual practices without necessarily implying dysfunction or deviance. Sexual feelings towards non-human sexual objects.

Predisposing factors:
* Parents who humiliate and punish the teenage boy for strutting around with an erect penis
* A young boy who is sexually abused
* Parental punishment–an individual who is dressed in a woman's clothes as a form of parental punishment
* Fear of sexual performance or intimacy
* Inadequate counselling
* Excessive alcohol intake
* Physiological problems
* Sociocultural factors
* Psychosexual trauma.

Causes

* Conditions represent a regression to or a fixation at an earlier level of psychosexual development resulting in a repetitive pattern of sexual behaviour that is not mature in its application and expression, i.e. individual repeats or reverts to a sexual habit arising early in life
* Expressions of hostility in which sexual fantasies or unusual sexual acts become a means of obtaining revenge for a childhood trauma
* Inability to erase the underlying trauma completely
* It is a process of conditioning, non-sexual objects can become sexually arousing if they are

frequently and repeatedly with a pleasurable sexual activity
* Poor self-esteem
* Difficulty in forming person-to-person sexual relationships
* Unstable relationships
* Loneliness or social isolation.

Categories Perversity

Perverse Acts

Which involve some other use of the genitals beyond the insertion of the penis into the vagina followed by ejaculation. For example, Masturbation, oral sex, stimulating clitoris for attaining female sexual satisfaction.

Perverse Objects

Getting enjoyment either by form fetisches and media objects. For example, by touching the under garments, shoes, gloves, nails, etc.

Forms of Paraphilia

I. Based on Severity

* Mild paraphilia is markedly distressed by the recurrent paraphilic urges, but has never acted on them
* Moderate paraphilia has occasionally acted on the paraphilic urge
* Severe paraphilia has repeatedly acted on the urge.

II. Based on Activity

* Optional paraphilia–alternative route to sexual arouses, e.g. wearing women's under garments
* Preferred paraphilia–a person prefers the conventional sexual activities, e.g. a man might prefer to wear women's under garments during sexual activity, or whenever possible
* Exclusive paraphilia–a person is unable to become sexually aroused in the absence of the paraphilia.

Common forms of Paraphilia

Exhibitionism

A recurrent or persistent tendency to expose the genitalia to the strangers or an unsuspecting person and gets excitement at the time of exposure and the act is commonly followed by masturbation. This tendency may be manifested mainly by male at the time of
- Emotional stress or crisis, e.g. shocked, frightened or impressed
- Conflicts in sexual relationships
- Women have more pleasure in displaying their body parts than male.

Pedophilia

Sexual arousal as a result of physical contact with prepubescent children. Men retain a preference of adult sex partners, but chronically frustrated in achieving right contracts, habitually turn to children as substitutes sexual activity often consists of looking and touching rather than intercourse.

Other Paraphilia

- Scatalogia–obscene phone calls.
- Zoophilia–involving in sexual activity or attaining sexual excitement through intercourse with animals.
- Loprophilia–feeling pleasure in handling faeces.
- Europhilia–urine.
- Emetophilia–sexual attraction to vomit.
- Sadomasochism–preference for sexual activity that involves bondage or the infliction of pain or humiliation. Sadomasochistic activity is the most important source of stimulation necessary for sexual gratification.
- Sexual masochism–receiving of humiliation or suffering or injury by others; the recurring urge or behaviour of wanting or infliction of pain or humiliation.

- Homosexuality–a desire to have sexual contact with the same sex.
- Adolescentilism–sexual pleasure from acting or dressing like an adolescent.
- Apodysophilia–desire to undress.
- Biastophilia–sexual pleasure from committing rape or being raped.
- Dacryphilia–sexual pleasure in eliciting tears from others or oneself.
- Faunoiphilia–sexual arousal from watching animals mate.
- Scoptophilia–sexual pleasure from watching others having sex.

Associated Problems with Paraphilia

Guilt, depression, shame, isolation and impairment in the capacity for normal social and sexual relationships.

Treatment

Once a diagnosis is established, appropriate education about possible behaviour therapies and use of psychopharmacological agents can improve the prognosis for these conditions
- Psychotherapy
- Utilization of behaviour modification techniques–desensitization procedure neutralizes the anxiety, provoking aspects of nonparaphilic sexual situations and behaviour by a process if gradual exposure
- Aversion imagery–involves pairing of a sexually arousing paraphilic stimulus with an unpleasant image
- Carrying relaxation exercises or therapy
- Orgasmic reconditioning–instruct a person to masturbate by using his paraphilia fantasy and to switch to a more appropriate fantasy just at the moment of orgasm
- Drug therapy, e.g. cyproterone acetate 50–200 mg/day, it inhibits testosterone directly at androgen receptor sites
- Serotonergies–Fluoxetine (serotonin derivatives) reduces anxiety and depression

- Open communication and mutual support can minimize or prevent disruptions or overcome barriers.

VOYEURISM (SCOPOPHILIA)

Voyeurism is a practice in which an individual derives 'sexual pleasure' from observing other people; who may be engaged in 'sexual acts' or 'nude' or in 'underwear' or dressed in whatever other way, the 'voyeur' find appealing. The word 'voir' is derived from French which means 'observer'. In DSM-IV, Voyeurism is classified as a 'Paraphilia' (with code 302.82) and described in ICD-10 $F_{65.3}$ and in ICD-9 302.82.

Characteristics

- Voyeur does not directly interact with the object of their voyeurism (often unaware that they are being observed), instead observing the act from a distance by peeping through an opening or using aids, e.g. Binoculars, mirrors, cameras. This stimuli sometimes becomes a part of a masturbation fantasy during or after the observation.
- The closer the voyeur is being discovered, the larger the thrill; this form of non-consensual voyeurism is considered as an invasion of 'privacy'.
- A recurrent or persistent tendency to look at people engaging in sexual or intimate behaviour or in naked which leads to sexual excitement.
- A subset of voyeurs derive sexual pleasure from looking under articles of clothing, an act known as, 'up skirt'.
- Some voyeur also derive pleasure by looking 'down shirts' and viewing 'breasts' particularly when women is bending over, commonly referred as, 'a down blouse'.

Treatment

- Behaviour therapy
- Psychoanalysis
- Drug therapy like antipsychotic medications.

Criminalization

- Some societies tolerate it depending upon circumstances, in some cultures, voyeurism is considered to be 'sexual deviant' and even a 'sex crime'. In UK nonconsensual voyeurism became a criminal offense on May 1st 2004 under 67 section of the Sexual Offences Act 2003; in Nov. 1st, 2005 under 162 section, the Canadian criminal code declared voyeurism as a sexual offense
- In USA, video voyeurism is crime in nine states
- Some institutions, gyms and schools have banned camera phones because of the privacy issues they raise in areas like change rooms.

FETISHISM

Sigmund Freud used the concept 'Fetishism' to describe a form of paraphilia, where the object of affection is an inanimate object or a specific part of a person.

Definition

'Fetishism is a fixation on an inanimate object or body part, i.e. not primarily sexual in nature and the compulsive need for its use inorder to obtain sexual gratification'. It is limited exclusively to males.

The object of a fetish is almost invariably used during masturbation and may also be incorporated into sexual activity with a partner in order to produce sexual excitation, non-living object usually intimately associated with the human body. Partialism refers to fetishes specifically involving non-sexual parts of the body.

Inanimate object fetishes are of 2 types

Form fetisches. For example, Undergarments (bras, panties) slips, stockings or panty hose, negligees, shoes, books, gloves and nails.

Media objects. For example, Leather, rubber, silk, fur.

In some cases drawings or photographs of the fetish object may arouse fetishists but more commonly the fetishist prefers or requires an object that has already been worn. The sexual acts of fetishists are characteristically depersonalized and objectified, even when they involve a partner. Sexual response may occur without the fetish, but usually at a diminished level; fetish objects enhance sexual excitements, poor developed social skills are quite isolated in their lives and have a diminished capacity for establishing intimacy.

Transvestic fetishism–sexual attraction towards the clothing of the opposite gender.

Causes

- Idiopathic: Early childhood experiences in which an object is associated with a particularly powerful form of sexual arousal or gratification.

Diagnosis

- If the fetish is the most important source of sexual stimulation or essential for satisfactory sexual response, then only fetishism is diagnosed.

Treatment

- Behaviour modification techniques
- Psychoanalysis.

SEXUAL PAIN DISORDERS/ DYSPAREUNIA

The term 'dyspareunia' is derived from Greek word, means 'badly mated'. It is quoted in ICD-10 N94.1 and ICD-9 625.0.

Definition

'A symptom, i.e. painful sexual intercourse or abnormal pain during coitus due to medical or psychological causes'.

It may be persistent or recurrent, occurs in both sexes; but the term will be used almost exclusively in women, as it is more common and considered to be primarily a physical, rather than an emotional, until proven otherwise.

Causes

In women

- Medical causes–infections, e.g. Candidiasis, Chlamydia, trichomoniasis, lower UTI, Herpes, Monilial, etc.
- Endometriosis, tumours, xerosis, rheumatoid arthritis, MI, CHD, DM
- Genital mutilation, PID, varicose veins in pelvis, Ectopic pregnancy
- Estrogen deficiency among post-menopausal women–due to less moisture in vaginal tissue and the low mucus secretions causes itching, dryness and painful discomfort during coitus
- Radiation therapy for pelvic malignancy due to the atrophy of vaginal walls and susceptibility for trauma.

In men

- Physical causes–infections of prostate, bladder or seminal vesicles can lead to intense burning or itching sensations following ejaculation
- Interstitial cystitis–may experiences intense pain at the moment of ejaculation
- Gonorrhoea infections–associated with burning or sharp pains during ejaculation
- Urethritis or prostatitis can make genital stimulation painful or uncomfortable
- Deformities of penis, e.g. peyronie's disease cause pain during coitus
- Too tight foreskin–painful retraction of foreskin
- During vigorous intercourse or masturbation, small tears may occur in the frenum of foreskin.

Psychological Causes

- Exposing to life stressors
- Dysfunctional Psychophysiologic reaction to sexual union, forcible coitus or incomplete sexual arousal
- Low self-esteem, inadequate use of coping techniques, cultural norms

- Psychiatric illness–depression, bipolar affective disorders, extramarital affairs, perceptual disturbances (psychotic conditions) schizophrenia, fear related to STD and AIDS
- Drugs–antihypertensive drugs may cause erectile difficulties, in turn dyspareunia.

Manifestations

- Burning, ripping, tearing, aching sensation associated with penetration
- When pain occurs, the women experiencing dyspareunia may be distracted from feeling pleasure and excitement
- Even after the original source of pain (e.g. Surgery) women may feel pain simply as she expects pain
- Anticipatory pain associated with a dry, tight vagina
- Three types of pain can be observed
  - Superficial dyspareunia occurs with attempted penetration usually secondary to anatomic or irritative conditions or vaginismus
  - Vaginal dyspareunia: pain related to friction including arousal disorders
  - Deep dyspareunia: pain related to thrusting often associated with pelvic disease or relaxation
- Bladder pain and discomfort during or after sex
- Painful spasms of pelvic floor muscles.

Diagnosis - According to DSM-IV (American Psychiatric Association)

- Client complaints of recurrent or persistent genital pain before, during or after sexual intercourse
- Vaginismus may occur secondary to a history of dyspareunia and even mild vaginismus is often accompanied by dyspareunia
- History of the client to identify stressor
- Careful examination of pelvis.

Treatment

- Identify and treat the underlying disorder or remove the stressor
- Usage of lubricants during intercourse, reduces discomfort, promotes ease, avoids friction
- Add pleasant, sexually natural lubrication, vaginal dilation, decreases friction and pain
- Positioning.

VAGINISMUS
Definition

'Involuntary painful spasms of the lower 1/3rd of vaginal muscles'.

Vaginismus occurs prior to sexual intercourse or interfering with coitus or sexual intercourse.

Incidence

Ten to Fifteen per cent of women are affected (1 out of every 10 women).

Classification

- Primary vaginismus–nothing has ever entered in vagina
- Secondary vaginismus–occurs after a particular event, an operation, serious illness, damage to the sexual organs or rape.

Causes

- Deep seated fear
- Concrete or other real experiences
- Traumatic experience (rape).

Manifestations

- Spasms includes not only the vaginal opening, but also the rest of the body, the legs close and the body does not allow anything to come near the genitalia
- Recurrent or persistent involuntary spasm of the vaginal muscles
- Marked distress

- Interpersonal difficulty
- It disturbs women's sexual freedom, enjoyment, disturbs coital functioning. In severe cases the women does not allow her partner to get near to her. Many times such women remain alone or it may lead to non-consummation of marriage.

Diagnosis

- Thorough history collection from the client
- Familiarization process–teaching about anatomical structure and its function; touching of vaginal muscles (contraction, relaxation, Kegel's exercises, vaginal floor muscle strengthening exercises)
- Gynaecological examination.

Treatment

- Vaginismus is a body-mind phenomenon, the symptom is expressed via the body (soma), its origin is in mind and body. An integrated approach is offered, inclusion of sufferer's partner in therapy is appropriate
- Cognitive behaviour therapy
- Psychosexual therapy
- Counselling.

GENDER IDENTITY DISORDER

Definition

'A condition in which a person assigned a gender on the basis of their sex at birth, but identifies as another gender and feels significant distress, discomfort or being unable to deal with their condition'.

Incidence

The feeling of transexualism, the person will have always been there since childhood; in some cases, it appears in adolescence or adulthood. It is a rare disorder.

Causes

- Idiopathic
- Prenatal hormonal imbalances
- Problems in the individual's family interactions or family dynamics or human bonding; defective child rearing practices
- Chromosomal abnormalities or genetic cause.

Manifestations

- Individual will have strong cross-gender identification
- Persistent uncomfortable with their biological sexual role and organs, may express a desire to alter their sexual organs
- Often attempts to pass socially as the opposite sex
- Transsexual alter their physical appearance cosmetically and hormonally and may eventually undergo a sex-change operation
- Refuses to dress and act in sex-stereotypical ways
- Significant interference in functioning because of their cross-gender identification
- Strongly believes that they will grow as an opposite sex
- Rejection by their peer groups
- Dressing and behaving typical of opposite sex (a girl wearing a boy's undergarment)
- May become severely depressed, anxious or socially withdrawn, isolated from social activities
- Distress, impairment in the functioning of an individual
- Disgust with their own genital (boys may pretend not to have a penis, girls may fear of growing breasts and menstruation).

Diagnostic Criteria

DSM-IV (302.85) has mentional criteria for the diagnosis of gender identity disorder can be given:

- A strong and persistent cross-gender identification
- Desire for any perceived cultural advantages of being the other sex
- Evidence of persistent discomfort about the one's assigned sex or sense of inappropriateness in the gender role of that sex
- Individual must not have a concurrent physical inter-sex condition, e.g. androgen insensitivity syndrome or congenital adrenal hyperplasia
- Evidence of clinically significant distress or impairment in social, occupational or other important areas of functioning
- A strong and lasting preference to play role playing games or stereotypical games as a member of the opposite sex or persistent fantasies that he or she is the opposite sex
- A strong preference for friends and playmates of the opposite sex
- Thorough history collection (sexual and social) the client and his family members will be interviewed in OPDs by psychologist or psychiatrist.

The current edition of the International Statistical Classification of diseases and Related Health Problems has different diagnoses for gender identity disorder: Transsexualism, Dual-role Transvestism, Gender identity disorder of childhood.

Transsexualism has the following criteria:
- The desire to live and be accepted as a member of the opposite sex, usually accompanied by the wish to make his/her body as congruent as possible with the preferred sex through surgery and hormone treatment
- The transsexual identity has been present persistently for at least 2 years
- The disorder is not a symptom of another mental disorder or a chromosomal abnormality.

Dual-role Transvestism has the following criteria:
- The individual wears clothes of the opposite sex in order to experience temporary membership in the opposite sex

- There is no sexual motivation for the crossdressing
- The individual has no desire for a permanent change to the opposite sex. Gender identity disorder of childhood has essentially 4 criteria:
  - The individual is persistently and intensely distressed about being a boy/girl, and desires to be of opposite sex
- The individual is preoccupied with the clothing, roles or anatomy of the opposite sex or rejects the clothing, roles, or anatomy of his/her birth sex
- The individual has not yet reached puberty
- The disorder must have been present for atleast 6 months.

Treatment

- Conversion therapies: To suppress their biological sex characteristics and acquire those of opposite sex, client must undergo extensive evaluation and transition period
  - Sex reassignment therapy/surgery
  - Hormone replacement therapy
- Treat secondary problems like depression, anxiety and to improve self-esteem, helping the individual to function as possible within his or her biological gender
- Psychosocial therapy
- Individual or family therapy
- Counselling and peer support.

Complications

- Poor self image
- Social isolation
- Emotional distress
- Depression and anxiety.

TRANSSEXUALISM (GENDER DYSPHORIA)

Gender and sex are separate entity, though the terms are often considered interchangeable by the less aware; sex is physical form and function while gender is a component of identity. Brain is structured in many sex-differentiated ways and the brain is the seat of identity. Transsexuals have always existed in the ancient world, it was both accepted and respected. Transsexuality occurs independently of sexual orientation and occurs in humans and in animals too. For example, apes, monkeys, etc. gender dysphoria, is the condition of being in a state of conflict between gender and physical sex. It is a condition in which a person identifies as the gender opposite to the sex assigned at birth. It is a syndrome with a physiological basis as a form of intersexuality.

Definition

'A transsexual is a person in which the sex related structures of the brain that define gender identity are exactly opposite, the physical sex organs of the body', i.e. 'a transsexual is a mind like literally, physically, trapped in a body of the opposite sex'.

'Transsexual is a person who believes that his or her body does not reflect his or her true 'inner gender''.

'The expression of desire to be of the opposite sex or assertion that one, is of the sex opposite from the one with which they were assigned at birth as sufficient for being transsexual'.   —*DSM*

'The desire to live and be accepted as a member of the opposite sex, usually accompanied by the wish to make his/her body as congruent as possible with the preferred sex through surgery and hormone treatment'.   —*ICD-10*

Incidence

- Occurs equally in both sexes.

Causes

- Critically timed hormonal release caused by stress in the womb of mother
- Presence of hormone mimicking chemicals present during critical development

- Alteration of the nervous system of developing foetuses.

Clinical Manifestation

- Transsexuals will be aware of their condition at preschool ages
- Depression
- Anxiety
- Change the physical body to match the mind
- If untreated it can lead to mental and emotional problem, self destruction and sometimes suicide.

Diagnosis

- Transsexuals present themselves for psychological treatment is 'gender identity disorder'. Transsexuality, homosexuality can occur in conjunction with each other, there is evidence that both are created by the similar mechanisms in utero.

Treatment

- Psychological treatment–sex reassignment therapy, a medical procedure will be carried out. It consists of
  - Hormone replacement therapy, to modify sex characteristics
  - Sex reassignment surgery, to later primary sex characteristics and permanent hair removal for trans women
- Transsexuals after therapy usually change their social gender roles, legal names and legal sex designation. The entire process of change from one gender presentation to another is known as 'transition'.

Prognosis

The conflict between gender identity and physical sex is almost always manifest from earliest awareness and is the cause of enormous suffering lead to self destruction unless treated. The absolute compulsion of classical transexualism is a matter of life and death, social oppression, cultural shame, self loathing of their condition. Almost all morbidity is attributed to the additional burden caused by the violent unacceptance of society, the rejection of family and friend, inability to find decent care. With treatment and support they are able to lead a successful life.

INTERSEXUALITY/DISORDERS OF SEX DEVELOPMENT

In most societies, intersexed individuals are expected to conform to either male or female gender role, whether or not they were socially tolerated or accepted by any particular culture. The terms Hermaphrodite and Pseudo-hermaphrodite or 'ambiguous genetalis' terms were used as synonyms, but now they are considered as problematic. A person with intersex, whose sex chromosomes, genitalia or secondary sex characteristics that are determined to be neither exclusively male or female.

Definition

'Conditions in which chromosomal sex is inconsistent with phenotypic sex or in which the phenotype is not classifiable as either male or female'.

Incidence

One per cent of live births exhibit some degree of sexual ambiguity.

Management

- Surgery on intersexed babies should wait until the child can make an infirmed decision
- Enhancements surgery–designed to create an advantage, e.g. breast enlargement surgery
- Restore functionality, e.g. treatment of a cleft palate.

PREMATURE EJACULATION/ RAPID EJACULATION

The word, 'premature ejaculation' derived from Latin term, 'ejaculatio praecox'. It is the most common sexual problem among men, (affecting 25-40%). Most men experience it atleast once in their life time, often adolescents and young men experience 'premature' ejaculation during their first sexual encounters, but eventually learns ejaculatory control. It involves a complex interaction of both psychological and biological factors.

Definition

'If man ejaculates sooner than his partner wish– such as before intercourse begins or shortly afterward'.

'Ejaculation before the completion of satisfactory sexual activity for both partners'.

Causes

- Genetic or inherited traits
- Biological factors: erectile dysfunction, abnormal hormone level, abnormal neurotransmitters levels, abnormal reflex activity of ejaculatory system, benign prostatic hypertrophy, Urethritis, inherited traits
- Neurological factors: trauma, nervous system damage, surgery
- Psychological factors: early sexual experiences may establish a pattern that can be difficult to change later in life, e.g. situations in which men may hurry to reach climax inorder to avoid being discovered, guilty feelings that will rush through sexual encounters
- Anxiety
- When lack of ejaculatory control interferes with sexual or emotional well being in one or both partners
- Narcotics drug abuse
- Temporary depression; marked distress
- Stress over financial matters, unrealistic expectations about performance, a history of sexual repression or overall lack of confidence
- Lack of interpersonal dynamics–lack of communication between partners, hurting feelings, unresolved conflicts which interferes with the ability to achieve emotional intimacy, interpersonal difficulties

- Premarital or extra-marital sexual relationships
- Prolonged noncoital stimulation to develop a degree of erection sufficient for intromission
- Cultural taboos.

Manifestations

- Persistent or recurrent ejaculation with minimal sexual stimulation before, on or shortly after penetration or before the person wishes it
- Concern or distress about his condition, as it may occur in all sexual situations during masturbation or it may only occur during sexual encounter with another person
- Perception of poor control over his ejaculation
- Interpersonal difficulties.

Screening and Diagnosis

- Detailed interview related to sexual history, from both partners is essential to identify the cause and suggest the best course of treatment collect health history and perform physical examination to exclude physical illness
- Enquire about frequency of premature ejaculation, sexual acts frequency, experience of premature ejaculation with partner or partners, quality of life they are leading, early, past, present sexual experiences
- History of drug abuse, interpersonal conflicts with this cause
- Consider age, novelty of sexual partner or situation, recent frequency of sexual activity in clinical enquiry.

Treatment

- Sexual therapy: Squeeze technique will be instructed for both couple
- Drug therapy: Tricyclic antidepressants based on cause ((Anafranil); topical anaesthetic creams (lidocaine or prilocaine); serotonin reuptake inhibitors (sertraline, paroxetine)
- Psychotherapy: counselling or talk therapy involves both couple, teaching them anatomical and physiological function of erectile function, factors contributing, coping-up techniques, relaxation techniques, open communication between couple and discussion about sexual function.

Complications

- Distress in personal life
- Strained relationship
- Fertility problems.

Sex Education

Sexuality is one of the most important aspects of life. Sexuality permeates the psychological and spiritual areas of a person's life. A decisive role in the formation of a family and if not understood properly can destroy families and the intimate relationship that should exist between members of family.

The great psychologist Sigmund Freud observed that until human beings learn to control their sexual instincts social life is impossible. Sexual relations are not only procreative but also recreative, they help to promote human fulfillment and satisfaction.

Differences in Sexuality

Men and Women exhibit–Physical sexual differences, emotional differences, intellectual differences and differences in sexual behaviour.

Physical Differences

- Prenatal
- At birth
- After puberty–physical changes
- At adolescence–boys/girls
- Growth/development
- Socialization
- Health and illness.

Emotional Differences

- Women are often considered to be bundles of emotions. Learn through observation, self reporting, measuring vital signs

- Anxiety and fear
- Menstrual cycle and emotions.

Components of Sex Education

- Physical aspects
  a. Anatomy and physiology of the repro-ductive organs, physical, emotional and psychological changes during puberty
  b. Conception, pregnancy and child birth
- Social aspects
  a. Sex drive or sexual feelings in childhood and adolescence
  b. Emotional development–teenage excite-ment and emotional stress (Teens 13–19)
  c. Personal identity (Self-esteem)
  d. Social relationship (with parents, siblings, peers members of either sex)
  e. Premarital sex
- Sex roles
- Gender roles
- STD/HIV.

Objectives of Sex Education

1. Sex education will focus on the total personality development of the individual
   It includes physical, social and psychological aspects of sex and sexuality. It will also create the power to make value judgment.
2. Factual, complete and honest information about sex and sexuality
   Sexual health education programme should aim at increasing awareness and insight regarding physical, social and psychological development. It will help clearing up myths and misinforma-tion that young people share among themselves. It will also prepare the adolescents to face the biological changes that would come about during puberty such as menstruation, seminal emissions, change of voice, enlargement of breasts, etc.
3. It enables young people to become responsible in making decisions, helping individuals to acquire and maintain responsible and caring

relationships and behaviour. Simultaneously it will prepare the children to recognize the beha-viour that is exploitative and self destructive.

4. Sexual health education will help the child to respect self and others
   Sexual health education will enable young boys and girls to become proud of their own sex while appreciating the attributes and capacities of the opposite sex.
5. Sexual health education will provide oppor-tunity to youngsters to imbibe human values, ethical, social and spiritual values which will serve as a guide to the individual in personal, family and social relationships.
6. Sexual health education should help the young boys and girls to understand that each part of the body and each phase of growth is good and has a purpose.
   This will give a holistic idea about human development and simultaneously. It will help the young people to nurture a feeling that sex is something beautiful, positive and is a creative part of life.
7. Sexual health education should help in the formation of an emotionally stable personality. By developing various skills, an individual will also become emotionally stable. Such an indivi-dual will be able to make rational decisions and will have judicious thinking. This is considered to be the ultimate outcome of sexual health education.

Content for Sex Education

Topics
PHYSICAL Reproductive systems of male and female, ovulation and menstruation, physical, emotional and psychological changes during puberty. The body clock, self awareness and self-esteem, conception, pregnancy and essential needs
SOCIAL ASPECTS Adolescents sexuality and behaviour, sexuality in childhood and adolescence, love, dating and relationship,

Contd...

adolescent pregnancy, moral code of ethics–their roles and functions

SEX ROLES
Role expectations, male and female roles, being masculine/feminine, stereotype

STDs
Sexually transmitted diseases

Sex Education to Adolescents

Sex education should be provided to all. However, our resources are limited. Priority is given to adolescents because:

- They have a maximum sex drive
- They form a high risk group
- They are eager to get information because of the physical and physiological changes
- Their common sources of misinformation are their friends, blue films and pornographic literature
- They are easily influence and therefore likely to go astray and land in problems of unmarried motherhood, abortions, STD/HIV infections, sexual abuse
- They are going to be the responsible citizens of tomorrow.

Adolescents gather information about sexuality from friends and through the print and electronic media. In India, talking about sex is taboo, educating children and adolescents about safe sex is one of the most effective way of postponing their onset of sexual activity and best investment to ensure people's future reproductive health and to prevent sexually transmitted diseases. There is rising rate of morbidity associated with sexual ignorance, poor decision making and inadequate sex education. The studies on the effects of sex education in schools show that sex and AIDS education often encourages young people to delay sexual activity and to practice safer sex, once they are active. Many women's organizations feel that the girls should not be ignorant about basic facts of life and become victims of sexual abuse, unwanted pregnancy and deception.

Aims of sex education to help children understand that each part of the body and each phase of growth is good and purposeful and helps in the following:

- To understand the process of reproduction
- To prepare children for the changes of developments which come with growing up
- To help young people see that sexual conduct involving other persons needs to be based upon a sincere regard for the welfare of the other
- To make children proud of their own sex and appreciate attributes and capacities of the other sex
- Responsible sex behaviour
- Build-up healthy attitudes to sex.

Sex education is

- *Information:* To provide accurate information about human sexuality, including growth and development, human reproduction, anatomy and physiology of genital organs, pregnancy, child birth, parenthood, contraception, abortion, sexual abuse, HIV/AIDS and sexually transmitted diseases (STD)
- *Attitude, values and insight:* Opportunity to question, explore and assess their sexual attitudes in order to develop their own values, increase self-esteem, develop insights concerning relationships with members of both gender, and understand their obligation and responsibilities to others
- *Relationships and interpersonal skills:* Help them to develop skills like communication, decision making, assertiveness, peer refusal skills and ability to create satisfactory relationships. Develop capacity for caring, supportive, non-coercive and mutually pleasurable intimate relationships
- *Responsibility:* To help young people exercise responsibility regarding sexual relationships, including abstinence; resist pressure to prematurely involve in sexual intercourse and encourage the use of contraception and other health measures.

Girls need to know about menstruation before it happens to them, and boys need to know about masturbation before they are experiencing the desire to masturbate. Boys experience nocturnal emissions from the age of about 14 years and girls attain menarche at the age of 11–13 years. Some boys and girls experience these events a year or two earlier. It is felt that the adolescent sex education should begin before these events take place. Ideally sex education for adolescents should be introduced from class VI (age 11 years) and continued through junior and senior colleges (age 20 years). The aim is to provide information and guidance before they become curious, face problems due to physical and psychological changes or become sexually active. Sex education should be offered as a part of overall comprehensive health education programme. It should include health promotion and disease prevention.

The sex education should be taught in a graded manner. The messages once introduced should be reinforced repeatedly at different levels. Age wise suitable curriculum should be available. Level–I: Std VI–X–age 11–15 years, to cover basics and essentials. Level–II: junior college and senior college age 16–20 years, to cover advanced studies and reinforcement of education. Give opportunity to discuss the concerned topics at length, avoid embarrassment while discussing the subject and overcome shyness and anxiety while listening and enable them to share doubts and views openly. Girls and boys have different problems. If the sex education programmes have to be made acceptable, girls and boys should be given sex education separately. The general topics of sexuality and health could be discussed in a male-female mixed group, while specific issues related to different sexes should be discussed separately in the respective groups.

The advantages of combined sessions are saving of time and repetition, fostering healthy interpersonal relationship between boys and girls, developing mutual respect and reducing inhibitions and anxiety about the subject in the presence of the opposite sex. Girls and boys feel more comfortable if the resource person is of the same sex as their's. Girls ask questions related to menstruation and gynaecological disorders. Boys ask questions related to virility, masturbation, wet dreams, size of penis and coitus. Teachers and students will feel more comfortable if they both are of the same gender. Therefore, it is preferable that the girls are given sex education by female teacher and boys by male teacher. There will be a necessity of having one male and one female educator in the school. These teachers should be trained by social workers, doctors, sexologists and psychologists.

Recommendations

- Sex education should be commensed before the onset of puberty.
- It should be provided in a graded manner and should be spread over a period of 8–10 years.
- It should be optional. This would help overall acceptance of the concept in the long run.
- Parent's permission should be obtained and their cooperation should be solicited.
- Sex education may be a part of the curricular or extracurricular activity.
- An evaluation of the programme should be done, feedback received, review and analysis done, and the programme should be modified from time to time.
- Teaching should have a social prospective.
- Answers have to be given truthfully.
- Use correct names for various organs.
- Parents/teachers should not be panic stricken or shocked if the child asks questions or indulges in sex play. Curiosity is normal. Such situation should be handled without rebuke, punishment or creating guilt feelings.
- Parents and teachers should inculcate a sound sense of values and ideals. They should help young people capture the vision that sex is not

a grimy secret between two ashamed individuals but divine impulse of life and love.

Teaching at School

Sex education in the school can be best extension of the sex education provided at home.
- Teaching should be scientifically correct
- It should be a two way dialogue
- The subject being emotionally charged, the language used and the manner of conducting the programme should be socially acceptable
- The group of students should be homogeneous in age and in cultural background
- If the teaching is round the year, 45 minutes to 1 hour session once in a week would be adequate. Half a day or full day workshop periodically 4 times a year would serve as an alternative
- Talks should be supported by audio-visual aids
- Group should not be over 50, otherwise two way communication is difficult to establish
- Should begin as a pilot project
  - At least one trained teacher
  - Support of administration
  - Support of parents and teachers. A talk should be arranged for them so as to give an idea of the contents of the programme. Prior permission of the parents of participating students would be obligatory
  - Informal experimental programme should be undertaken on a modest scale and carefully planned to avoid culture-based sensational and needlessly controversial topics.

Ethics of Sex Education

- No body contacts
- No slang language
- No vulgar jokes
- No use of naked photographs/pornography
- No late hours
- No individual training
- Non-judgemental
- No religious, cultural criticism
- No sharing of and asking for personal experiences
- No emotional involvement
- No advertisement or promotion of any commercial product
- Confidentiality about the communication on sexual and personal matters. Be honest and answer truthfully all the questions posed by children.

Planning Curriculum

Sex educators and teachers create their own curriculum for sex education. Some include anatomy and physiology of sex organs, physical, emotional changes at puberty, STD and AIDS, nutrition and hygiene and family planning; while some include family life issues such as relationship between family members, gender role, socialization and child development; few provide information about cultural and social aspects of human sexuality, sexual values, attitudes, beliefs, sexual activities and functioning. Very few include information on sexual behaviour. However, there can be a document containing guidelines on topics that may be presented to the adolescents in a developmentally appropriate manner and to suit their needs. Community attitudes, developmental differences in children, local socio-economic influence, parents' expectations, students' needs and expectations and religious and other perspectives should be paramount in designing the local sex education programme. Sex relationships are most sensitive of all human relationships. A programme will not be effective if there is no understanding of moral, ethical, aesthetic and religious sensibilities of the people for whom the curriculum is designed. Apart from accepting a few basic principles on which general agreement is reached, planners would be wise to adopt a flexible approach and avoid stereotypes. The programme will require modification from time to time depending upon the feedback, the need, the acceptance and the changing circumstances.

REVIEW QUESTIONS

1. Sexual Dysfunction. (5M, MGRU, 03).
2. Write in detail about Sexual Deviant Behaviour. (15M, GULB, 98).
3. Four types of Sexual Perversions. (2M, RGUHS, 00).
4. Trans Sexualism. (2M, RGUHS, 04, 05, Oct, 07).
5. What is Voyeurism. (2M, RGUHS, 04, 5M, RGHUS).
6. Gender Identity Disorder. (2M, MSc, RGUHS, 07).
7. Importance of Sex Education. (2M, MSc, RGUHS, 04).
8. Sexual Disorders. (5M, RGUHS, 04, 07).
9. Classification of sexual disorders. (5M, RGUHS, 00).
10. Paraphilias. (5M, RGUHS, 03).
11. Sex eduction. (2M, RGUHS, 07).

19

Substance Abuse

ALCOHOLISM

Alcoholism is not only detrimental to the health and welfare of the individual, family, community and society at large. The word 'alcoholism' was first coined by 'Magnus huss'. It was derived from Arabic word, 'alkuhl' means 'essence'.

Definitions

"The use of alcoholic beverages to the point of causing damage to the individual, society or both."
—*Alphonse Jacob*

"It is a chronic disease manifested by repeated drinking that produces injuring to the drinker's health or to his social or economic functioning."
—*S Nambi*

"Chronic dependence of alcohol characterized by excessive and compulsive drinking, that produces disturbance in mental or cognitive level of functioning, which interferes with social and economic functioning."

Properties of Alcohol

Alcohol is a clear liquid with a strong burning taste. Rapid absorption of the alcohol is more into the blood stream rather than its elimination. Slow absorption takes place when food is there in the stomach. Elimination of alcohol is through urine and by exhalation.

A concentration of:
- 80–100 mg of alcohol/100 ml blood is intoxication
- 200–250 mg of alcohol/100 ml of blood is loss of consciousness
- 500 mg of alcohol/100 ml of blood is fatal.

All the symptoms can change according to the tolerance.

Process of Alcoholism

Alcoholism is the excessive consumption of alcohol and become addicted to it. It starts with
- Experimental
  Due to peer pressure and curiosity individuals starts to consume alcohol.
- Recreational
  Gradually the frequency of alcohol consumption will increase during cultural meets as an enjoyment.
- Relaxational
  During weekends or on holidays individuals start enjoying and continue it. If consumed small

quantities may not cause problem. It may work out to release the tension, relaxes the mind and sedates the brain from painful emotions and promotes a sense of well-being and pleasure.

- Compulsive
  Once used to drinking, tendency to develop as compulsive and becomes as an addicts to overcome the discomfort of withdrawal symptoms.

Types of Drinkers

1. Moderate drinkers
   Moderately consuming alcohol and does not cause much problem.
2. Problem drinkers
   As a result of drinking the health will be impaired, affects peace of mind, family disrupted, loss of reputation and drinking will become as a routine.

Causes

- To forget miseries and problems of life
- Physical exhaustion
- Hard physical labour
- Certain occupations such as heavy vehicle drivers, labourers, manual workers
- Unhealthy environment
- Ignorance
- Sudden loss in property or close ones
- *New ethics*: Suddenly if a person become rich, consumes alcohol to show the status
- *Chronic stage*: Even for small amounts of alcohol a person will start begging, borrowing, stealing. Alcohol takes priority over family or job
- Common in cyclothymic personalities
- Disorders like depression, anxiety, phobia are prone to consume as an escape
- *Biochemical factors*: Role of dopamine and nor epinephrine affects neurotransmitter mechanism
- *Psychological factors*: E.g. injustice, inferiority, low self-esteem, poor impulse control. Poor

stress management skills, loneliness, desire to escape from reality, a sense of adventure, pleasure seeking etc.

- Sexual immaturity
- Social factors like over-crowding, influence of bad company, cinemas, literature, peer pressure, urbanization, religious reasons, unemployment, poor social support, fashion–a sign of modernity, social inadequacy, isolation.

Pathogenesis in Alcoholism

- Pre-alcoholic symptomatic phase
  In conventional social situations an individual starts drinking alcohol but soon experiences tension relief, gradually tolerance for tension decreases such as extent he resorts to alcohol almost daily.
- Prodromal phase
  Sudden onset blackouts, signs of intoxication, loss of memory or events.
- Crucial phase
  Loss of control over drinking, increased isolation, decrease in sexual drive, centering the behaviour around alcohol.
- Chronic phase
  Marked impairment in thinking process leading to alcoholic psychosis, delirium tremen occurs. Develops rationalization and amenable to treatment.
- Casual to habitual drinker
  Elliott and Merrill has described five stages through which a person has to pass till he becomes complete disorganization of personality.

1. *Morning drinking*: Person starts drinking of alcohol in the morning and he feels it is necessary to push him throughout the day.
2. *Escape drinking*: It starts, when a person is not able to face reality of problems without the help of alcohol.
3. *Increasing consumption*: Consumption of alcohol increase in amount leading to personal

disorganization and decreased social values and feels without alcohol he cannot survive.

4. *Drinking and social function*: Absolute necessity in social gatherings.

5. *Extreme behaviour*: Drinks excessively and behaves indiscriminately, e.g. fighting, abusing, throwing away things, beating wife and children, absurd and dangerous behaviour.

Clinical Features

- Blackout–amnesia of events
- Indigestion–anorexia
- Loss of self-control
- Outbursts of aggressive behaviour
- Sweating
- Unsteady gait, lusterless eyes and haggard look
- Malaise, tremors
- Weakness in feet and legs
- Pain in upper abdomen
- Insomnia.

Evil Effects of Alcoholism

Alcoholism is a social evil and as far as possible every individual should avoid it. Continuous consumption of alcohol adversely affects the brain and its efficiency. Alcoholism is a main cause of family unhappiness, tensions and total disorganization. Individual will waste lot of money on alcohol and economic life of family also suffers. Poverty, quarrels, violence and abusive behaviour develop. Children may become delinquents; alcoholic may commit crimes, anti-social activities. It may also associate with gambling, prostitution and at least one-forth of the income are wasted on alcoholism.

Complications of Alcohol Dependence

A. Medical

a. Gastro-intestinal Tract

- Gastritis
- Dyspepsia
- Vomiting
- Peptic ulcer
- Cancer
- Reflex esophagitis
- Carcinoma of stomach and oesophagus, larynx, liver, colon
- Fatty degeneration of the liver, interferes with absorption of vitamin B-complex
- Cirrhosis of liver
- Hepatitis, Jaundice
- Liver cell carcinoma
- Acute and chronic pancreatitis
- Malabsorption syndrome.

b. Cardiovascular System

- Cardiomyopathy
- Hypertension
- Heart failure or stroke
- High risk for myocardial infarction.

c. Blood

- Folic acid deficiency anaemia
- Decreased WBC production causes infections.

d. Nervous System

- Confusion, numbness of hands, feet, disordered thinking
- Depression, depresses vital centres of the brain
- Peripheral Neuropathy, Dementia
- Epilepsy
- Head injury
- Cerebellar degeneration
- Wernick's encephalopathy, coma.

e. Hormonal

- Hypoglycemia.

f. Muscle

- Peripheral muscle weakness
- Wasting of muscles.

g. Bones

- Interferes with the production of bone
- Thinning of bones, osteoporosis
- Fractures.

h. Skin

- Spider angioma
- Acne.

i. Reproductive System

- Sexual dysfunction in male
- Failure of ovulation in female
- Interruption in menstruation.

j. Nutritional Deficiency Diseases

- PEM
- B complex deficiency–Pellagra, Beriberi.

k. Pregnancy

- Fetal abnormalities
- Developmental disabilities - Mental retardation, Growth retardation
- Low birth weight
- Still births
- Birth defects
- Foetal alcohol syndrome.

l. Social Complications

Domestic abuse, divorce, poor performance in school and at work, prone for motor vehicle accidents, susceptible for accidental injuries, violence acts, e.g. murder, reduced productivity.

Acute Intoxication

During or shortly after alcohol ingestion characterized by maladaptive behaviour. For example, aggressive behaviour, inappropriate sexual behaviour, mood lability, poor judgement, slurred speech, unsteady gait, and nystagmus.

WITHDRAWAL SYNDROME

Any rapid decrease in the amount of alcohol content in the blood will produce withdrawal symptoms.

1. Simple Withdrawal Syndrome

- Mild tremors
- Nausea and vomiting
- Weakness
- Irritability
- Insomnia
- Anxiety
- Tachycardia
- Hypertension
- Impaired attention.

2. Delirium Tremens

The term derived from Latin means 'trembling madness'. It occurs within 2–4 days of complete or significant abstinence from heavy alcohol drinking.

Definition

'A severe form of withdrawal that involves sudden and severe mental or neurological changes'.

Causes

- After a period of heavy alcohol drinking, especially when the person does not eat enough food
- Head injury
- Infection or illness
- Habitual excessive consumption of major tranquilizers, e.g. Benzodiazepines or Barbiturates.

Manifestations

- *Mental status changes*: Mood changes, confusion, disorientation in time and place, psychomotor agitation, restlessness, excitement, decreased attention span, irritability, disorderly behaviour, clouding of consciousness, altered sensorium,

- Hallucination–visual is common
- Shouting
- Fear
- Severe uncontrollable tremors of the extremities, secondary to anxiety, panic attacks, paranoia
- Truncal ataxia
- Autonomic disturbances like sweating, fever, tachycardia, dilated pupils, hypertension
- Insomnia
- Fear
- Fever, in some cases individuals experiences convulsions
- Dehydration
- Leucocytosis
- Impaired liver function
- Autonomic hyperactivity
- Adrenergic storm–tachycardia, hypertension, hyperthermia, hyper reflexia, diaphoresis, cardiac arrhythmia, stroke, anxiety, panic attacks, paranoia, agitation
- Symptoms of alcohol withdrawal.

3. Delirium

Diagnosis

It is a medical emergency.

Based on symptoms, the investigations like ECG, EEG.

Toxicology screening has to be carried out.

Treatment

Aims

To save life
- To relieve from symptoms
- To prevent complications
- Hospitalization may be required
- Check and record the vital signs
- Maintain fluid and electrolyte imbalances
- Control environmental stimuli
- Correct symptomatology by administrating appropriate medications as per prescription, supportive treatment

- Counselling
- Aid from supporting groups, e.g. self help groups like Alcoholic Anonymous.

4. Alcoholic Seizures

Tonic-clonic seizures occur 12–48 hours after a heavy bout of drinking; status epilepticus may result.

5. Alcoholic Hallucinations

Auditory hallucinations during abstinence.

6. Alcoholic Psychosis

- Behavioural problems
- Thought disturbances
- Delusion
- Hallucination
- Impairment of mental functions
- Morbid jealousy.

Depression: Suicide and attempt to suicide are more common.

Criminality: Reduces inhibition and increases hostile behaviour, violence and anti-social behaviour.

7. Korsakoff's Syndrome

Korsakoff's psychosis, amnesic-confabulators syndrome is a degenerative brain disorders caused by thiamine deficiency in brain. The syndrome is named after Sergei korsakoff, Neuropsychiatrist, who popularized the theory.

Causes

Conditions resulting in the vitamin deficiency and its effects includes.
- Alcohol abuse (neurotoxic effects of alcohol)
- Severe malnutrition
- Hyperemesis gravidarum results in inflammation of stomach lining results into thiamine deficiency
- Eating disorders

- Effects of chemotherapy
- Mercury poisoning
- Patients undergoing dialysis
- Post-operative cases, who are given vitamin free fluids for a prolonged period of time.
  The affected parts of the brain are: Diencephelon-mamillary bodies and the thalamus.

Symptoms

- Anterograde and retrograde amnesia or severe memory loss; the main area of memory affected is the ability to learn new information. Usually the intelligence and memory for past events is relatively unaffected, so that an individual may remember what occurred 20 years ago, but is unable to remember what happened 20 minutes before. This memory defect is referred to as 'anterograde amnesia'.
- Confabulation, invented memories which has to be taken as true due to gaps in memory with fabricated or imagined information, sometimes associated with blackouts meager content in conversation.
- Lack of insight and apathy (the client looses interest in things quickly and generally appear indifferent to change).
- Neuronal loss.
- Gliosis-result of damage to supporting cells of CNS.
- Haemorrhage in mamillary bodies.
- Damage to the dorsomedial nucleus of the thalamus.
- Ataxia.
- Tremors.
- Paralysis of eye muscles.
- Coma.

Diagnosis

- Whenever someone have a possible diagnosis of alcoholism, sudden onset of memory difficulties, it is important to seriously consider the diagnosis of Korsakoff's syndrome

- A careful exam of the individual's mental state
- Checking the patient's retention of factual information along with the patient's ability to learn new information
- Physical examination.

Treatment

- Immediate administration of thiamine (I.V or I.M)
- Vitamin supplementation
- Providing proper nutrition and hydration
- Drug therapy to alleviate symptoms
- Supervised living situation may be needed.

Prevention

- Treating the underlying alcohol addiction
- Adequate vitamin supplementation along with balanced diet.

TREATMENT OF ALCOHOLISM

Through Assessment

A thorough assessment includes:
- An appraisal of current medical, psychological and social problems
- History taking: drinking pattern, work spot, family pattern, environmental conditions
- Diagnose the extent of habit formation and effects of alcohol over the body
- Formulate nursing diagnosis.

Goal Setting

Short term goals related to:
- Health
- Marital relationship
- Efficiency in job performance
- Social adjustment
- Healthy family pattern.

Long term goals: such as changing the factors that precipitate or maintain excessive drinking.

Therapeutic Modalities

Psychotherapy

1. *Motivational interviewing*
   - Explaining the complications and personal risks of consuming the alcohol
   - Availability of treatment options to change their behaviour related to alcohol consumption.

2. *Individual psychotherapy*
   Educate each affected individual the detrimental effects of alcohol consumptions and the coping strategies to overcome the habit; precautionary measures, diversional activities to prevent these occurrence of complications with alcohol consumption.

3. *Group therapy*
   Observe the problems of alcoholic, provide an opportunity to observe others problems and discuss with each other and explain them to workout in better ways of coping with these problems.

4. *Counselling*
   The therapist has to counsel the client to find out the problem and shows the ways to solve the same. And also guides the individual the various methods to relax the mind and engaging themselves in productive activities.

5. *Aversive conditioning*
   It is based on the principle of classical conditioning. The therapist has to explain the behaviour patterns which are pleasurable, pros and cons of alcoholism, maladaptive behaviour, show the clients who are with the complications of alcoholism, and their family problems. The client is exposed to adverse effects of excessive alcohol consumption like chemical induced vomiting, shock, etc. thereby develops aversion towards the evil habits.

6. *Cognitive therapy*
   Help the client to identify the maladaptive thinking patterns; evil effects of alcoholism and guide the individual to slowly reduce the dose of alcohol intake and by understanding the evil effects of alcohol.

7. *Relapse prevention technique*
   It helps the client to
   - Identify high-risk relapse factors and develop strategies to deal with them
   - Learn the methods to cope up with cognitive distortions.

8. *Cue Exposure Technique*
   Repeated exposures to desensitize the clients to the effects of alcohol and thus improve their ability to remain abstinent.

9. *Supportive Psychotherapy*
   Symptomatic treatment along with educating the individual about preventive measures against complications.

10. *Behaviour Modification Techniques*
    Systematic desensitization, relaxation techniques, operant-conditioning techniques can be used.

11. *Family Therapy*
    If the head of the family develops alcoholism the total members of the family will be affected with economic crisis, maladjustment, children are prone to develop this bad habit thus family disorganization occurs hence it is necessary and responsibility of health personnel to educate the social evil effects of alcoholism, care of the clients and preventive measures to adopt.

Treatment of the Client with Withdrawal Effects

a. *Detoxification*

It is the process by which an alcohol dependent person recovers from the intoxication effects in a supervised manner.

Benzodiazepines–Chlordiazep oxide 80–200 mg/day.

Diazepam 40–80 mg/day to control anxiety, insomnia, agitation and tremors.

Thiamine 100 mg intramuscular for 3–5 days followed by vitamin-B administration 100 mg OD for atleast 6 months.

If necessary anti-convulsants, close observation for 5 days, maintenance of intake and output chart. Strict monitoring of vital signs, observation of level of consciousness and orientation, assess fluid and electrolyte balance, if necessary administer I.V fluids. High protein diet (if the liver is not damaged) provision of calm and safe environment.

b. *Alcohol Deterrent Therapy*

Deterrent agents like disulfiram are given to desensitize the individual from alcohol effects and to maintain abstinence.

Deaddiction Centres

To generate awareness of the evils of addiction is absolutely essential for creating alcoholic and drug free society. The information has to be provided in simple, local language and in an interesting manner. Awareness Programmes has to be organized in the form of street plays, awareness lectures, film shows, etc. in slum area, at various other community platforms, e.g. low income families situated places, drug/alcohol addiction prone areas, educational institutes, industrial areas, etc. to bring a total change in attitudes and to bring meaningful recovery among addicts, to improve personality pattern and coping pattern of individuals, a multi dimensional approach will be adopted. In awareness campaigns the common emotional and behavioural issues, stress management, value of good health and its maintenance, vocational guidance, evil effects of alcoholism and drug addiction over the individual, family and society. Motivates the target groups to spread message to others in the community to use in their day-to-day lives.

Activities

- Deaddiction activities will be organized for target and focus groups within the community, e.g. day care centres, half way homes.

- Narcotic Anonymous and Alcoholic Anonymous meetings are conducted regularly.
- *Major activities in deaddiction centres are*: OPD services, Inpatient services, occupational therapy, Community Outreach Programmes, Group Therapies for alcoholics and narcotics, Self help groups, Drug monitoring, Psycho therapeutic activities, Disulfiram Clinics, Community Awareness Programmes, Community Drug Deaddiction Development Pro-gramme and recreational activities.
- *Special activities are*: Demand Reduction and or harm minimization, Community group meetings for families of alcoholics and substance abusers.
- The patient's validated history is collected from numerous resources, clinical observation of the client, numerous psychological tests of the client will be conducted.
- Patients are encouraged to cultivate interests and regain physical and mental health. Facilities like a well equipped gymnasium, a well stocked library with books in different languages, musical instruments, art material, play equipment to play different indoor and outdoor games, etc. are provided. Patients are encouraged to contribute in an in-house monthly magazine. Yoga and Meditation is taught to all patients. Every effort is made to fill up the vacuum which is left after leaving addiction. Thus the patient is guided towards a new way of living and thinking.
- The patients will be guided towards a new way of living and thinking, to regain self-esteem and confidence.
- The patient is taught vocational skills and helped in being assimilated into society.
- Helps the clients to take their own decisions.
- Motivates them to spread the message to others in the community.

NURSING MANAGEMENT OF THE CLIENT WITH ALCOHOLISM

1. Nursing Assessment

History

Collect brief history of the client

- Developmental aspects–milestones pattern, educational status, scholastic environment and any problems associated with it
- Employment history and details about stressors in working environment, work load
- *Marital history*: Marital life pattern, any history of conflicts between life partners/couple, deprivation, disparities
- *Sexual history*: Satisfactory pattern/dissatisfactory life/difficulties in sexual life
- Transitional periods in life–any life events influencing alcoholism or drug abuse
- Any positive family history–history of alcoholics or drug addicts among parents and relatives
- *Social history*: Social environment-peer group influence, influence of western culture, social gathering, broken family, deprivation of love, school environment, life style pattern
- Psychological factors, e.g. feeling of aloofness, isolation, exposed to extreme stress in life, e.g. death of loved one; separation/divorce, failure in life
- *Forensic history*: Previous court cases, any imprisonment, or pending court case.

Physical Examination

- *Inspection or observation*: General appearance, behaviour pattern, evidence of malnutrition manifestations, tremors, etc.
- *Percussion*: Tenderness-epigastric region
- *Palpation*: Hepatomegaly, splenomegaly, cardiomegaly
- *Auscultation*: Look for cardiac murmurs, respiratory sounds.

Mental Status Examination

- General appearance and behaviour
- Psychomotor activity
- Thought, content, mood, perception
- *Cognitive function:* orientation, memory, intelligence, abstractibility, judgement insight
- General information.

Mini Mental Status Examination

- Orientation, registration, attention, concentration, recall, language perception.

Psychosocial Assessment

- *Family*: Environment, interaction and relationship, pattern, bondage, healthy/unhealthy living pattern
- *Work environment*: Regularity in job, performance, responsibilities, workload, change of job relationship with superior and colleagues
- Social environment- peer group, social relationship, social functions, accidents, friends and relatives influence
- *Crime:* History of committing criminal acts and violence
- Religion, caste, cultural functions, social gatherings, motivating or stimulating factors.

Lab Investigations

Drug Analytical Testing

- Chromatographic tests
- Competitive binding/immuno-reactive tests.

1. Nursing Diagnosis

Alteration in sleep pattern.

Goal

Enhances adequate sleeping pattern.

Interventions

- Provide a calm and quiet environment

- Advice the family members to stay along with the client to promote comfort and security
- Never leave the client alone
- Observe the sleeping pattern
- Ask the client to cultivate the habit of taking bath before going to bed
- Give a glass of warm milk at hour of sleep and back care before going to bed
- Provide dim light, soft music, if the client is having the habit of reading books, allow him to do so
- Administer the medications as per doctors prescription.

2. Nursing Diagnosis

Potential for self injury and injury to others related to alcohol withdrawal, seizures and confusion.

Goal

Protect the client from self injury and others.

Intervention

- Provide safe environment, if the client exhibits violent or withdrawal behaviour
- Administer medications as per prescription
- Assist for self care activities and ambulation
- Observe and document, if the client is having seizures
- Provide care for the client during and after seizures
- Observe the gait and assist, if the client needs help
- Assess the emotions of the client, e.g.: depression, violence; counsel the client, utilize behavior modification techniques, cognitive, assertiveness techniques.

3. Nursing Diagnosis

Alteration in physical health.

Goal

Promotes and maintains good physical health.

Interventions

- Observe and record vital signs, physical complaints
- Provide symptomatic care and needed assistance
- Provide care to the client during and after seizures, if any
- If the client is too calm during withdrawal period, observe or check for any possession of alcohol.

4. Nursing Diagnosis

Negligence in meeting physical needs related to depression, insecurity.

Goal

Calm-up the mind and maintain good personal hygiene.

Interventions

- Promote a sense of well-being to the client
- Motivate the client to be self sufficient and independent
- Make the client to understand about the importance of maintenance of good personal hygiene
- Insist on hygienic habits and maintaining it
- Assist the client for self care activities, if the client is in depressive mood.

5. Nursing Diagnosis

Addiction to alcohol, knowledge deficit related to adverse effects of alcoholism.

Goal

Make the client to adopt the normal life without alcohol, slowly and gain knowledge over the adverse effects of alcoholism.

Intervention

- Educate the client on adverse effects of alcoholism; show the case, who are suffering with complications of alcoholism, how their families are affected due to this problem

- Counsel the client to utilize behaviour modification techniques to get aversion towards alcoholism
- Motivate the client to have change in life style, social group gathering pattern.

6. Nursing Diagnosis

Altered sensory perception related to disturbances like hallucinations, altered consciousness, fear, psychomotor retardation.

Goal

Reduction in fear, anxiety, hallucination, depression.

Intervention

- Maintains good emotional status and improved sensory perception pattern
- Assess the level of consciousness and behavioural responses
- Accept the clients emotions pattern and altered levels
- Note onset and pattern of hallucination and document it
- Provide emotional/moral support; counsel the client, explore the stressors and teach the strategies to overcome the problems
- Provide calm and quiet environment
- Encourage family members to provide emotional support to the client at the need of hour
- Be nonjudgemental; observe the clients' behaviour
- Motivate the client to talk about his feelings openly without any inhibitions
- Never leave the client alone, always motivate someone who is close to him
- Provide stress free environment
- Protect the client from self-injury

- Explain to the relatives, not to show their emotional disturbances to the client; not to discuss about the client, on bedside.

7. Nursing Diagnosis

Impaired socialization due to alcoholism

Goal

Enhances socialization, slowly withdraws from alcohol.

Intervention

- Provide social support, let the client enjoy socialization without the use of alcoholism
- Promote self concept, socialization
- Help the client to try out with new social group to adjust and accommodate
- Assist the family members to develop confidence over the client
- Motivate the client to live happy and comfortable life and to regain insight into life and to have hope and pleasure without alcohol
- Mobilize the client to engage his mind in interested activities like spiritual activities, reading books, playing games
- Motivate the client to lead tension free life.

8. Nursing Diagnosis

Prone for altered respiratory function due to confusion, restlessness and withdrawal.

Goal

Maintains effective breathing pattern.

Interventions

- Monitor and record vital sings
- Elevate the head end of the bed
- Demonstrate deep breathing and cool down exercises

- Review the investigations, if needed like blood gas analysis can be done
- If needed, administration of oxygen may be required.

Nursing Diagnosis

Potential for decreased cardiac output.

Goal

Maintains normal cardiac output and homeostasis.

Intervention

- Inform the client to follow the instructions
- Monitor and record vital signs, breath sounds, heart sounds
- Maintain intake and output chart
- If necessary, provide CPR
- Assess blood electrolyte levels and administer medications as per prescriptions
- Change of positions, deep breathing exercises are taught to the client
- Insist for follow-up and continuity of care.

DRUG ABUSE/DRUG ADDITION

Substances have deleterious effects over the individual. Substance abuse includes alcoholism and drug abuse. People will opt substance abuse for varied reasons like tensions release, solvation of problems, to fulfill their needs like to overcome anxiety, pressure or fatigue, experimental use, recreational use or circumstantial phase. No single factor can be identified as a cause for drug addition.

Progressive changes in a drug addict are:

Drug Use

People will use drugs to relieve physical and psychological problems and for mood alteration effects.

Tolerance

When a person uses drug for first time, even for a small dose, drug is very effective, whereas on repeated use increasing doses are required as the individual lost his sensitivity to a particular drug.

Drug Dependence

Person may be dependent upon one or more drugs. Craving for the drug becomes more and more. To experience drugs psychic effect and to avoid discomfort, compulsion to take the drug on a continuous or intermittent basis.

Definition

'It is a maladjustive pattern of substances use leading to significant impairment or distress'.

—S Nambi

'Pathological or indiscrimination use of drugs, which impairs social and occupational functioning of an individual by minimal duration (atleast one month)'.

'Drug dependence is a detrimental factor for individual and society, due to tolerance, compulsion to take the drug in increase doses'.

Habituation

It results from the repeated consumption of the drug, a desire to continue taking the drug for the sense of improved well being; it will have some degree of psychic dependence on the drug effect, but absence of physical dependence. It will have detrimental effect over the individual.

Drug Abuse

Taking a drug for other than medical reasons, and increased frequency, dose or manner that damages the physical or mental functioning.

Drug Addiction

The risk of addiction is more in mentally ill persons than physically ill. It is 'a state of periodic or chronic intoxication produced by the repeated consumption of a drug'.

Characteristics

- An overpowering desire or need (compulsion) to continue taking the drug and to obtain it by any means
- A tendency to increase the dose
- A psychic and physical dependence on the effects of the drug
- A detrimental effect both on the individual and on the society.   *—WHO 1957*

Withdrawal Syndrome

If drug use is suddenly stopped, client will develop a group of clinical manifestations.

Incidence of Drug Abuse

It is commonly seen in the age group of 16–30 years; unmarried people and the individuals belonging to low socio-economic strata.

Causes for Drug Addiction

Social Environment

- To gain acceptance in a group to belong
- Peer group pressure or influence of bad company
- Too much pocket money/loose availability of money
- Escape from social, economic pressures
- Defiant gesture against authority
- Broken families, unhappy home conditions
- Lack of parental control
- Homelessness
- Industrialization
- Unemployment
- Low socio-economic conditions
- To get relief from strenuous activities
- Relaxed legal systems
- Social prestige
- Social pressures, insisting on consumption of drugs to achieve status
- Low religiosity

- Social deprivation
- Problems within the family
- Lack of recreational facilities
- Easy availability of drugs.

Iatrogenic (Doctor Induced)

Medical officers in their practice prescribing over dosage, high frequency of drugs.

Individuals with Vulnerable Personality

- Emotional immaturity
- Sensation seeking
- Impulsivity
- Emotional frustrations
- To overcome depression, anxiety
- Psychopath personality
- Suffering with psychiatric disorders like anxiety, neurosis, schizophrenia
- Low frustration tolerance
- Inability to cope-up with tension or difficult situations
- Low self-esteem
- Excessive freedom
- Anti-social personality traits
- Psychological traumatic experiences during early childhood
- Feeling boredom, loneliness
- To express hostility
- Reaction to neglect
- To get thrill or pleasure seek
- Escape from problematic situations
- Deep psychological need
- For curiosity purpose.

Clinical Manifestations

Emotional Manifestations

- Euphoria (A sense of well-being)
- Deterioration in moral and ethical sense
- Moodiness
- Dull
- Physiological depression
- Irritability

- Purposefully avoids interaction and communication with family members
- Withdrawal from family activities
- Lethargy
- Lack of motivation, curiosity, enthusiasm, energy and vitality
- Stealing money and valuable items
- Erratic behaviour, confused thoughts.

Physical Symptoms

- Reddening of eyes
- Glazed dull eyes
- Pin-point pupils
- Puffiness under the eyes
- Slurring of speech
- Ataxic gait
- Anorexia
- Weight loss
- Presence of pricks and injection marks all over the body
- Sleep disturbances.

Long term Effects of Drug Usage

Tolerance

User needs more and more of the drug to experience the same effect.

Psychological dependence

Drug becomes central to the user's thoughts, emotions and activities.

Physical dependence

The body functions normally only if the drug is present and if it stopped suddenly withdrawal symptoms will appear.

Social cost

Alienation from family, friends, user becomes withdrawn and uncommunicative with the societal members.

Personal cost

User needs money to support the habit and is caught in a vicious circle, goes to any length to procure money by borrowing, stealing and lying.

Physical Cost

- Loss of weight
- Loss of physical stamina
- Unkempt appearance.

Diagnosis of Drug Misuse

In early stages, we have to diagnose drug use by the following

a. Physical Signs

Needle tracks, vein thrombosis especially in the anti-cubital fossa, wearing garments with long sleeves in hot weather also, scars.

b. Behavioural Manifestations

- Absence from school or work
- Occupational decline
- Neglect in personal appearance
- Loneliness
- Minor criminal offenses.

c. Medical Presentation

Drug addicts will declare different types like
- Some may present that they are dependent on drugs
- Some may conceal their dependency and ask for drugs to control or for relief of pain, e.g. renal colic or dysmenorrhoea
- Some may present with drug related complications like cellulites, pneumonia, serum hepatitis, accidents.

Laboratory Tests

- Raised gamma-glutamine transpeptidase
- Raised mean corpuscular volume
- Urine test for drug concentration.

Management

- Hospitalization
- Create realistic goals with the client, incorporate positive attitude

- Detoxification
- Supplementation of vitamins, minerals
- Supportive psychotherapy
- Counselling
- Family therapy
- Rehabilitation facilitated through daycare centres.

Rehabilitation

- To enable the drug dependents to leave the drug sub-culture
- To develop new social contracts
- Provide social support when the person makes the transition to normal work and living
- Inculcate responsibility in protecting themselves Facilities for rehabilitating drug abusers by Government and other voluntary organizations.

Counselling Centre

- Clients are screened for residential treatment and motivating them for withdrawal of drugs
- Extended care after discharge
- Family therapy
- Supportive psychotherapy.

Deaddiction Centre

- Keep all lives of communication open
- Medical care–detoxification, primary care
- Educational measures for healthful living, discipline and value of time
- Speak to addicts' friends, teachers, family members in supportive measures.

After-care Centre

Plan for long term therapeutic community programme (6–9 months) depending upon individual's progress. It consists of structured environment to encourage the members to develop positive peer pressure and to establish healthy relationships, sound values and a productive life style in drug free environment.

Day-care Centres for Women

Provides support to women narcotics and alcoholics who has completed detoxification treatment. In day-care centres, one-year course is offered in which *yoga, sadhana*, meditation, work therapy, individual and group sessions, etc. activities will be performed.

Out-reach Services

Family Therapy

- Conducting family association meetings
- Domicilliary visits
- Joint sessions with addicts and family members for holistic approach and therapeutic modalities
- Awareness campaigns in form of seminars, workshops, exhibition, etc. will be organized to improve the knowledge of public about drug addition.

Relapse in Drug Addiction

In few cases, drug addicts will resume their habit within six months. It is due to poor follow-up and rehabilitative services, easily availability of drugs, persistent pressure from peer group.

PREVENTIVE MEASURES IN DRUG ADDICTION

Primary Prevention

- Provide healthy and happy family environment
- Loving, tender-care, establish healthy child-parent relationship
- Give mutual respect for the child
- Taking timeout for fun
- Openly talk to the child and communicate love
- Show interest in child's activities
- Share problems of child, talk to the child and teach how to solve the problems and handle the situations
- Counselling, inform career options and motivate the child to set goals in life

- Parents should not be sarcastic, accusatory or blaming of the child for his behaviour
- Avoid influencing factors like companion which promotes the child for bad habits
- Promote mass-media activities and prepare IEC modules, organize awareness campaigns to improve the knowledge of public, special attention to focus group about the dangers associated with drug abuse and coping strategies to overcome stressors
- Insist in general meetings, celebrations at college level that students should not misuse the available freedom.

Related to Drugs

- Limit the availability of drugs
- Legislation measures to be formulated to control the production, supply, sale, possession and export of drugs
- Physicians should be careful, not to prescribe drugs of powerful action and if needed they have to advice to take drugs on prescription
- Drug should be made available for genuine use and safeguard to prevent illicit use.

Secondary Prevention

- Observe closely change in the behaviour of the individual and avail medical assistance as early as possible
- Establish deaddiction centres, after-care centres, day-care centres which will assist the individual and their family members in over-coming the problem of drug addition
- Early identification of the drug abusers
- Treat promptly by specified therapies to prevent the complications of disease.

Tertiary Prevention

- Includes the treatment in the state of severe dependence
- Identify the social agencies which will assist in rehabilitative activities

- Rehabilitation measures has to be planned based on severity of the problem
- Family has to be involved in the restorative and rehabilitative activities.

NURSING MANAGEMENT OF THE CLIENT WITH DRUG ABUSE

Nursing Assessment

Collect Brief History of the Client

- Developmental aspects–milestones pattern, educational status, scholastic environment and any problems in it
- Employment history and details about stressors in working environment, workload
- *Marital history*: Marital life pattern, any history of conflicts between life partners/couple, deprivation, disparities
- *Sexual history*: Satisfactory pattern/dissatisfactory life/difficulties in sexual life
- Transitional periods in life–any life events influencing alcoholism or drug abuse
- Any positive family history–history of alcoholics or drug addicts among parents and relatives
- *Social history*: Social environment-peer group influence, influence of western culture, social gathering, broken family, deprivation of love, school environment, life style pattern
- Psychological factors, e.g. feeling of aloofness, isolation, exposed to extreme stress in life, e.g. death of loved one; separation/divorce, failure in life
- *Drug history*: Nature of drug consuming, age of first drug use, age for regular drug use, age of dependent drug use, route of consuming drug, abstinence period, Ist injecting episode, site of injection, source and use of sterile equipment, HIV risky behaviour, any treatment history
- *Forensic history*: Previous court cases, any imprisonment, or pending court case.

Physical Examination

- *Inspection or observation*: General appearance, behaviour pattern, evidence of malnutrition manifestations, tremors etc.
- *Percussion*: Tenderness-epigastric region
- *Palpation*: Hepatomegaly, Splenomegaly, cardiomegaly
- *Auscultation*: Look for cardiac murmurs, respiratory sounds.

Mental Status Examination

- General appearance and behaviour
- Psychomotor activity
- Thought, content, mood, perception
- Cognitive function–orientation, memory, intelligence, abstractibility, judgement insight
- General information.

Mini Mental Status Examination

- Orientation, registration, attention, concentration, recall, language perception.

Psychosocial Assessment

- *Family*: Environment, interaction and relationship, pattern, bondage, healthy/unhealthy living pattern
- *Work environment*: Regularity in job, performance, responsibilities, workload, change of job relationship with superior and colleagues
- Social environment-peer group, social relationship, social functions, accidents, friends and relatives influence
- Crime–history of committing criminal acts and violence
- Religion, caste, cultural functions, social gatherings, motivating or stimulating factors.

Lab Investigations

Drug analytical testing
- Chromatographic tests
  Competitive binding/immuno-reactive tests.

Nursing Diagnosis

Alteration in nutrition less than body requirement evidenced by manifestations of malnutrition.

Goal

Maintains adequate nutrition.

Nursing Interventions

- Motivate the client to take regular and adequate balanced diet
- Educate the client and his family members the importance of high protein diet, high protein, high caloric and high vitamin rich diet and its sources, uses of nutrients, deficiencies and its manifestations; cultivation of good dietary habits
- Provide small and frequent food, provide an opportunity to choose liking foods among rich sources, serve the food of their choice as per dietary plan
- Weekly check and record the weight
- Give more fluids, maintain fluid and electrolyte balance, maintain intake and output chart.

2. Nursing Diagnosis

Disturbances in sleep related to emotional disturbances.

Goal

Enhances good sleeping pattern.

Nursing Interventions

- Motivate the client to have sleep for 6-8 hours per day
- Provide safe environment
- Ask the client to take warm water bath, a glass of warm milk before going to bed
- Permit one family member to stay with the client for continuous monitoring of the client

- Encourage the client to divert his mind from stressors and utilize relaxation measures like yoga and meditation
- Prepare the clients' mind to attend for deaddiction therapeutic sessions
- Keep light music to have to have smoothening effect over the client's mind
- Motivate the client to attend for spiritual prayers (if they are interested)
- Promote the client to develop positive ideas in life and join in deaddiction group.

3. Nursing Diagnosis

Impaired social interaction.

Goal

Enhances socialization.

Nursing Interventions

- Motivate the client to interact with peer group other than drug addicts
- Encourage them to discuss their difficulties to the significant personalities
- Assist the client to identify their abilities, strengths
- Permit the relatives and friends to take care of the client and visits frequently, motivate them to support the client
- Promote the client to develop positive and friendly attitude, insist for clear and direct language
- Encourage the client to perform activities to get efficiency and to develop skills.

4. Nursing Diagnosis

Inadequate coping evidenced by restlessness and anxiety.

Goal

Relieves from emotional disturbances and utilizes positive coping strategies.

Nursing Interventions

- Establish and maintain therapeutic nurse-patient relationship
- Accept the clients' feelings
- Never criticize the client in front of others by labeling
- Assess the emotional pattern, motivate the client to ventilate his feelings openly viz. fear, anxiety, hopelessness, powerlessness, worth-lessness
- Observe the client's interaction pattern with others
- Check whether the client is possessing any money
- Encourage the family members to provide moral, emotional support
- Ask the client whether he has any problems with their family members and relatives
- Explain to the client, how the maladaptive behaviour affects health, effect of the drugs on individual's health
- Advise the family members not to upset because of withdrawal symptoms of client
- Permit the family members to involve in clients' care
- Provide factual information and discuss current life situations and pattern, provide positive feedback
- Motivate the client to take responsibility for their recovery
- Review the coping strategies, set limitations for maladaptive behaviour, grant special privileges, appreciate for exhibiting adaptive behaviour
- Motivate the client to use peer support in utilizing coping strategies
- Demonstrate relaxation exercises and strategies to relax the mind
- Identify the triggers or stressors that promotes relapses and try to avoid them
- Administer the drugs as per order or prescription
- Encourage the client to utilize support of self help groups and community resources for their welfare.

5. Nursing Diagnosis

Low self-esteem related to the feelings of powerlessness and hopelessness.

Goal

Develops optimistic ideas and positive interest in life.

Nursing Interventions

- Utilizes crisis intervention techniques to develop adaptive behaviour and to overcome the problem of drug addiction.
- Suggest alternative solutions and methods to tackle the stressors.
- Identify the supportive group, encourage the client to ventilate his/her feelings openly to the people, whom they have confidence. Motivate the supportive members to be with the client and show their concern.
- Motivate the client to divert the mind by engaging in productive activities and relaxation activities.
- Encourage the client to interact with others and to follow assertiveness techniques.
- Involve the client in group therapy and utilize coping techniques.

6. Nursing Diagnosis

Impairment in family functioning manifested by family discord.

Goal

Maintains normal functioning pattern within the family.

Nursing Interventions

- Assess the interaction of family members, supportive system, level of functioning, sharing of responsibility and concern
- Demonstrate the coping strategies that has to be utilized by family members in meeting emotional needs of the client in reducing stressors or other stimuli that provokes drug abuse
- Involve the family members actively in provision of care to the client
- Provide educational opportunity and counselling to the client along with family members
- Provide information related to the activities of helping organizations like self help groups, deaddiction groups and rehabilitation groups
- Teach the family members the effects of specific drugs used for addiction, withdrawal symptoms and coping behaviour, deaddiction, rehabilitation measures and role of family members in provision of care, preventive aspects etc.
- Promote safety and security.

7. Nursing Diagnosis

Risk for injury related to intoxication effects.

Goal

Adapts safety measures.

Nursing Interventions

- Assess behaviour pattern, psychological functioning and cognitive abilities of the client
- Assist him in self care and health maintenance
- Promote Ego strengthening measures through counselling and adapting behaviour modification techniques
- Demonstrates coping strategies to be adopted in handling emotional imbalances or disturbances.

BRIEF DESCRIPTION OF COMMON DRUGS USED FOR DRUG ADDICTION

1. Opioids (Narcotics)

For Example, morphine, pethidine, fortwin, tidigesic and Heroin (Brown sugar, Smack)

Route of administration: Injection

Cinical Picture

Acute intoxication, apathy, bradycardia, hypotension, respiratory depression, sub-normal temperature, pinpointed pupils, thready pulse, coma.

Withdrawal symptoms: Begin within 12 hours of the last dose peak in 24–36 hours, disappear in 5–6 days.

Watery eyes, running nose, anorexia, irritability, tremors, sweating, cramps, nausea, diarrhoea, insomnia, fever.

Complications

Parkinsonism, peripheral neuropathy, transverse myelitis.

Treatment

Opoid overdose can be treated with narcotic antagonists like naloxone, naltrexone.

Maintenance therapy: Behaviour therapy, family therapy.

2. Morphine

Action

On the cortex, increasing its inhibitory effect on thalamic centres of sensation and raising the pain threshold.

Effected on pain sensation: Depress sensation of all kinds, although itching may be present. If it is taken orally, morphine is quickly absorbed through the intestinal mucosa and is slowly oxidized in the liver. Stimulates parasympathetic nervous system, increased bronchial secretions, respiratory centre failure.

Intoxication effects: Spinal reflex are increased, urinary retention is frequent, constipation and respiratory centre failure.

The tendency of morphine to cause addiction depends on its analgesic and euphorizing effects, also on the fairly rapid tolerance development.

Clinical Picture of an Addict

Miosis, scars or abscesses at the site of carelessly given injections, trophic disturbances of the skin, loss of hair, poor appetite, malnutrition, hepatitis, anxiety, depression, restlessness are banished only to return with the hang-over.

Chronic Abuse

Increasing inactivity, laziness, wasting of time in day-dreams, indecisiveness, paralysis of the ability to make strong and persistent effort. As a secondary consequence, due to need to conceal the habit and to overcome social and other barriers in the way of regular supply the client is likely to become fraud, the falsification of prescriptions, embracing insincerity to family, friends, colleagues and doctors, dishonest maneuvers of all kinds and flagrant breaches of the law.

Withdrawal

Abstinence syndrome, euphoria, calm and content give way to depression, restlessness, physical and mental irritability, habitual constipation changes to diarrhoea, anorexia, trembling, malaise and sleeplessness.

Diagnosis

- Papillary changes when the client is under the influence of a dose
- Small injection scars in the skin at accessible sites
- When the client is trying to conceal the addiction a change in mood, debility, tremor, apathy, depression at one time followed, after an absence from the room, at a short interval by alertness and a cheerful humour.

Treatment

Pre-hospital phase

When the patient is persuaded to enter the hospital; avoid over-prescription of drugs.

Hospitalization

- *Withdrawal phase*: Total abstinence by substituting drugs, Lethidrone-N is the most effective antagonist
- *Rehabilitation phase*: Physical and Emotional rehabilitation
- *Transitional phase*: Making the client able to manage his affairs outside hospital
- *Prolonged after-care phase*: Psychotherapy, family therapy, social therapy, guidance and counselling.

3. Lysergic Acid di-ethylamide (LSD-25)

After administration of LSD-25 within 15–20 minutes, autonomic effects occur like rise in body temperature, hypoglycemia, mydriasis and pilo-erection, psychological changes are delayed for 40–60 minutes, most intense after 1 or 2 hours, e.g. intense mood effects, euphoria, profound depression, anxiety, unmotivated giggling or laughter, sometimes accompanied by tears, sense of oppressive malaise, perceptual disturbances, visual hyperaesthesia is common, hallucination, some may experience intense somatic discomfort or pain, feeling themselves crushed, twisted or stretched.

Intoxication, depersonalization, de-realization, illusions, synthesis, autonomic hyper-activity, marked anxiety, impaired judgement.

Withdrawal syndrome: Flashbacks
Compilations
Anxiety, depression, psychosis, visual hallucinations.

Treatment

Symptomatic management by anti-depressants or anti-psychotic agents.

4. Cannabis Sativa

The flowering tops of the female plant of *cannabis sativa* have a pleasant intoxication effect. It may be eaten, drunk or smoked (ingestion or inhalation).

The drug is always taken in company hence the spread of habit.

Intoxication Effects

Mental phenomon arise 2–3 hours after ingestion or almost immediately after inhalation of the drug; floating of air sensation; falling on waves; lightness or dizziness in the head; ringing in the ears; heaviness in the limb; euphoria; increased psycho-motor activity; confused lassitude; elevated moods, mental status–hyperactive, apprehensive, loquacious, suspiciousness; lowered educational activities; psychosis; unreality feeling; double personality; thought disorder–fragmentation of thought process, memory disturbances, perplexity and immobility, frequent and sudden interruption of the stream of thought.

Withdrawal symptoms occur between 72–96 hours.

Complications

Acute anxiety, paranoid psychosis, hysterical fugue state like hypomania, schizophrenia, memory impairment.

Treatment

Supportive therapy; symptomatic treatment.

5. Cocaine

Local anaesthetic, it acts centrally as an excitant and euphorizing agent, stimulates sympathetic nervous system causing pupil dilatation, skin-pallor, raise in pulse rate, sweating, raise in body temperature.

If cocaine administered subcutaneously or inhale as a snuff, quickly absorbed through the mucus membrane. Immediate elation with mental ability feelings, greater precision of though and action, fatigue, excited, restless, likes to take and mixes well in society. He may make the impression of a brilliant conversationalist, witty and full of ideas, superficial thinking, over-activity, and lacks direction.

Prognosis and Treatment

Physical and mental ruin–treat with *barbiturates;* if the drug is withdrawn immediately and completely delirium and sub-acute paranoid episode pass off.

Intoxication–amyl nitrate is anti dose, diazepam, and propranolol

Withdrawal symptoms: Antidepressants like imipramine, psychotherapy.

6. Barbiturates

- The doctor should be careful in prescribing drugs of powerful action, such as barbiturate as placebos. These are cortical depressants acts on autonomic nervous system through hypothalamic centres.
- To relieve general restlessness and tension
- To mitigate some physical pain
- To procure a deeper sleep and obviate early morning wakening
- To protect the client against an excessive sensitivity to noises and other sensory stimuli.

Acute Intoxication

Depend on the amount of drug and on its nature and speed of action.

Suicidal attempt, drowsiness, ataxia, asynergia, nystagmus, and hypotonia, slow pulse, respiration and peristalsis, fall in body temperature, paresis, disseminated sclerosis or pre senile dementia, renal respiratory failure, coma and death.

Withdrawal Symptoms

Delirium tremens, anxiety, terrifying hallucination, tremulous withdrawal psychosis, convulsions, paranoid reaction, impairment of consciousness.

Complications

Intravenous use can lead to skin abscesses, cellulites, infections, embolism, hypersensitivity reactions.

Treatment

An unhurried regime must be pursued, rehabilitation–contact with the family, plan diligent, systematic, social and medical follow-up services, use of activated charcoal can reduce the absorption, symptomatic managements.

7. Cyanide

When large doses are taken, the client loses consciousness within 10 seconds and dies in convulsion in 5 minutes, the symptoms are vertigo, headache, palpitations, drowsiness, severe Dyspnoea, convulsions, loss of consciousness, death is due to asphyxia and due to paralysis of respiratory centre, medullary centre.

8. Inhalants or Volatile Solvent Use

For example, Petrol, aerosol, vanish remover, industrial solvents.

Intoxication

Euphoria, excitement, slurring of speech, apathy, impaired judgement
Withdrawal symptoms
Anxiety, depression
Complication
Peripheral neuropathy, liver and kidney damage, brain damage, perceptual disorders.

Treatment

Reassurance, tab, diazepam 5–10 mg at HS.

9. Carbon Monoxide Poisoning

The symptoms are lowering of efficiency and of self-control without insight, neuritis, disoriented, clouded consciousness, absent-minded, loss of consciousness, sometimes Parkinson syndrome with akinesia, rigidity and a mask-like facial expression, symptoms of aphasia, Apraxia and agnosia are more frequent, vascular damage to the cortex is irreversible.

Treatment

Pure oxygen administration, assistance form an efficient mechanical respirator, hypothermia, CPR technique.

10. Lead Poisoning

Acts on central nervous system, easily absorbed from the mucous membranes of respiratory or alimentary tract. Confusional state with signs of meningeal irritation, focal signs. For example, apraxia, transient paresis and convulsions and coma.

Slow cases, client manifests a retarded depression, dullness, failure of concentration and memory, headache, deafness, transient speech defect, visual disturbances.

11. Amphetamine

Powerful CNS stimulants with peripheral symptomatic effects. For example, Pemoline, methylphenidate.

It increases verbal and motor activity elevates the mood and prevents drowsiness in sleep, to combat apathy, tension, fatigue, depression and hunger and it is useful when heightened confidence and decisiveness are needed.

Euphoria state with excitement, which readily erupts into violence. Deterioration in social adjustment, depression, psychosis attempted suicide after abrupt withdrawal, to enable them to get through work under pressure, to control obesity among female.

Acute Intoxication

Tachycardia, hypertension, cardiac failure, seizures, tremors, hyperpyrexia, pupillary dilatation, panic, insomnia, restlessness, irritability, psychosis, paranoid hallucinatory syndrome.

Withdrawal Symptoms

Agitation, depression, apathy, fatigue, hypersomnia or insomnia.

Complication

Seizures, delirium, arrythmias, aggressive behaviour, coma.

REVIEW QUESTIONS

1. Prevention of substance abuse. (5M, RGUHS, 2000; 5M, MGRU, 2002).
2. Addictions. (5M, GULBU, 1995; 5M, MGRU, 1995, 97).
3. Substance abuse. (5M, GULBU, 2002; 2M, 2001, 5M, 2002, RGUHS; 10 M, MSc N, 2006).
4. Alcoholism. (5M, RGUHS, 1999, 2000, 03).
5. Abuse of alcohol and drugs. (10M, MGRU, 2002).
6. Write about the psychopathology and management of substance abuse. (10M, MGRU, 2002).
7. Drug dependence. (5M, MGRU, 2003; 2M, 5M, RGUHS, 2003).
8. Alcoholic psychosis. (5M, MGRU, 1992).
9. Prevention of drug abuse. (5M, MGRU, 1992).
10. Explain the nursing care of patients who depend on alcohol. (15M, MGRU, 1990).
11. a. Define addiction.
    b. What are the causes for an individual to consume alcohol?
    c. Describe the effects of alcohol.
    d. What are the methods of treatment for alcoholic addicts?
    (2+3+5+5M, MGRU, 1990).
12. Four causes of alcoholism. (2M, RGUHS, 1999).
13. Define drug addiction. List the drugs that are commonly abused and explain nursing management of patient with drug addiction. (10M, RGUHS, 2001).
14. Define substance abuse. Describe in detail the nursing management of alcoholic patient. (10M, RGUHS, 2001).
15. Alcohol dependence syndrome. (5M, RGUHS, 2003).
16. Management of alcohol dependence syndrome. (5M, RGUHS, 2004).
17. Drugs commonly used for addiction. (2M, RGUHS, 2003).

18. De-addiction. (2M, RGUHS, 2003).
19. Kosakoff's syndrome. (2M, RGUHS, 2006).
20. Define substance abuse. List the substance which can be abused. Describe the withdrawal systems. (6M, IGNOU, 1999).
21. Toxins affecting brain. (2M, PCBSc, 2000).
22. Effect of toxins on behaviour. (5M, PCBSc, 2001).
23. Differentiate between abuse and intoxication in relation to alcohol use. Describe the role of nurse in management of alcoholic client. (15 M, MSc(N), RGUHS, 2004).
24. Delirium tremens. (5M, RGUHS, 2004, 2M, RGUHS, 1999; 05; 4M, 1997, 2000).
25. Prevention of substance abuse. (5M, RGUHS, MGRU, 00, 02).
26. Addictions. (5M, GULB, 94).
27. Outline the social management of mental health problems of drug dependence. (5M, RGUHS, 02).
28. Abuse of alcohol and drugs. (10M, MGRU, 03).
29. Write about the psychopathology and management of substance abuse. (10M, MGRU, 02).
30. Prevention of drug abuse. (5M, MGRU, 92).
31. Explain the nursing care of patients who depend on alcohol. (15M, MGRU, 90).
32. Define addiction. What are the causes for an individual to consume alcohol? Describe the effects of alcohol. What are the methods of treatment of alcoholic addicts. (2+3+5+5M, MGRU, 00).
33. Four causes of alcoholism. (2M, RGUHS, 99).
34. Define drug addiction. List the drug that are commonly abused and explain nursing management of patient with drug addiction. (10M, RGUHS, 01).
35. Define substance abuse. Describe in detail the nursing management of alcoholic patient. (10M, RGUHS, 01).
36. Alcohol dependence syndrome. (5M, RGUHS, 03).
37. Drugs commonly used for addiction. (2M, RGUHS, 03).
38. Deaddiction. (2M, RGUHS, 03).
39. Kosakfoff's syndrome. (2M, RGUHS, 06).
40. Define substance abuse. List the substance which can be abused. Describe the withdrawal systems. (6M, IGNOU, 99).
41. Sociopath reactions. (5M, RGUHS, 05).
42. Poisons and brain damage. (5M, RGUHS, 02).
43. Opoid use disorders. (5M, RGUHS, 2007).
44. Nursing Management for substance use disorder. (10M, 2000, 01, 02, 03, 04).
45. Outline the rehabilitation programme for an alcoholic patient, who is on antabuse therapy. (10M, RGUHS, 2003).
46. Esperol. (2M, RGUHS, 2006).
47. Define substance abuse and explain the complications of Alcohol abuse, Discuss the Nurse's role in rehabilitation of alcoholic patients. (15M, RGUHS, 2006, MSc(N).
48. Detoxification. (2M, RGUHS, 2007).
49. Substance abuse. (5M, RGUHS, 2007).
50. Mention types of substance abuse, explain the nursing care of a patient with alcohol abuse. (10M, RGUHS, 2007).
51. Drug Addiction. (5M, RGUHS, 2000).
52. Drug abuse. (2M, RGUHS, 2002, 04).
53. Drug Dependence. (2M, 2003, RGUHS).
54. Drug Tolerance and Withdrawal. (2M, RGUHS, 2000).
55. Dependency producing drugs. (5M, RGUHS, 2000).
56. Aetiology of substance abuse. (5M, RGUHS, 1999).
57. Complications of Alcohol dependence. (5M, RGUHS, 2005).
58. Prevention of Alcohol abuse. (5M, RGUHS, 2000).
59. Treatment of Alcohol Dependence. (5M, RGUHS, 2000).
60. Alcohol Anonymous groups. (5M, RGUHS, 2003).
61. Alcohol Dependent syndrome. (5M, RGUHS, Oct, 07).

Bibliography

1. ACOG technical bulletin. 'Sexual dysfunction' Washington DC. American College of Obstetricians and Gynecologists 1995.
2. Akhtar S. 'Schizoid Personality Disorder: A System of Developmental, Dynamic and Descriptive Features'. 'American Journal of Psychotherapy'. 1987;151:499-518.
3. Alphonsa Jacob. 'Hand Book of Psychiatric Nursing'. New Delhi. Vikas Publishing House Private Limited 1996.
4. American Association on Intellectual and Developmental Disabilities. 'Mental Retardation'. Washington DC 2002.
5. American Psychiatric Association Work Group on Eating Disorders': 'Practice Guide line for the treatment of patients with eating disorders.' American Journal of Psychiatry' 2000;1-39.
6. American Psychiatric Association. 'DSM For Mental Disorders'. Washington DC. American Psychiatric Press 1994.
7. Apple RF, et al. A Cognitive Behavioural Treatment For Eating Disorders'. San Antonio. Harcourt Brace and Company 1997.
8. Avinash De souza. 'Notes in Psychiatry'. Bombay. Vikas Medical Publishers 2001.
9. Baby R. 'Psychiatric Nursing'. Pondicherry. NR Brothers Publishers House 2001.
10. Barbara Schoen Johnson. 'Psychiatric Mental Health Nursing'. Philadelphia. Lippincott Company 1997.
11. Barlow DH, Durand VM. 'Essentials of Abnormal Psychology'. California. Thomson Wads Worth 2006.
12. Barsky AJ, Ahern DK. 'Cognitive Behaviour Therapy For Hypochondriasis: A Randomized controlled Trial'. JAMA 2004.
13. Batshaw ML. 'Children with disabilities'. Baltimore. Paul H Brookes Publishing Co 1997.
14. Beers Mark H, Robert Berkow. 'The Personality Disorders'. 'The Merck Manual of Diagnosis and Therapy'. White House 1999.
15. Benjamin JS, Virjinia AS. 'Synopsis Of Psychiatry Behavioural Sciences/Clinical Psychiatry'. Philadelphia. Lippincott Williams and Wilkin's Company 2003.
16. Benjamin H. 'Trans-sexualism and sex reassignment.' Baltimore. The John Hopkins Press 1999.
17. Bhatia MS. 'A Concised Text Book On Psychiatric Nursing- Comprehensive Theoretical and Practical Approach'. New Delhi. CBS Publishers and Distributors 2001.
18. Bhatia MS. 'Short Text Book of Psychiatry'. New Delhi. CBS Publishers and Distributors 2002.
19. Bimla Kapoor. 'Text Book of Psychiatric Nursing – volume I and II'. New Delhi. Kumar Publishing House 2005.
20. Carter K. 'Obsessive-compulsive personality disorder'. Oxford College of Emory University 2006.
21. Charks E Skinner. ' Educational Psychology'. New Delhi. Printice-Hall of India Private Limited 2004.

22. Chaube SP. 'Educational Psychology'. Agra. Lakshmi Narain Agarwal Educational Publishers 1999.

23. Chauhan SS. 'Advanced Educational Psychology'. New Delhi. Vikas Publishing House 1994.

24. Clark DM, et al. 'Two Psychological Treatments for Hypochondriasis, a randomized controlled trail'. Br J Psychiatry. 1998;218-25.

25. Clifford T Morgan, et al. 'Introduction to Psychology'. New Delhi. Tata McGraw Hill Publishing Company Limited 1993.

26. Comer RJ. 'Fundamentals of Abnormal Psychology'. New York 1996.

27. Coolidge FL, et al. 'Heritability of Personality Disorders In Childhood: A Preliminary Investigation.' 'The Journal of Personality Disorders.' 15.No.1. 2001;33-40.

28. Coryell W, et al. 'The enduring social consequences of mania and depression'. 'American Journal of psychiatry' 1993.

29. DM Hambridge. 'Post-traumatic Stress Disorder'. London 2003.

30. Diamond M, HK Sigmundson. 'Management of intersexuality'. 'Archives of Paediatrics and Adolescent Medicine' 1997.

31. DSM-IV TR. 'Diagnostic criteria for gender identity disorder'.

32. Eisendrath Stuart J. 'Psychiatric Disorders'. Stanford 1998.

33. Elizabeth MV. 'Foundations of Psychiatric Mental Health Nursing, A clinical Approach'. New York. Saunders Company 2002.

34. Elizabeth B Harlock. 'Developmental Psychology'. New Delhi. Tata McGraw Hill Publishing Company Limited 2005.

35. Endicoff J, Coryell W Keller. 'Affective syndromes, psychotic features and prognosis – mania'. Arch Gen Psychiatry 1990;437.

36. Ernest R Hilgard, et al. 'Introduction to Psychology'. New Delhi. Oxford and IBH Publishers 1996.

37. Faedda GC, Tando L, et al. 'Outcomes after rapid versus gradual discontinuation of lithium treatment in bipolar disorders' Arch Gen Psychiatry 1993.

38. Fallon BA, et al. 'Hypochondriasis and its relationship to OCD.' 'Psychiatry Clinical North America' 2000;605-16.

39. Folstein MF, Folstein SE. 'Mini Mental State- A Practical Method For The Clinician' 'Journal of Psychiatric Research' 1975;185-98.

40. Frank GK: ' Oxytocin and Vasopressin Levels after recovery from eating disorders'. 'Biological psychiatry' 2000;315-18.

41. Freud Sigmund. 'The standard Edition of The Complete Psychological Works of Sigmund Freud.' London. Trans James Starchey 1974;24.

42. Gail Wiscarz Staurt, MT Laria. 'Principles and Practice of Psychiatric Nursing'. Philadelphia CV Mosby Company 2005.

43. Gail Wiscarz Staurt, Sandra J Sundeen. 'Principles and Practice of Psychiatric Nursing'. Philadelphia. C. V. Mosby Company 1979.

44. Gelder, et al. 'New Oxford Textbook of Psychiatry'. New York. Oxford University Press 2004.

45. Hare RD. 'Psychopathy and Anti social Personality disorder. A case of Diagnostic Confusion' 'Psychiatric Times' 1996;41-45.

46. IGNOU Manuals. 'BNS-108 Series on Mental Health Nursing'. New Delhi 2006.

47. Intersex Society Of North America. 'What Evidence is there that you can grow up Psychologically health with intersex genitals' 2006.

48. Jauch DA, et al. Toward Reformulating the Diagnosis of Schizophrenia'. 'American Journal of Psychiatry' 2000;1041-50.

49. Jayaswal SR. 'Foundations of Educational Psychology'. Lucknow. Prakashan Kendra 2004.

50. Jerry M Wiener, Nancy A Bresline. 'NMS (National Medical Series for Independent Study) The behavioural Sciences in Psychiatry'. New York. Williams and Wilkins Company 1995.

51. Johansson P, et al. 'Linking adult psychopathy with childhood hyperactivity'. 'Journal of Personality Disorders' 2005;19(1):94-101.

52. Jung CG. 'Psychological Types, Collected Works'. Princeton. N J Princeton University Press 1971.

53. Jung CG. 'Memories, Dreams, Reflections.' New York. NY Vantage Books 1989.

54. Karlawish J, Clark C. 'Diagnostic Evaluation Of Elderly Patients With Mild Memory Problems'. Ann Intern Med 2003;138(5):411-9.

55. Keithlcheng, KM Myers. 'Child and Adolescent Psychiatry'. Philadelphia. Lippincott Williams and Wilkin's Company 2005.

56. Kernberg PF. 'Personality Disorders in Children and Adolescents'. New York 2000.

57. Kozier Erb, et al. 'Fundamentals of Nursing'. Singapore. Pearson Education Limited 2003.

58. Lalitha K. 'Mental Health and Psychiatric Nursing'. Bangalore. Gajanana Book Publishers 1999.

59. Lalitha K, 'Mental Health and Psychiatric Nursing, An Indian Perspective'. Bangalore. VMG Book House 2007.

60. Leibenluft E. 'Women with bipolar illness: clinical and research issues'. 'American Journal of psychiatry 1996.'

61. Lesley Stevens, Ian Rodin. 'Psychiatry an Illustrated Colour Text'. London. Churchill Livingstone Company 2001.

62. Lundberg SC, et al. 'Nicotine Treatment of Obsessive Compulsive Disorder'. Prog Neuro Psycho Pharmacol. Biol. Psychiatry 2004;28(7).

63. Mac Donald JM. 'The Threat To Kill'. American Journal of Psychiatry' 2003;125-30.

64. Mangal SK. 'Abnormal Psychology'. Sterling Publishers Private Limited. Ludhiana 1999.

65. Mangal SK. 'Educational Psychology'. Sterling Publishers Private Limited. Ludhiana 1999.

66. Mangal SK. 'Advanced Educational Psychology'. New Delhi. Prentice- Hall of India Private Limited 2002.

67. Marshall W, Serin R. 'Personality Disorders- Adult Psychopathology and Diagnosis.' New York 2002;508-41.

68. Mary C Townsend. 'Psychiatric Mental Health Nursing - Concepts of Care'. Philadelphia. FA Davis Company 2003.

69. Master VA, Turck PJ. 'Ejaculatory Physiology and Dysfunction'. Urol Cli North Am 2001;363-75.

70. Mertz, Michael E. 'Coping with Premature Ejaculation'. Oakland. SCA. New Harbinger Publications 2003.

71. Michael Gelder. 'Oxford Textbook of Psychiatry'. Melbourne. Oxford University Press 1996.

72. Millon, Theodore. 'Disorders of Personality: DSM IV and Beyond'. New York 1995.

73. Murphy CC, et al. 'Epidemiology of MR in children'. MR and Developmental Disabilities Research Reviews. 1998;6-13.

74. Namboodiri VMD. 'Concise Textbook of Psychiatry'. New Delhi. Elsevier Company 2005.

75. Nancy Burns, Susan K Grove. 'Understanding Nursing Research'. Philadelphia. WB Saunders Company 1995.

76. Neeraja KP. 'Text book of Growth and Development'. New Delhi. Jaypee Brothers Medical Publishers (P) Ltd 2006.

77. Noreen CF, Lawrence EF. 'Psychiatric Mental Health Nursing'. Australia. Delmar Thomson Learning Company 2002.

78. Norman L Munn, et al. 'Introduction to Psychology'. Calcutta. Oxford and IBH publishing Co. Pvt Ltd 1972.

79. Ochberg FM, et al. ' Psychopathic, sadistic and sane'. International Journal of Emergency Mental Health' 2003;121-36.

80. Ogden Cl, et al. 'Prevalence of Obesity and Over Weight in USA 1994-2004 JAMA. 2006;295(13).

81. Phil Barker. 'Psychiatric and Mental Health Nursing, the Craft of Caring'. London. Oxford University Press 2003.

82. Phillips NA. 'The clinical evaluation of dyspareunia.' Int J Impot Res 1998;117-20.

83. Potter A, Patricia, Perry AG. 'Basic Nursing Theory and Practice'. Chicago. CV Mosby Company 1995.

84. Potter Perry. 'Fundamentals of Nursing'. Chicago. CV Mosby Company 2005.

85. Raju SM. 'Introduction to Psychiatric Nursing' New Delhi. Jaypee Brothers .Medical Publishers Pvt Ltd 2004.

86. Read S, Watson J. 'Sexual dysfunction in primary medical care: prevalence, characteristics and detection by the general practitioner' 'Journal of Public Health Medicine' 1997.

87. Ringold MD, Warren J. 'The ABC's of Premature Ejaculation'. Department of Chief of Family Medicine 2004.

88. Robert AB. 'Psychology'. New Delhi. Prince Hall of India Pvt Ltd 1996.

89. Rosen JB, Schulkin J. 'From Normal Fear to Pathological Anxiety'. Psychological Review 1998;105(2).

90. Sandra M Nettina. 'The Lippincott Manual of Nursing Practice'. Philadelphia. Lippincott Company 1991.

91. Satoskar, et al. 'Pharmacology and Pharmaco Therapeutics'. Mumbai. Popular Prakashan Pvt Ltd 2005.

92. Sax Leonard. 'How common is the Intersex? A Response to Anne Fausto Sterling' . 'Journal of Sex Research' 2002;174-78.

93. Scott J. 'Psychotherapy for bipolar disorders' 1995;581-88.

94. Seligman MEP, et al. 'Personality Disorders'. 'The Merck manual of diagnosis and therapy'. 17th (Ed). White House Station. Nj. Merck Research Laboratories 1999.

95. Shah LP, Ham Shah. 'A Handbook of Psychiatry'. Mumbai. Vora Book Centre 1997.

96. Sheila LV. 'Psychiatric Mental Health Nursing'. Philadelphia. Lippincott Williams and Wilkin Company 2004.

97. Sheldon J Korchin. 'Modern Clinical Psychology. Principles of Intervention in the Clinic and Community' New Delhi. CBS Publishers and Distributors 1986.

98. Sims Andrew. 'Symptoms in the Mind: An Introduction to Descriptive Psychopathology'. Philadelphia. WB Saunders Company 2002.

99. Sreevani R. 'A Guide to Mental Health and Psychiatric Nursing'. New Delhi. Jaypee Brothers Medical Publishers Pvt Ltd 2007.

100. Stampfer MJ, et al. 'Effects Of Moderate Alcohol Consumption on Cognitive function In Women'. Journal of Medicine.' New England 2005.

101. Stephen, et al. 'Pharmacology Principles and Applications'. New Jersey. Printice Hall International Ltd 2005.

102. Strakowski SM, et al. 'The co-occurrence of mania with medical and other –psychiatric disorders'. 'International journal of psychiatry medicine' 1994.

103. Sullivan PF. 'Mortality in Anorexia Nervosa'. 'American journal of psychiatry'. Tandon Publications 1995;1073-74.

104. Wanda R Mohr. 'Psychiatric Mental Health Nursing'. London. Lippincott Williams and Wilkins Company 2006.

105. Web CT, DF Levinson. 'Schizotypal and paranoid personality disorder in the relatives of patients with Schizophrenia and affective disorders. A Review. 'Schizophrenia Research' 1993;81-92.

106. Weismann MM. 'The Epidemiology Of Personality Disorders'. 'The Journal of Personality Disorders' 1993;44-62.

107. WHO. 'The ICD-10 Classification of Mental and Behavioural Disorders'. Geneva 1992.

108. WHO. Technical Report Series: Obesity: Preventing and managing the Global Epidemic 2000.

109. Winokur G, et al. 'Alcoholism in bipolar illness' 'American Journal of Psychiatry' 1995;365-72.

110. Wlfley DC, Cohen CR. 'Psychological Treatment Of Bulimia Nervosa and Binge Eating Disorder'. 'Psycho pharmacology Bulletin' 1997;437-54.

111. Zucker KJ, Spitzer RL. 'Was the gender identity disorder of childhood diagnosis introduced into DSM-III as a back door maneuver to replace homosexuality? A historical note. 'Journal of sex and marital therapy' 2005;31(1).

112. Basavanthappa BT. 'Psychiatric Mental Nursing'. New Delhi. Jaypee Brothers Medical Publishers (P) Ltd 2007.

113. Neeraja KP. 'Textbook of Sociology for Nursing Students'. New Delhi. Jaypee Brothers Medical Publishers (P) Ltd 2005.

Index